Aging Medicine

Robert J. Pignolo, MD, PhD; Mary Ann Forciea, MD;
Jerry C. Johnson, MD, Series Editors

For other titles published in this series, go to
www.springer.com/series/7622

Robert J. Pignolo • Mary Ann Keenan
Nader M. Hebela
Editors

Fractures in the Elderly

A Guide to Practical Management

Humana Press

Editors
Robert J. Pignolo
Departments of Medicine and Orthopaedic Surgery
Director Ralston-Penn Clinic for Osteoporosis and Related Bone Disorders
University of Pennsylvania School of Medicine
Philadelphia, PA
USA
pignolo@mail.med.upenn.edu

Mary Ann Keenan
Professor, Department of Orthopaedic Surgery
Hospital of the University of Pennsylvania
Philadelphia, PA
USA
maryann.keenan@uphs.upenn.edu

Nader M. Hebela
Assistant Professor of Orthopaedic Surgery
Department of Orthopaedic Surgery
University of Pennsylvania School of Medicine
Philadelphia, PA
USA
nader.hebela@uphs.upenn.edu

ISBN 978-1-61779-718-7 ISBN 978-1-60327-467-8 (eBook)
DOI 10.1007/978-1-60327-467-8
Springer New York Dordrecht Heidelberg London

Softcover reprint of the hardcover 1st edition 2011

Printed on acid-free paper

Humana Press is part of Springer Science+Business Media (www.springer.com)

Preface

According to the National Osteoporosis Foundation, one in two women and one in four men over age 50 will have an osteoporosis-related fracture in their lifetime, accounting for more than 1.5 million fractures annually. In the USA, a women's risk of hip fracture is equal to her *combined* risk of breast, uterine, and ovarian cancer. Although not all fractures in the elderly are related to osteoporosis, the vast majority of them are, and the risk of fracture from both low- and high-impact trauma is increased in the setting of osteoporosis.

Only about 40% of hip fracture survivors are able to return to their prior level of activities of daily living, and even fewer return to their prefracture level for instrumental activities. A nontrivial proportion of patients with hip fractures will require long-term institutional care. Despite these sober statistics, currently less than 15% of those with recent fragility fractures are evaluated and treated for osteoporosis, dramatically increasing the likelihood of future fractures.

This book is an acknowledgement that fractures in the elderly are common, very often multifactorial, and are best approached by the collaborative efforts of orthopaedic surgeons and specialists in geriatric medicine. Other medical disciplines, including anesthesiology, rehabilitation medicine, psychiatry, endocrinology, and rheumatology also play key roles in the care of the elderly fracture patient. Because of the potentially devastating consequences of fractures in the elderly, their presentations should be viewed as opportunities to reduce future morbidity and mortality as well as to preserve function. This book is dedicated to these goals.

The specific aims of *Fractures in the Elderly* are (1) to provide geriatricians and other medical specialists who provide care for older adults with the necessary information and most current data and opinions regarding the treatment of elderly patients who sustain a variety of fractures, and (2) to provide orthopaedic surgeons with the necessary information and most current data and opinions regarding assessment and management of geriatric conditions that predispose the elderly to fracture, perioperative complications, and subsequent functional decline. The scope of the book will encompass the etiologies of fracture in the elderly, perioperative management, the surgical treatment of common fractures in the elderly, as well as rehabilitation and prevention in the older patient.

It was the intention of the editors to have the content of each chapter be both readable and appealing to both of the two major target audiences, as well as to all disciplines that have contact with elderly patients who have sustained or are at high risk of sustaining a fracture. We hope to illustrate that although in some cases pre- and postoperative care in elderly fracture patients may proceed as it does in younger individuals, often there are considerations owing to functional status, preexisting conditions, and age-related physiological declines that require specialized knowledge and alternative approaches. This book serves to provide this specialized knowledge and approaches to care, and it is intended to be a valuable reference for clinicians as well as fellows and residents in training.

Contents

Contributors

Jaimo Ahn
Assistant Professor, Department of Orthopaedic Surgery, University of Pennsylvania School of Medicine, Philadelphia, PA 19104, USA

Keith Baldwin, MD/MSPT/MPH
Department of Orthopaedic Surgery, Hospital of the University of Pennsylvania, 2 Silverstein Pavilion, 3400 Spruce Street, Philadelphia, PA 19104, USA

Karen Boselli, MD
Shoulder and Elbow Fellow, Department of Orthopaedic Surgery, Columbia University, New York, NY 10032, USA

David J. Bozentka, MD
Department of Orthopaedic Surgery, Hospital of the University of Pennsylvania, 34th and Spruce Streets, 2nd Floor, Silverstein Building, Philadelphia, PA 19104, USA
and
Department of Orthopaedic Surgery, Penn Presbyterian Medical Center, Cupp 1, 39th and Market Streets, Philadelphia, PA 19104, USA

John Bruza, MD
Division of Geriatric Medicine, University of Pennsylvania School of Medicine, 3615 Chestnut Street, Philadelphia, PA 19104-2676, USA

Amy M. Corcoran, MD
Department of Medicine, Division of Geriatrics, University of Pennsylvania, Penn-Ralston Center, 3615 Chestnut Street, Philadelphia, PA 19104, USA

Derek J. Donegan, MD
Department of Orthopaedic Surgery, Hospital of the University of Pennsylvania, Philadelphia, PA 19104, USA

John L. Esterhai, MD
Department of Orthopaedic Surgery, Hospital of the University of Pennsylvania, 2 Silverstein, 3400 Spruce Street, Philadelphia, PA 19104, USA

Jonathan R. Gavrin, MD
Department of Anesthesiology and Critical Care, Department of Medicine, Hospital of the University of Pennsylvania, Dulles 6, 3400 Spruce Street, Philadelphia, PA 19104, USA

Albert O. Gee
Instructor, Department of Orthopaedic Surgery, University of Pennsylvania School of Medicine, Philadelphia, PA 19104, USA

Nader M. Hebela, MD
Department of Orthopaedic Surgery, University of Pennsylvania School of Medicine, Penn Presbyterian Medical Center, 1 Cupp Pavilion, 51 N 39th Street, Philadelphia, PA 19104, USA

G. Russell Huffman, MD/MPH
Department of Orthopaedic Surgery, University of Pennsylvania, 3400 Spruce Street, 2 Silverstein Pavilion, Philadelphia, PA 19104, USA

Jerry C. Johnson, MD
Division of Geriatric Medicine, Department of Medicine, University of Pennsylvania School of Medicine, 3615 Chestnut Street, Philadelphia, PA 19104-2676, USA

Atul F. Kamath, MD
Department of Orthopaedic Surgery, Hospital of the University of Pennsylvania, Philadelphia, PA 19104, USA

Mary Ann Keenan, MD
Professor, Department of Orthopaedic Surgery, Hospital of the University of Pennsylvania, Philadelphia, PA 19104, USA

Jung-Hoon Kim, MD
University of Pennsylvania, Department of Medicine, Division of Geriatric Medicine, 3615 Chestnut Street, Ralston-Penn Center, Philadelphia, PA USA

Bruce Kinosian, MD
Associate Professor of Medicine, Department of Medicine, University of Pennsylvania Health System, Philadelphia, PA 19104, USA

Andrew F. Kuntz
Instructor, Department of Orthopaedic Surgery, University of Pennsylvania School of Medicine, Philadelphia, PA 19104, USA

Richard D. Lackman, MD
Department of Orthopaedic Surgery, Sarcoma Center of Excellence at the Abramson Cancer Center of the University of Pennsylvania, Hospital of the University of Pennsylvania, Philadelphia, PA 19104, USA

Gwo-Chin Lee, MD
Department of Orthopaedic Surgery, University of Pennsylvania,
3400 Spruce Street, 2 Silverstein Pavilion, Philadelphia, PA 19104, USA

Samir Mehta
Orthopedic Trauma and Fracture Service, Department of Orthopaedic Surgery,
Hospital of the University of Pennsylvania, Silverstein 2, 3400 Spruce Street,
Philadelphia, PA 19104, USA

J. Stuart Melvin, MD
Orthopaedic Trauma Fellow, Department of Orthopaedic Surgery,
Carolinas Medical Center, Charlotte, NC 28203, USA

Nick D. Pappas, MD
Department of Orthopaedic Surgery, Hospital of the University
of Pennsylvania, Philadelphia, PA 19104, USA

Robert J. Pignolo, MD/PhD
Departments of Medicine and Orthopaedic Surgery,
University of Pennsylvania School of Medicine, 424B Stemmler Hall,
36th Street and Hamilton Walk, Philadelphia, PA 19104-6081, USA

Kathleen Walsh Reyes, DO
Staff Physician, Jefferson Regional Medical Center
and University of Pittsburgh Medical Center,
Philadelphia PA, USA

Andrew Rosenzweig, MD
Staff Geriatrician and Internal Medicine Core Faculty Member,
Division of Geriatics and Department of Medicine, Abington Memorial Hospital,
Abington, PA 19001, USA;
Clinical Assisstant Professor of Medicine, Drexel University College of Medicine,
Philadelphia, PA 19102, USA

John Alan Scolaro, MD
Department of Orthopaedics, Hospital of the University of Pennsylvania,
Philadelphia, PA, USA

Jesse T. Torbert, MD, MS
Department of Orthopaedic Surgery, Hospital of the University of Pennsylvania,
Philadelphia PA, USA

Ejovi Ughwanogho, MD
Department of Orthopaedic Surgery, Hospital of the University of Pennsylvania,
Philadelphia, PA 19104, USA

Joan Weinryb, MD/CMD
Division of Geriatric Medicine, University of Pennsylvania Health System, Philadelphia, PA, USA

Laura C. Wiegand, MD
Department of Orthopaedic Surgery, Hospital of the University of Pennsylvania, Philadelphia, PA 19104, USA

Part I
The Aging of Bone and Etiologies of Fractures

Chapter 1
Osteobiology of Aging

Andrew Rosenzweig and Robert J. Pignolo

Abstract The goals of this chapter will be to give a brief overview of bone biology, describe the molecular mechanisms of bone remodeling and pathologic uncoupling, and provide a general survey of the multiple pathways leading to aging bone and osteoporosis.

Keywords Bone • Remodeling • Osteoporosis • Osteoblast • Osteoclast • Cellular senescence

1.1 Introduction

The human skeleton is a dynamic organ that serves multiple functions including support, protection, storing metabolic building blocks, and providing insertion points for tendons and ligaments. A tightly coupled mechanism known as remodeling exists in the skeleton which allows for the constant turnover of bone, even after longitudinal growth has ceased. Osteoclasts reabsorb old bone and osteoblasts follow closely, laying down new structural units of bone. There is a complex interplay between these cells mediated by many endogenous local and systemic factors as well as exogenous mechanical stresses [1]. Peak bone mass usually occurs in the third decade of life in humans after which there is a period of relatively stable bone mass followed by progressive decline. As the body ages, the mechanism of bone remodeling becomes more dysfunctional, leading to an uncoupling of bone formation and resorption and a net loss of bone density and structural integrity, causing osteoporosis and increasing the risk of fractures.

R.J. Pignolo (✉)
Departments of Medicine and Orthopaedic Surgery, University of Pennsylvania School of Medicine, 424B Stemmler Hall, 36th Street and Hamilton Walk, Philadelphia, PA 19104-6081, USA
e-mail: pignolo@mail.med.upenn.edu

R.J. Pignolo et al. (eds.), *Fractures in the Elderly*, Aging Medicine,
DOI 10.1007/978-1-60327-467-8_1,

It has been estimated that only 31–36% of people greater than 70 years of age have normal bone mass [1]. The lifetime risk for fracture in men ranges from 13 to 25% and approaches 50% for Caucasian women [2, 3].

1.2 Basic Anatomy of Bone

1.2.1 Bony Matrix

The bony matrix is composed of mineral crystals associated with type I collagen fibers and noncollagenous proteins. The predominant mineral composition of bone (95% of its mineral weight) is $Ca_{10}(PO_4)_6(OH)_2$, hydroxyapatite, with carbonate and other small impurities. Type I collagen accounts for about 90% of the total protein in bone with absorbed plasma proteins and proteins synthesized by bone-forming cells accounting for the remaining noncollagenous component. Bony matrix glycoproteins and proteoglycans serve to stabilize the mineral crystal [4].

1.2.2 Cortical Bone

The mammalian skeleton is made up of two types of bone: cortical (or compact) and trabecular (or cancellous) bone. Cortical bone is composed of an outer layer (periosteum) and an inner surface (endosteum) [5]. Grossly, cortical bone makes up about 80% of the adult skeleton and is the outer casing while trabecular bone is the inner, spongy meshwork of bone that makes up the remaining approximate 20% [6]. Individual bones are made up of varying proportions of cortical and trabecular tissue, depending on location, and reflect specific structural and functional differences.

Cortical bone is found primarily in the shaft of long bones, at the end of joints, and in the vertebrae. Microarchitecturally, it is organized into different types of structures classified by porosity. In humans, this includes woven and lamellar bone [7]. Woven bone is made up of osteocytes and type I collagen laid down in a relatively disorganized fashion, often in the face of fracture or trauma. It may be mineralized rapidly which leads to increases in brittleness [7]. Woven bone may be formed de novo in the absence of previously formed bone or cartilage or in the presence of fracture or trauma [8]. In the developed adult cortical skeleton, remodeling takes place in the intracortical or Haversian layer [5].

Lamellar bone is mature bone with collagen fibers arranged in sheaths within cortical bone and in parallel sheets on flat surfaces. This layer of cortical bone is made of osteons, discrete units of concentric bone surrounding a central blood supply, or "Haversian canal." Primary osteons are likely formed by mineralization of cartilage, thus being formed where bone was not present [6]. Secondary osteons are formed by replacement of existing bone through the remodeling process, the complex mechanism by which osteoclasts clear the central tunnel/Haversian canal and then osteoblasts lay down lamellae of new cortical bone [7]. In addition to osteoblasts, Haversian canals contain blood vessels and nerve fibers. Lacunae are spaces between layers of matrix that contain bone cells called osteocytes. Osteocytes evolve from osteoblasts that become entrapped in bone matrix during the mineralization process. These cells extend cytoplasmic processes within the canaliculi of the bony matrix and form a network of communicating cells. This network functions to sense mechanical stressors and transmit signals to surface cells to trigger bone remodeling when necessary [9].

1.2.3 Trabecular Bone

Trabecular bone fills the medullary cavity of long bones and also makes up the majority of vertebral bodies. Trabecular bone, although more porous, has a substantially greater surface area than cortical bone [10]. It also has a much larger interface with soft tissue such as bone marrow, vascular, and connective tissue. Trabecular bone is more affected by metabolic processes, and those conditions predisposing to bone loss tend to affect trabecular bone more severely than cortical bone [9, 11]. With aging, as in cortical bone, the balance of remodeling favors bone resorption over formation leading to a net thinning of trabecular bone over time [9].

1.3 Basic Multicellular Units

The process of bone resorption followed by formation, which produces newly remodeled bone, is carried out by discrete clusters of osteoclasts and osteoblasts known as basic multicellular units (BMUs) (also known as bone remodeling units). These units make up the building blocks for bone resorption and formation. The BMUs are found in cortical bone as Haversian systems or in trabecular bone as Howship lacunae and are accompanied by a blood supply along with supporting connective tissue [12, 13]. It is important to note that the new bone initially laid down is not as strong as mineralized, "old" bone. Fracture of BMUs, increased resorption rate, or decreased formation rate will alter the remodeling balance and this leads to decreased bone density and strength and predisposes the elderly to fracture [5]. The lifespans of osteoclasts and osteoblasts are short compared to the lifespan of BMUs and these cells must be continually replenished for the BMUs to successfully resorb old bone and replace it with new bone [14].

Aging bone is subject to intrinsic (genetic) and extrinsic (environmental) factors which predispose it to fracture. Decreases in tissue mineral density, bone size, trabecular number, thickness and connectivity, and cortical thickness over time play a role in this process [15]. Aging in and of itself leads to discordance in the remodeling process, whereby osteoblasts do not lay down new bone at a rate proportional to the resorption by osteoclasts. This leads to a net negative balance in each bone multicellular unit with reductions in trabecular and cortical number and thickness as well as increased porosity, manifested as increased buckling, microdamage, and fracture [16, 17]. This net negative bone balance probably begins in young adulthood and well before menopause [17]. Current drug therapies to treat age-related osteoporosis and prevent fracture work to reduce resorption and increase bone formation. This may preserve bone density by minimizing bone loss and preventing thinning, but may not restore the damaged microarchitecture that plays an equally important role in age-related bone loss [17].

1.3.1 Osteoclasts

The formation of osteoclasts and osteoblasts involves a complex interplay of stem cell production, amplification, and commitment to differentiated cell fates. Osteoclasts are large, multinucleated cells derived from macrophage/monocyte precursors of hematopoetic lineage (CFU-GM and CFU-M) that originate in the bone marrow [5]. These cells are found on the bone surface within Howship's lacunae where they resorb old bone in preparation for new bone formation [18]. The estimated lifespan of these cells is 2–3 weeks and is dictated by the onset of programmed cell death (apoptosis).

In response to various factors released by damaged, aged, or otherwise resorbed bone, e.g., insulin-like growth factors (IGFs), transforming growth factor β (TGF-β), bone morphogenic proteins (BMPs), support cells, including bone marrow stromal cells, pre-osteoblasts and osteoblasts, express macrophage-colony stimulating factor (M-CSF) and receptor activator of nuclear factor κβ Ligand (RANKL) to promote osteoclast differentiation and maturation. Osteoblasts secrete osteoprotegerin (OPG), a circulating decoy receptor, which regulates RANK/RANKL-induced osteoclast formation and activity by preventing excessive bone resorption [5, 19, 20]. Multiple hormones and cytokines including parathyroid hormone (PTH), 1,25-vitamin D3, IL-1, IL-6, IL-11, and tumor necrosis factor (TNF) influence osteoclast differentiation [5]. In addition to the interaction between hematopoetic precursors and cells of the osteoblast lineage, inflammatory cells, particularly T cells, may also be involved in osteoclast differentiation [21]. Once the osteoclast is activated, resorption occurs in regions where the osteoclast creates an acidic milieu conducive to mineral degradation [19] (see Fig. 1.1).

1.3.2 Osteoblasts

Mesenchymal stem cells (MSCs) or marrow stromal fibroblasts are responsible for the derivation of osteoblasts and are subject to the influence of local growth factors including BMPs, IGFs, and TGF-β [1, 22, 23]. Multiple transcriptional regulators

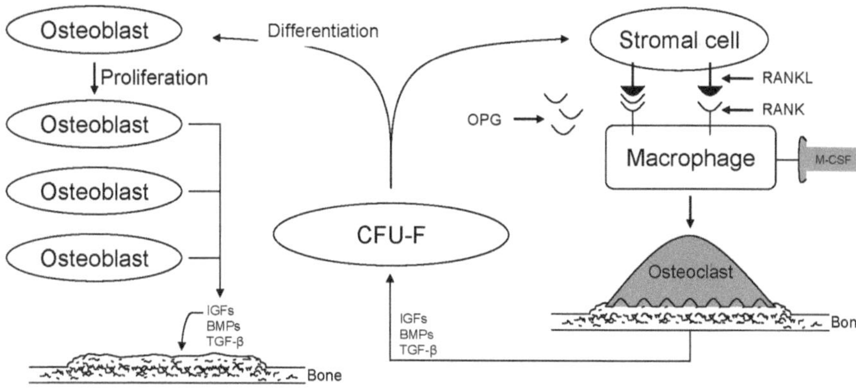

Fig. 1.1 Regulation of osteoblast formation and the coupling of bone resorption to formation. Osteoclastogenesis depends on the association of M-CSF and RANKL, produced by stromal cells and osteoblasts, with their receptors on monocytes/macrophage cells. This process is inhibited by OPG secreted by osteoblasts. The differentiated osteoclast polarizes on the bone surface, forming a ruffled membrane that acidifies the extracellular microenvironment, mobilizes the mineral phase of bone, and provides the milieu for organix matrix degradation. Bony dissolution releases various hormones and growth factors including IGFs, TGF-β, and BMPs. In a process that couples bone formation to resportion, these signaling molecules stimulate osteoblast differentiation and proliferation

are involved in perpetuating an osteoprogenitor phenotype including the homeodomain proteins (e.g., Msx-2, Dlx-2, Dlx-5, BAPX1), steroid receptors, as well as the helix-loop-helix (HLH) proteins Id, Twist, and Dermo [24]. The HLH proteins play important roles in the proliferation of osteoprogenitor cells, but repress osteoblast differentiation and must be downregulated before differentiation into a mature bone cell occurs [24] (see Fig. 1.2).

Bone marrow MSCs are multipotent and may differentiate into fibroblasts, osteogenic cells, chondrocytes, myocytes, and adipocytes in the formation of bone, cartilage, or other connective tissues [1, 25]. Multipotent stem cells have been isolated in vitro and can be induced to differentiate into multiple cell lineages [25]. Subpopulations of these cells, in response to systemic growth factors, play an integral role in fracture healing [1].

Osteoblast-mediated bone remodeling is influenced by a multitude of factors including PTH, 1,25-dihydroxyvitamin D, PTH, glucocorticoids (GCs), sex hormones, growth hormones (GHs), thyroid hormone, interleukins, TNF-α, prostaglandins, IGFs, TGF-β, BMPs, fibroblast growth factors (FGFs), platelet-derived growth factors (PDGFs), vascular endothelial growth factors (VEGFs), and interferon-γ (IF-γ) [26–28].

The BMPs and the Wnt signaling pathway are critical inducers of bone formation, the later through the expression of Runx2 [29]. The osteoblast-specific factor runt-related transcription factor 2/core binding factor α1 (Runx2/Cbfa1) is required for commitment of mesenchymal progenitors to the osteoblast lineage and is a key transcription factor in osteoblast differentiation [30–32]. Osterix (Osx), expressed

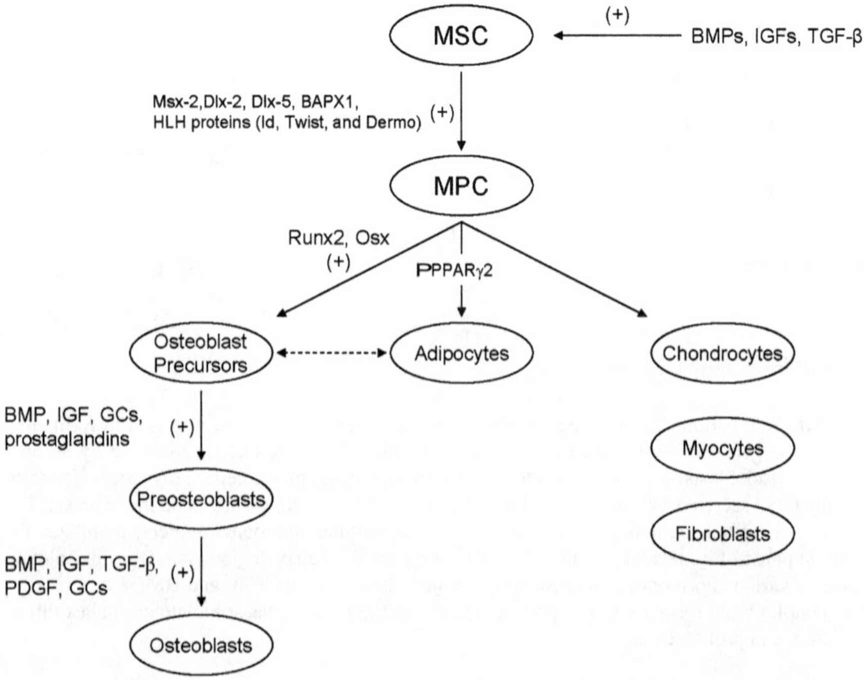

Fig. 1.2 Osteoblast differentiation. MSCs are responsible for the derivation of osteoblasts and are subject to the influence of local growth factors including BMPs, IGFs, and TGF-β. Multiple transcriptional regulators are involved in perpetuating an osteoprogenitor phenotype including the homeodomain proteins (e.g., Msx-2, Dlx-2, Dlx-5, BAPX1) and the helix-loop-helix (HLH) proteins (e.g., Id, Twist, and Dermo). BMPs and Wnt pathway signaling induce Runx2, which is required for commitment of multipotent progenitors (MPCs) to the osteoblast lineage. Runx2 is followed by downstream expression of Osterix (Osx). Glucocorticoids (GCs) and prostaglandins also play a role in osteoblast differentiation. PPARγ2 causes termination of osteoblastogenesis by downregulation of Runx2 and induction of adipocyte differentiation. Increasingly, MSC differentiation may shift from osteoblast to adipocyte formation with age. Although more controversial, a mature osteoblast may potentially undergo adipogenic transdifferentiation (*stipled, double-headed arrow*). MPCs may differentiate into other lineages including chondrocytes, myocytes, and fibroblasts

downstream of Runx2, is essential for the later stages of osteoblast differentiation [33]. Osterix is a zinc-finger containing transcription factor that is expressed in osteoblasts of all endochondral and membranous bones [33]. Mice lacking the *Osx* gene still do express the *Runx2/Cbfa1* gene but do not form cortical or trabecular bone because there is no endochondral or intramembranous bone ossification [33]. Runx2 knockout mice have incompletely differentiated osteoblasts and develop unmineralized cartilaginous skeletons [31, 33–35]. Nakashima et al. hypothesized from these findings that both Runx2 and Osx are required for formation of the functional osteoblast [33].

In humans, mutations in Runx2 lead to alterations in skeletal formation and growth (both endochondral and intramembranous), resulting in a disorder known as cleidocranial dysplasia [34, 35]. It is characterized by hypoplasia/aplasia of clavicles, patent fontanelles, supernumerary teeth, and short stature [36]. Vaughan et al. found that alleles of the Runx2 gene, specifically mutations in the polyQ/polyA repeat sequence preceding the "runt" domain, are associated with decreased bone mineral density and risk of fractures [31]. Runx2 is also expressed in mature osteoblasts and activates proteins involved in matrix deposition including type I collagen, osteocalcin, and osteopontin [37, 38].

The VEGFs are known to be important regulators of angiogenesis during endochondral ossification and may also exert a direct effect on osteoblasts [39]. Zelzer et al. has shown that Runx2 deficient mice lack expression of VEGFs [40]. In addition to its known role in angiogenesis during bone formation, VEGFs act as chemotactic agents for migration of osteoclasts and stimulate bone formation by upregulating osteoblast activity [39, 41].

1.3.2.1 Osteoblast Versus Adipocyte Differentiation

An inverse relationship exists between age-related bone loss and increased bone marrow adipose tissue accumulation [22]. This concept of increased marrow adiposity at the expense of bone volume has been observed in conditions leading to bone loss, such as ovariectomy, immobilization, and treatment with GCs [22]. The balance of MSC differentiation may shift from osteoblast to adipocyte formation with age, increasing the number and size of marrow adipocytes in a linear fashion over time [42]. In vitro studies have also provided some evidence that a mature osteoblast can undergo adipogenic transdifferentiation, indicating possible "plasticity" among cells of stromal lineage [22]. This potential transition from osteogenesis to adipogenesis, either by transdifferentiation or by a preferential shift of MSC differentiation to favor adipocyte over osteoblast production, may be an important contribution to fragility in aging bone.

Recent attention has been focused on the peroxisome proliferator-activated receptor γ2 (PPARγ2), a member of the nuclear receptor superfamily of ligand-activated transcription factors that is known to be expressed early in adipocyte differentiation [43]. Stimulation of PPARγ2 has been shown in mouse models to cause termination of osteoblastgenesis and induction of adipocyte differentiation [30, 42, 44]. PPARγ2 suppresses the osteoblast phenotype through downregulation of Runx2 [30, 45]. Lecka-Czernik et al. have shown that ligands which activate expression of PPARγ2 ligands downregulate Wnt-10b expression, which in turn may negatively modulate Runx2 expression [29, 46].

Ogawa et al. showed an association between PPARγ2 polymorphisms and changes in bone density in postmenopausal women, implicating PPARγ2 in postmenopausal bone loss [47]. Local factors including IGF-I, TGF-β, BMPs and hormonal factors including vitamin D and estrogen are also involved in this process [44]. Thiazolidinediones, insulin sensitizers with clinical applications in the management of type II diabetes mellitus, are known inducers of adipocyte differentiation and exert their influence through the PPARγ2 pathway [22, 48, 49]. Jennermann et al.

demonstrated that the administration of the thiazolidinedione pioglitazone to rats mediated both a reduction in osteoblast progenitors and bone mass [50].

1.3.3 Osteocytes

Osteocytes are osteoblasts that have become embedded in the bony matrix they produce. These cells extend long cytoplasmic processes that interconnect and make up a network of canaliculi that allow for cell-to-cell communication. Osteocytes are the most abundant cell type in bone. Once thought to be inactive, mature osteocytes have been shown to have a role in transduction of signals of mechanical loading, thereby acting as the mechano-sensors in bone [51, 52].

Recent work has elucidated a link between polymorphisms in the *SOST* gene and age-related changes in bone mineral density in postmenopausal women [53]. The protein product of the *SOST* gene, sclerostin, is a secreted glycoprotein related to BMP antagonists and most distantly to the BMP antagonist noggin [53, 54]. Sclerostin, released from osteocytes, controls the proliferation and differentiation of osteoprogenitor/pre-osteoblasts as well as the activity of mature osteoblasts by downregulating BMP activity [53]. Defects in the *SOST* gene lead to decreased production of this BMP antagonist and clinically manifest as dysregulated bone overgrowth (sclerosteosis) [55]. This is attributed to dysregulation of the anabolic phase of bone remodeling [53]. Thus, sclerostin may prove to be an appropriate therapeutic target in metabolic bone disorders [53].

1.4 Bone as a Mineral Reservoir

The human skeleton is made up of inorganic ions (30%) as well as collagen and noncollagenous proteins (70%). Calcium and phosphorus make up the main portion of mineral content, with smaller amounts of magnesium, sodium, and bicarbonate present. Bone serves as the body's reservoir for these minerals [56]. These minerals are not only critical for bone health and skeletal structural stability but also play important roles in normal functioning of all other tissues and organs. A complex interplay exists between bone and endocrine/exocrine regulators to maintain homeostatic regulation of circulating levels of these minerals.

Approximately, 97% of the body's calcium and 70% of the body's phosphorus are maintained in the skeleton [56]. The majority of calcium and phosphorus in the body is stored as hydroxyapatite, $Ca_{10}(PO_4)_6(OH)_2$, the main mineral component of bone. Calcium is maintained within a narrow physiologic range and must be persistently conserved and replaced. It is lost through the gastrointestinal (GI) tract, urine, sweat, and skin. In humans, exogenous calcium is taken in through the GI tract under the influence of vitamin D. The renal system regulates calcium and phosphorus homeostasis through urinary excretion/reabsorption. Vitamin D (cholecalciferol),

PTH, and calcitonin are the predominant hormones responsible for calcium and phosphorus homeostasis in the bone. To a lesser extent, thyroid hormone, GH, and the adrenal GCs play a role in calcium/phosphorus balance in the body.

Mineral homeostasis is skewed towards a negative balance with aging. Disorders of the GI system leading to malabsorption and of the renal system (renal failure or renal tubular disorders) leading to disregulated excretion of minerals may contribute to this net loss. Negative mineral balance is defined as mineral loss (fecal plus urine) exceeding mineral retention as seen in men >65 years of age and in postmenopausal women [57]. Examples of conditions that lead to negative mineral balance include chronic GC excess, hyperthyroidism, and vitamin D deficiency [57]. With aging, the skeleton uptakes less of these circulating minerals and bone ion efflux exceeds bone ion influx [57].

1.5 Skeletal Maintenance and Remodeling

The dynamic properties of bone are exemplified by remodeling, the process of continual rejuvenation after skeletal growth is completed whereby old bone is resorbed and new bone is formed. Uncoupling of this process is the general premise for age-related bone loss. There are four well described and unique phases of remodeling: activation, resorption, reversal, and formation.

1.5.1 Activation (Phase 1)

Activation refers to recruitment of mononucleated osteoclast precursors from the circulation to sites on the bone surface where they coalesce to form multinucleated pre-osteoclasts [58]. In response to signals released by damaged bone, marrow stromal cells are released from sclerostin inhibition and pre-osteoblasts are formed [59]. Osteoblasts and marrow stromal cells (and possibly T cells) provide signals to recruit and stimulate differentiation of the pre-osteoclast and initiate a BMU [60]. As described below, systemic factors such as GH, PTH, vitamin D; local factors including IL-1, IL-6, RANKL; and colony stimulating factors, specifically M-CSF play a role in the interaction between osteoblast and osteoclast [9, 19, 58, 61].

1.5.1.1 Osteoprotegerin/RANK/RANKL

Along with M-CSF, RANKL is a major factor in recruitment and differentiation of the osteoclast. It is produced by and expressed on the cell surfaces of osteoblasts and marrow stromal cells and interacts with the RANK receptor on pre-osteoclasts. This interaction leads to the differentiation and maturation of osteoclasts which coalesce and become capable of resorbing bone. OPG is a peptide member of the TNF receptor super-family that is synthesized by osteoblasts [62]. OPG is a free-floating, soluble decoy receptor that binds to RANKL and inhibits osteoclastgenesis and bone resorption [62]. Serum concentrations of OPG increase with age and may be a compensatory response to enhanced bone resorption in the estrogen deficient state or to age-dependent bone loss [63]. Vitamin D_3, PTH, prostaglandin E2 (PGE2), IL-1, IL-4, IL-6, IL-11, IL-17, and TNF-α all appear to stimulate osteoclastgenesis through the dual action of inhibiting production of OPG and stimulating production of RANKL [62, 64]. Estrogens, on the other hand, appear to inhibit production of RANKL and RANKL-stimulated osteoclastgenesis [64].

1.5.2 Resorption (Phase 2)

During resorption, an erosion cavity is created across the bone surface. Mononuclear precursors migrate to the bone surface, coalesce and form larger, activated, multinucleated osteoclasts [5]. These activated osteoclasts transfer protons to the resorbing compartment and lower the pH by secreting hydrogen ions via proton pumps [9, 65]. Surrounding the osteoclast is a "ruffled border," where the plasma membrane is folded into finger-like projections and contains the lysosomal enzymes that digest the mineral matrix [65]. Tight adherence to the surface is maintained by a "clear zone" that surrounds the ruffled border and contains only actin-like filaments [65]. Matrix and mineral is dissolved in the erosion cavity by secreted proteases and the local acidic milieu, respectively [9]. Absence of the ruffled border and clear zone has been shown in osteopetrotic rats [66]. The enzymes TRACP, cathespin K, and matrix metalloprotein MMP-9 (also known as collagenase or gelatinase) aid in resorption of the collagen and noncollagen matrix components [9, 41, 67]. When resorption is complete (after approximately 2 weeks), osteoclasts undergo apoptosis and phase three or reversal begins.

1.5.3 Reversal (Phase 3)

The reversal phase, which can last take up to 5 weeks, occurs once osteoclast resorption is complete. In this stage, mononuclear cells prepare the newly exposed bone surface for new osteoblasts to begin laying down bone. Initially, the lacunae are populated with liberated osteocytes, monocytes, and pre-osteoblasts [68]. Osteoblasts attracted to the surface synthesize a protein matrix primarily made up of type I collagen known as osteoid, which provides the scaffold for mineralized bone and subsequently undergoes mineralization. Sclerostin, produced by the osteocytes, inhibits the Wnt signaling pathway and thus regulates bone formation. As stated previously, the Wnt pathway stimulates bone formation by stimulating Runx2 as well as OPG [59, 69].

Also, at this time, the "cement line" is laid down. This is a layer between secondary osteons and the surrounding cortical bone [70]. It was previously thought to be an area of reduced mineralization relative to surrounding bone, but recent work has questioned this hypothesis and the exact composition of this line is still unclear [71, 72]. The cement line is a malleable surface that interfaces with surrounding bone matrix and is able to transfer energy in a manner that slows fracture growth in cortical bone [71]. The protein osteopontin is thought to be a key regulator of this process [73]. It has been hypothesized that the cement lines in aged bone have altered mechanisms of "crack arrest" and "energy dispersal" suggesting a decreased ability to reduce or prevent fracture [74].

Recruitment activity prior to bone formation is known as coupling, a poorly understood mechanism by which resorption and formation remain in equilibrium for bone mass to be maintained. Factors involved in coupling include TGF-β, IGF-1 and II, BMPs, PDGF, and FGFs (see Sect 1.6-Regulation of Bone Remodeling) [9, 75–77]. TGF-β is a potent inhibitor of osteoclast differentiation that acts by reducing RANKL production and limiting bone resorption [78].

1.5.4 Formation (Phase 4)

Bone formation is a two-step process whereby osteoblasts form layers of osteoid that then serves as a framework to promote mineralization. Enzymes that degrade mineral are inhibited and calcium and phosphorus are concentrated in the lacunae and canaliculi [79]. As bone formation continues, a portion of the early osteoblasts become imbedded in the new bone and become osteocytes. By poorly understood mechanisms, communication among osteocytes transmits information about mechanical changes, affecting the bone surface and remodeling. Mineralization begins when the lacunae are nearly filled with osteoid and the process may last for months, providing strength and density to the new bone [80].

Once the remodeling process is complete, osteoblasts are subject to several fates [9]. Some undergo apoptosis, some become osteocytes, and a portion goes on to become bone-lining cells. These lining cells serve to regulate ion (predominantly calcium) flux into and out of the bone, may modulate local bone formation and remodeling, and may reactivate from a quiescent to active state in the setting of mechanical loading (in vitro data) [81, 82].

Remodeling occurs in both cortical and trabecular bone but, with aging, differences in remodeling balance on the periostial and endostial surfaces lead to a decrease in cortical thickness and thinning of trabecular plates [9]. Bone loss is greater in trabecular than cortical bone. Consequently those areas of the skeleton with larger surface area, namely vertebrae and distal radius, are more prone to fracture [83]. Uncoupling and increased bone turnover lead to loss of trabeculae and increased porosity in bone [84]. Bone turnover in the elderly leads to a net loss of bone. The product of this is osteoporosis.

1.6 Regulation of Bone Remodeling

Proper bone remodeling and coupling is mediated by a complex regulatory system of both local and systemic factors.

1.6.1 Vitamin D and Osteomalacia

Vitamin D (cholecalciferol) is a fat-soluble hormone which humans acquire from the diet as well as synthesize in the skin from 7-dehydrocholesterol in the presence of ultraviolet light [85]. The main role of vitamin D is to facilitate absorption of calcium and phosphate for bone mineralization and to prevent low serum levels of these minerals. Vitamin D must be modified in the liver and kidney to become metabolically active, regardless of its source. The hepatic enzyme 25-hydroxylase places a hydroxyl group in the 25 position of the vitamin D molecule, forming calcidiol (25-hydroxyvitamin D). Calcidiol is transported in circulation attached to the vitamin D-binding protein [86]. Calcidiol is further modified by kidney tubular cells where 1-alpha-hydroxylase and 24-alpha-hydroxylase produce 1,25-dihydroxyvitamin D (calcitriol), the most active form of vitamin D or 24,25-dihydroxyvitamin D, an inactive metabolite [85, 87, 88].

Renal hydroxylation is enhanced by PTH, hypocalcemia, and hypophosphatemia but inhibited by 1,25-dihydroxyvitamin D [87]. Of note, the principal effect of estrogen on vitamin D is the synthesis of binding protein that carries it in serum [88]. Active 1,25-dihydroxyvitamin D stimulates intestinal Ca^{2+} absorption in inverse proportion to the amount of Ca^{2+} circulating in the extracellular compartment to maintain homeostatic levels.

Defective bone mineralization at sites of remodeling is known as osteomalacia and leads to an increased risk of osteoporosis and fracture [89]. In the setting of inadequate calcium and phosphorus due to deficient Vitamin D, osteoid is not mineralized and osteomalacia occurs. Histological studies have shown that 15–20% of patients with hip fractures have some element of osteomalacia [90, 91]. Polymorphisms in the vitamin D receptor, independent of bone density, may also alter calcium homeostasis and impact frequency of falls [92].

1.6.1.1 Vitamin D and Aging

Vitamin D deficiency is produced by decreased exposure to sunlight and decreased GI intake and absorption. Many older adults are bed or home bound, institutionalized or have limited access to the outside environment. In addition, many elderly do not receive adequate exogenous vitamin D either from diet or supplementation. These factors precipitate a deficient state which, as described above, leads to a decrement in bone mass and increase risk for osteomalacia and osteoporosis. Age-related changes in normal physiology as well as increased prevalence of chronic comorbidities lead to decreased amounts of active vitamin D. Elderly patients have less subcutaneous fat which may decrease vitamin D production (conversion) and storage. In addition, chronic kidney disease (CKD) leads to impairment in the hydroxylations necessary to produce the active form of vitamin D.

1.6.1.2 Vitamin D-Related Myopathy

Not only does vitamin D deficiency lead to decreased bone mineralization, but it also causes neuromuscular impairment, which contributes to increased fall rates [21, 93, 94]. Secondary hyperparathyroidism has also been shown to negatively affect skeletal muscle function [95]. Skeletal muscle expresses the vitamin D receptor and vitamin D stimulates myocyte uptake of inorganic phosphates necessary for ATP and creatine kinase production [96, 97]. Pfeifer et al. treated 122 ambulatory women aged 63–99 with 800 IU per day of Vitamin D combined with 1,200 mg calcium and reported reduced secondary hyperparathyroidism, body sway, and number of falls after 1 year [98]. Although conflicting data exists, the weight of evidence suggests that vitamin D supplementation reduces the risk of falls among ambulatory or institutionalized older individuals by at least 20% [93].

1.6.1.3 Vitamin D and Risk of Falls and Fracture

Some studies suggest that vitamin D supplementation along with calcium (but not vitamin D alone) may prevent osteoporotic fractures in community dwellers known to be deficient in vitamin D as well as in postmenopausal women [89, 99, 100]. Cummings et al. showed that a low level of 1,25-dihydroxvitamin D (57 pmol/l) was associated with an increased risk for hip fracture (adjusted risk ratio = 2.1) [101]. A meta-analysis of relevant pooled data also demonstrated a significant reduction in hip fracture (26%), as well as any nonvertebral fracture (23%) with calcium and vitamin D supplementation [102]. In one study, long-term supplementation in ambulatory older women found that long-term calcium and vitamin D supplementation in ambulatory older women reduced the odds of falling by 46%, and in sedentary women by 65%, but had a neutral effect on men regardless of their physical activity level [103].

1.6.2 Parathyroid Hormone and Secondary Hyperparathyroidism

The PTH is a polypeptide synthesized by the parathyroid glands and is negatively regulated by serum calcium and calcitriol [104]. It is released in response to decreases in plasma Ca^{2+} which is sensed by a specific Ca^{2+}-sensing protein [105]. Excessive stimulation is prevented by the rise in plasma Ca^{2+} itself and by negative feedback regulation involving PTH. Conversely, elevations in extracellular calcium activate this sensing receptor leading to the inhibition of PTH secretion and renal calcium reabsorption [104, 106]. The PTH maintains serum calcium by stimulating bone resorption, increasing vitamin D activity by renal conversion of 25-hydroxyvitamin D to 1,25-dihydroxyvitamin D, enhancing intestinal Ca^{2+} and phosphate absorption, and augmenting active renal Ca^{2+} reabsorption. Secondary hyperparathyroidism emerges when levels of circulating 25-hydroxyvitamin D fall below approximately 30 ng/ml and bone mineral density (at the hip) decreases when this level drops below this threshold [21, 107].

Serum levels of PTH increase with age leading to increased bone turnover [108, 109]. This may be due to decreased GI calcium absorption as well as significantly decreased circulating levels of calcitriol [108]. Enhanced secretion of PTH with aging increases the number of bone remodeling units and, with age-related uncoupling, leads to increased bone loss.

1.6.3 Gonadal Hormones

Estrogen and testosterone in women and men are necessary for proper maintenance of both cortical and trabecular bone [6, 110]. Estrogen functions as an anabolic agent in bone by inhibiting both osteoclastgenesis and osteoclast function [6]. Hypogonadism, as exemplified by postmenopausal osteoporosis, leads to accelerated bone resorption and osteoporosis. Estrogen is also known to increase osteoblast differentiation, proliferation, and function [14]. The loss of estrogen prolongs the resorption phase and shortens the formation phase. Estrogen deprivation also increases the frequency of resorption cycles [14].

In addition to directly effecting osteoclast and osteoblast function, estrogen (or lack thereof) may play a role in age-related bone loss by regulating production of various local cytokines and growth factors (including IL-1, TNF-α, and TGF-β) during T cell activation [111–113]. RANKL, a potent stimulator of osteoclast differentiation and function as described above, may also be produced by T cells and has been shown to increase in estrogen deficient (early postmenopausal) women [21, 114].

The role of estrogen deficiency in osteoporosis and osteoporotic fractures in postmenopausal women has been well documented. There is also accumulating evidence that estrogen may also play a key role in regulating bone turnover in men [115]. Osteoporosis in older men has been shown to be more closely correlated with low estrogen than testosterone levels [116]. Khosla et al. looked at longitudinal changes in bone mineral density in young versus elderly men and accumulated data to support a role of estrogen both in the acquisition of peak bone mass in young men and in bone loss in elderly men [117]. They were able to show that aging men with levels of bioavailable estrogen below the 50th percentile were at the greatest risk for bone resorption and bone loss [117].

1.6.4 Thyroid Hormone

Hyperthyroidism is associated with increased excretion of calcium and phosphorous in the urine and stool, which results in a loss of bone mineral. This loss is reflected in lower bone densitometry and leads to an increased risk of fractures [118]. Excess thyroid hormone has been shown to directly stimulate osteoclast resorption although the exact mechanism is not known [119, 120]. Britto et al. found that thyroid hormone stimulated increased osteoclast activity only in the presence of osteoblasts [120]. They hypothesized that thyroid hormone may work indirectly through osteoblasts which in turn mediate osteoclastic bone resorption [120]. Patients with hypothyroidism treated with exogenous thyroxine have been shown to lose bone mineral from the spine more rapidly than those without known thyroid disease [121, 122].

The TSH itself has been shown to display physiologically relevant effects on both the bone formation and bone resorption phases of remodeling [123]. This process is mediated via the TSH receptor on osteoblast and osteoclast precursors [123]. TSH inhibits osteoclast formation and survival by attenuating signals initiated by RANKL and TNF-α [123]. TSH inhibits osteoblast differentiation through the Runx-2 and osterix pathways by downregulating Wnt and VEGF signaling [123].

1.6.5 Growth Hormone/Insulin-Like Growth Factors

Growth hormone, IGF-1, IGF-2, and IGF binding proteins play a crucial role in skeletal growth as well as maintenance of bone mass in adults [77]. The catabolic effects of GH on bone are mediated through IGF-1 [77]. IGF exerts its influence on bone remodeling through the OPG/RANK/RANKL pathway. GH and IGF-1 in vivo stimulate osteoblasts to express OPG and RANKL, promote osteoclast activity directly, and also expand the pool of osteoblasts needed to equalize bone resorption [77]. The GH/IGF-1 axis also stimulates IL-1, IL6, and TNF-α production, which supports osteoclastgenesis and a negative remodeling balance. Serum levels of GH and IGF-1 decrease with age and are associated with the loss of bone density [124]. However, studies have shown that short-term treatment with GH, in a dose-dependent fashion, increases biomarkers of bone resorption in elderly, osteopenic, postmenopausal women [125]. The efficacy of long-term use of this hormone as a treatment for low bone mineral density is still in question. Friedlander et al. showed that 1 year of treatment with IGF-1 raised serum levels to a "normal" range but had no effect on improving bone density in older women [126]. In contrast, Langois et al. showed that higher IGF-1 levels were associated with higher BMD in very old men and women (aged 72–94) [127].

1.6.6 Interleukins

Cytokines have multiple regulatory actions on bone formation and resorption [128]. IL-1 and IL-6 play a role in origination of the BMU and osteoclast recruitment [129]. IL-1 is a potent stimulator of osteoclast activity and recruitment and may also serve to regulate stromal cell production of IL-6 and M-CSF [129]. Inhibition of IL-1 and IL-6 reduces the increase of osteoclast number seen after ovariectomy [111, 130]. IL-6 is under the regulatory control of TNF-α, a known potent stimulator of osteoclast recruitment and activity. In addition to their effects on osteoclasts, IL-1 and TNF-α can also inhibit osteoblast activity [131]. IL-11 has a biological profile similar to IL-6 and induces formation of osteoclasts by upregulating RANKL on marrow stromal cells and immature osteoblasts [132].

Interferon-γ (IF-γ) is produced by activated T cells and has been shown to block RANKL-induced osteoclast differentiation [133]. Replicative senescence of CD8 T-cells is associated with the reduced ability to produce IF-γ, which would favor disinhibited osteoclast formation and increased bone resorption [134]. It has also been suggested that increased production of TNF-α and IL-6 by senescent CD8 T-cells could promote osteoclast maturation and activation, influencing age-related bone alterations [131]. For example, increased proportions of CD8 T-cells expressing senescence-related surface markers have been correlated with osteoporotic fractures in older women [135].

1.6.7 Calcitonin

Calcitonin is a 32-amino acid peptide hormone produced by thyroid parafollicular C cells. It functions to reduce serum calcium and inhibit bone resorption when serum Ca^{2+} levels go above a certain level. Zaidi et al. have shown that osteoclast sensitivity to this peptide exists in vitro and serves a mechanism of skeletal conservation [136]. At the cellular level, calcitonin inhibits extracellular Ca^{2+} sensing which serves as an antiresorptive signal [137].

1.6.8 Fibroblast Growth Factors and Transforming Growth Factor-β

Fibroblast growth factors and TGF-β play a prominent role in osteoprogenitor cell commitment to the osteoblast lineage [138]. Both FGFs and TGF-β have been shown to exert anabolic effects on bone formation in animals and to reduce bone loss in experimental models of osteoporosis [138, 139]. FGFs are produced by the osteoblast and stored in the matrix [138]. FGFs interact with four distinct cell-surface receptors that are ubiquitous in bone. FGFs increase the number and functionality of osteoblasts by increasing Runx2 expression and cause increased matrix mineralization [138]. These results have been shown both in vitro and in vivo and suggest a role for FGFs in bone formation on endosteal and trabecular surfaces [140]. Mutations in this group of proteins and their receptors result in abnormal skeletal phenotypes, including achondroplasia [141].

It has been postulated that decreased responsiveness to FGF might account for the reduced bone formation by aged osteoblasts [142]. Pfeilshifter et al. looked at cultures of osteoblast-like cells from outgrowths of human trabecular bone and exposed them to various local and systemic factors, including FGF [143]. Increases in DNA synthesis were significantly negatively correlated with donor age and approximately tenfold higher concentrations of growth factors and hormones were required to yield comparable increases in DNA synthesis in cells derived from the oldest age group [143]. Mayahara et al. administered intravenous human basic FGF for 2 weeks to both young and old rats and showed that this intervention stimulated osteoblast proliferation and new bone formation, suggesting a potential role for FGF in treating osteoporosis [144].

TGF-β is an important growth factor in bone and is also secreted by osteoblasts. It is found in large amounts within the bone matrix and functions in the proliferation and recruitment of osteoblasts and marrow stromal cells, chemotaxis of osteoblasts, and induction of several bone matrix proteins [138]. TGF-β regulates osteoblast differentiation and downstream effects on Runx2 expression through the Smad protein-signaling pathway [145]. Studies in animal models have shown an anabolict effect of TGF-β in bone formation [138]. Marrow from aged and ovariectomized rats expresses less TGF-β and presumably have less osteogenic potential (due to decreased size and osteogenic potential of marrow osteoblast progenitor cells) [146, 147].

1.7 The Pathophysiology of Bone Loss in the Elderly

1.7.1 Age-Related Bone Loss

It is clear that bone remodeling is under the control of endogenous hormonal and local regulators as well as external mechanical loads secondary to physical activity. As the skeleton ages, it become less responsive to these factors and the final common pathway is a net increase in bone resorption but no change in or a decrease on bone formation [5]. This uncoupling of the remodeling process leads to a net loss of bone and increase in skeletal fragility, the major hallmarks of osteoporosis [148].

Markers of bone turnover are seen in higher concentrations in older patients. The EPIDOS trial showed the highest levels of osteocalcin, N-telopeptide, C-telopeptide, and bone-specific alkaline phosphatase in those elderly women with the lowest BMD [149]. In contrast to these elevated markers of turnover with age, indicators of bone formation such as procollagen peptide are not proportionally elevated [150].

It has been well documented that bone mass decreases in the skeleton with aging but it is crucial to note that the risk of fracture also climbs with age, regardless of bone mineral density [151, 152]. Clinically, this increase in bone loss (quantity) along with alterations in skeletal micro-architecture (quality) leads to a propensity toward fracture. Dual energy X-ray absorptiometry (DXA) provides a measure of bone mass but lacks the ability to measure architectural changes related to fracture risk, changes in the cellular make up of marrow (e.g., increased adipocity), and the periosteal response to trabecular bone loss [44, 153]. Reductions in both trabecular and cortical bone have been demonstrated in older bone [154, 155]. As discussed above (see Sect. 1.3.2.1), pluripotent MSCs favor adipogenesis over osteogenesis with aging in vitro and the subsequent decrement in numbers of committed cells to the osteoblast lineage may contribute to age-related bone loss [156].

Age-related osteoporosis should be considered a unique entity and must be contrasted with other causes of bone loss seen in advancing age. Mechanistically, age-related bone loss is characterized predominantly by decreased bone formation (secondary to decreased osteoblast numbers and activity) in the presence of persistent resorption [156]. This is in contrast to postmenopausal osteoporosis, for example, whereby estrogen deprivation leads primarily to an increase in osteoclast initiation events and accelerated bone resorption [84, 148, 157, 158]. Multiple factors in the geriatric population, including hormonal changes, comorbidities (such as CKD), immobility, nutritional factors, and drug interactions, influence bone metabolism. These mechanisms will be described below. Taken collectively, all forms of age-related osteoporosis constitute an international epidemic.

1.7.2 Postmenopausal Osteoporosis

The reduction of ovarian hormone production seen in menopause is a well-accepted contributor to age-related bone loss in women. Estrogen exerts an anabolic effect directly on bone by promoting the differentiation of osteoblasts in preference to other mesenchymal cell types, increasing the number of functional osteoblasts, and increasing several secreted proteins involved in the formation phase including IGF-1, procollagen type 1, TGF-β, and BMPs [84, 154]. Estrogen also prevents bone resorption by increasing osteoclast apoptosis and decreasing osteoblast and osteocyte apoptosis [159–161]. It also reduces the activity of IL-1, IL-6, TNF-α, cytokines known to stimulate osteoclast activity [110].

In vitro studies have provided data suggesting that endogenous nitric oxide (NO) present in osteoclast cultures regulates resorption activity [162, 163]. Endothelial NO prevents osteoporosis by inhibiting the activity of osteoclasts [163]. Estrogen, either endogenous or supplemental, enhances endothelial NO production, which inhibits osteoclast activity and prevents osteoporosis [163].

Estrogen deficiency, conversely, leads to absence of these mechanisms, which may play a role in the dysregulation of bone remodeling [158]. Estrogen deprivation leads to reductions in osteoclast apoptosis and increases in osteoblast apoptosis,

Table 1.1 Bone remodeling abnormalities in age-related bone loss and postmenopausal osteoporosis

	Age-related bone loss	Postmenopausal osteoporosis	Remodeling phase
Number of remodeling sites	↓	↑	Activation
Formation of multinucleated osteoclasts	↔	↔	
Osteoclast activity	↔	↑	Resorption
Size of erosion pit	↔	↑	
Disappearance of osteoclasts	↔	↔	
Appearance of MSCs	↔	↔	Reversal
Proliferation and differentiation of MSCs	↓	↔	
Osteoblast maturation	↔	↔	Formation
Osteoblast activity/ osteoid formation	↓	↔	
Matrix mineralization	↔	↔	
Pit restoration	↓	↓	Quiescence

↑ increased; ↓ decreased; ↔ no change

leading to a net loss of bone. In addition, estrogen deficiency is known to induce osteocyte apoptosis that may cause microarchitectural damage [5, 161]. The effects of estrogen deprivation are more pronounced in trabecular bone. The increase in bone resorption seen in perimenopausal women results from an increase in activation frequency during phase 1 of remodeling (mediated by pre-osteoblasts) and the extended recruitment of osteoclasts leading to a prolonged resorptive phase [84, 148]. Changes in the levels of locally acting growth factors and cytokines (including IL-1, IL-6, and TNF-α) that also impair osteoblast function may be mediated by estrogen withdrawal [164].

Menopause is also associated with decreasing levels of circulating vitamin D and decreased renal tubular calcium absorption, even in the presence of fluctuating PTH levels [84, 165, 166]. These factors may contribute to an overall negative calcium balance, a subsequent increase in bone resorption, and further bone loss (see Table 1.1).

1.7.3 Somatopause

Aging is associated with a progressive decrement of lean body mass, increased fat mass, reduced exercise tolerance, decreased strength and mobility, as well as an increased catabolism [167, 168]. These factors are associated with a progressive decline in independence and quality of life [169].

Somatopause refers to the gradual and progressive fall in spontaneous GH secretion that occurs with increasing age, which may lead to the aforementioned physiologic changes. GH secretion depends on hypothalamic stimulation and its effects on bone homeostasis are regulated primarily through IGF-1 [170]. GH and IGF-1 both stimulate bone formation and enhance bone turnover (see Sect. 1711.6.5). In vivo, GH and IGF-1 activate osteoclasts and are crucial factors in osteoclastgenesis and osteoclastic resorption, possibly through the RANK/RANKL/OPG pathway [171]. The positive effects of GH and IGF-1 on osteoblast development and function have been validated [77, 172–174]. Impaired osteoblast function with aging is mediated in part by low levels of circulating and/or local IGF-I levels [168]. GH and IGF-1 appear to influence osteoblast and osteoclast activation and function at various levels, but the significance and exact mechanisms are still being elucidated [77].

The in vitro and in vivo data pertaining to the efficacy of somatotrophic treatment in the elderly vary widely. GH treatment of older adults with low bone mineral density results in only small changes in lean body mass, musculoskeletal function, and overall quality of life [175].

1.7.4 Androgen Decline in the Aging Male Syndrome and Andropause

Andropause is a phenomenon characterized by increase risk for fracture, sexual regression, erectile dysfunction, lower urinary tract symptoms, increased atherosclerosis, cognitive decline, loss of energy, sarcopenia, and decreased physical agility in men over the age of 40 due to dropping testosterone levels [176]. ADAM syndrome is a term used to describe the same clinical scenario but includes not only a drop in serum testosterone, but also a decrement in GH, melatonin and dehydroepiandrosterone, in aging males [177]. Circulating plasma testosterone levels decrease by 0.5–1% per year after the age of 40 in men [170, 178]. Andropause mimics a hypogonadal state reflected in low testosterone and other androgen levels. The cause of late-life hypogonadism is multifactorial and may be related to defects at the level of the hypothalamus, pituitary, and/or testes as well as increases in serum hormone binding globulin [176].

Androgen deficient men are at an increased risk of osteoporosis. BMD decreases by approximately 1% per year after age 40 [179]. Androgens have a major role in the growth and maintenance of both cancellous and cortical bone mass in men. Studies by Tenover et al. and Snyder et al. assessed BMD by DXA scans and found significant increases in men treated with intramuscular testosterone when compared with placebo [180, 181]. Androgen receptors are expressed in osteoblasts, osteoclasts, and bone marrow stromal cells. Androgens have been shown to control bone formation and resorption by regulating the expression and activity of several cytokines and growth factors including IGF-1, IL-1, IL-6, TGF-β, and OPG/RANKL [182]. A recent study by Nair et al. showed that men who received testosterone therapy had a slight increase in bone mineral density at the femoral neck and women who received DHEA had an increase in BMD at the ultra distal radius. Neither treatment, though, improved quality of life [183].

1.7.5 Renal Osteodystrophy

Research from the United States Renal Data System estimates that nearly half of all new CKD patients are over the age of 65 and this subset of the population is three times more likely to have CKD [184]. CKD stages 3 and 4 (GFR < 60 ml/min/1.73 m^2), known risk factors for fracture, is present in 17% of all comers from this age group [185]. These values are even more pronounced in the institutionalized setting. In a large, retrospective, cross-sectional analysis of 9,931 long-term care residents aged 65 or older, Garg et al. found that approximately 40% had a GFR < 60 ml/min/1.73 m^2 [186].

The skeletal complications and aberrations of bone and mineral metabolism that accompany CKD are grouped under the phenomena of renal osteodystrophy. The National Institute of Diabetes and Digestive and Kidney Diseases (NIDDK) reports that 90% of hemodialysis patients are affected with renal osteodystrophy [184]. This disease is associated with increased morbidity, including bone pain, fractures, deformity, myopathy, soft tissue calcification and tendon rupture, as well as increased mortality [187].

The pathologic abnormalities that take place in renal osteodystrophy encompass a range of mechanisms which may lead to bone loss. Bone turnover may be excessively high, as manifested by elevated levels of circulating PTH, or abnormally low in the state of "adynamic bone" disease [187]. Broadly, renal osteodystrophy is classified as osteitis fibrosa, osteomalacia, or adynamic bone disease according to histologic features [188]. Mixed combinations along this spectrum may also be seen. All entities result in defects in bone mineralization.

Secondary hyperparathyroidism, due to hyperplasia of the parathyroid glands seen in CKD, is the main mechanism involved in high turnover renal osteodystrophy [189]. Virtually all stage V CKD (GFR < 15 ml/min/1.73 m^2) patients will develop secondary hyperparathyroidism. Phosphorus is retained, less calcitriol is produced by the failing kidney, less calcium is absorbed in the GI tract, and calcium homeostasis is dysregulated [187]. In addition, decreased expression of the vitamin D receptor and/or the calcium-sensing receptor in the setting of parathyroid hyperplasia leads to altered calcium homeostasis [104].

The PTH and calcitriol are important factors in the differentiation of preosteoclasts during activation as well as in osteoblast proliferation during bone formation [190, 191]. The PTH works in concert with IGF-1, IL-1, IL-6, IL-11, and TNF-α to stimulate activation [192]. Secondary hyperparathyroidism in CKD patients manifests in the skeleton as osteitis fibrosa, characterized by marrow fibrosis and increased bone resorption [188]. Increased osteoclast number and activity are seen and nonlamellar bone is laid down. This process occurs mainly in the cortical portions of long bones, leading to increased porosity and decreased strength as lamellar bone is replaced by weaker, woven bone [188].

Osteomalacia in CKD is characterized by low rates of bone turnover, defective mineralization, and increased osteoid [188]. This is due to aluminum deposition/toxicity related to treatment with aluminum-based phosphorus binders in end-stage renal disease (ESRD) and has decreased in prevalence with the decreased use of these agents [193].

Adynamic bone disease is the most common renal osteodystrophy in those without secondary hyperparathyroidism, in addition to those on hemodialysis or peritoneal dialysis [188]. This process may also be caused by aluminum intoxication, although nonaluminum intoxication cases do exist [192]. Deficiency of BMP-7 (also known as osteogenic protein-1), a growth factor that has been shown to induce osteoblastic cell differentiation of pluripotent mesenchymal cells, has been hypothesized to play a role in adynamic bone disease [188, 192, 194]. Mineralization is low and the osteoid thickness never increases [192].

Another important factor in the pathogenesis of CKD related bone disease is the presence of metabolic acidosis. Bone is dissolved as hydrogen ions are buffered by bone carbonate [187]. Acidosis has been shown to alter the cellular effects of PTH and vitamin D on osteoblasts, as well as affect the RANKL/OPG pathway, IL-6 and IL-1 [187, 195].

Patients with ESRD have been shown to be at risk for fracture secondary to reduced bone mineral density and Alem et al. demonstrated an overall increased risk of hip fracture in ESRD patients as compared with the general population [196]. The overall relative risk for hip fracture was 4.44 (95% CI, 4.16–4.75) for male dialysis patients and 4.40 (95% CI, 4.17–4.64) for female dialysis patients compared to controls [196].

1.7.6 Skeletal Unloading/Immobilization

Weight bearing contributes to the maintenance and development of bone mass and it is well known that lack of gravitational or mechanical loading of the skeleton leads to a rapid loss of bone and osteoporosis [197–200]. Nishimura et al. demonstrated that immobilization has an immediate and significant effect on bone loss by placing 20 healthy young adults on bed rest for 20 days and showing that, after this time, BMD as measured by DXA was decreased at both lumbar and metacarpal bones by 4.6 and 3.6%, respectively [201]. The elderly population is particularly susceptible to chronic immobility due to lack of physical activity for a variety of reasons. This may be related to immobilization from prolonged bed rest [following orthopedic injury, spinal cord injury (SCI), stroke, systemic illness], pain, fear of falling, lack of sufficient supportive care in the home, or neglect. Immobilization leads to increased osteoclast-mediated bone resorption and reduced bone formation [199]. Lack of stress on bones decreases osteoblast recruitment as well as proliferation and bed rest triggers increased recruitment of osteoclasts that lasts until the end of the bed-rest period [202–204].

Rapid loss of bone in the setting of skeletal unloading has also been studied extensively in the arena of weightlessness related to the zero gravity environment encountered by astronauts in space. Studies of bone atrophy during space travel indicate that urinary calcium levels increase immediately and the negative calcium balance peaks at approximately 200 mg/day [205]. Studies from the Mir space station revealed that space travelers loss on average 1–2% of bone mass with each month in space [205]. Bone loss was noted to be most significant in the lumbar vertebrae and legs of astronauts [205].

Urinary calcium increases with immobilization or skeletal disuse and calcium imbalance favoring loss occurs within days, peaking at about 5 weeks [206]. In bed rest, the average urinary calcium loss at its peak is approximately 150 mg/day, which corresponds to 0.5% of total body calcium [206]. In patients with SCI, there is an immediate loss of calcium through the urine with a negative balance of approximately 100 mg/day. Although calcium balance reverts back to normal within 6–18 months, up to 1/3 of cortical bone and 1/2 of trabecular bone may be lost [206, 207]. Bone loss is enhanced in SCI patients from lack of muscle traction on bone as well as impaired GI absorption of calcium, both of which occur acutely after injury. In patients with injury within 1 year of measurement, reduction in bone mineral densities has been noted in the femoral neck (27%), midshaft (25%), and distal femur (43%), as compared with controls [208]. Over 50% of bone in these regions may be demineralized at 10 years postinjury [208]. The net effect in the upper extremities and trunk is a 10–21% loss of bone at the 10-year point [208].

The main consequence of this bone loss is progression to fracture. In 2002, the Model Spinal Cord Injury System produced figures on fracture rates based on time following SCI, with incidences of 14% at 5 years, 28% at 10 years, and 39% at 15 years postinjury [208, 209].

1.7.7 Tobacco- and Alcohol-Related Bone Loss

The National Institute on Alcohol Abuse and Alcoholism (NIAAA) defines excessive alcohol intake in individuals over age 65 as more than one drink per day [210]. The 2001 National Household Survey on Drug Abuse found that 33% of adults age 65 and older report consuming alcohol during the preceding month [211]. A large national cross-sectional survey of community-dwelling elders demonstrated that 25% of individuals over age 65 who reported alcohol consumption reported daily drinking (31% of men, 19% of women) [212]. Approximately 10% of elders reported "binge drinking," defined as drinking five or more drinks on one occasion at least 12 times in the previous year [212].

Alcohol consumption is a risk factor for osteoporosis based on the frequent finding of low bone mass, decreased bone formation rate, and increased fracture incidence in alcoholics [213, 214]. Negative effects of ethanol are seen both directly on bone and indirectly by modulating vitamin D and calcium homeostasis [215, 216]. Alcohol has been shown to reduce bone formation in healthy humans and animals and to decrease proliferation of cultured osteoblastic cells [213]. Alcohol has also been shown to increase indices of bone resorption in isolated osteoclasts and decrease indices of osteoblast differentiation (e.g., alkaline phosphatase activity) in osteoblast-like cells [215].

Fractures were reported to be approximately four times as common in a series of 107 chronic alcoholics as in age-matched random controls [217]. Alcoholism is known to decrease the amount of available and active vitamin D by influencing intestinal absorption and liver metabolism, respectively [213]. Turner et al. showed in a rat model that alcohol affected bone mass primarily by reducing indices of bone formation and found that PTH-induced bone formation was blunted by alcohol [218]. Malnutrition commonly seen in alcohol drinkers leads to metabolic derangements in calcium, magnesium, and phosphorus. The known neurologic effects of alcohol (imbalance, ataxia, altered judgment, etc.) may be more pronounced in the elderly (due to increased volume of distribution of alcohol with aging) and may predispose this population to falls. Coupled with the pathologic effects of alcohol on bone described above, falls and fractures in elderly subjects who consume alcohol constitute a dangerous problem.

Tobacco exposure (smoke, smokeless, passive) has been linked to decreased bone mass and increased risk of osteoporotic fractures [219, 220]. Active tobacco smoking is associated with reduced bone density and increased risk of fractures in postmenopausal women [221]. Blum et al. showed that individuals exposed to household tobacco smoke had a mean adjusted BMD that was significantly lower at the total hip ($p = 0.021$) and femoral neck ($p = 0.018$) compared with subjects who were not exposed [220]. Smoking in women from the time of the menopause onwards increases the risk of hip fracture in old age by about 50% [221]. Tobacco's pathologic role in bone loss may be attributable to the effects of nicotine on bone collagen synthesis, alterations in the level of circulating estrogens, and decreased calcium absorption [220].

1.7.8 Drug-Induced Osteoporosis

Many classes of drugs have been implicated in the alteration of bone metabolism and the induction of osteoporosis. These include GCs, anticonvulsants, antimetabolic agents (i.e., chemotherapy drugs for prostate and breast cancers), cyclosporine, excessive vitamin A intake (from supplemental nutritional products), heparin, warfarin, thiazide diuretics, beta-blockers, exogenous thyroid hormone, proton pump inhibitors, medroxyprogesterone acetate, statins, and SSRI antidepressants. Many of these are used frequently in the geriatric population.

1.7.8.1 Glucocorticoid-Induced Osteoporosis

Glucocorticoid-induced osteoporosis (GIO) is the most well studied prevelant and debilitating drug side effect in the elderly population and one of the main causes of fractures in the elderly [148]. GIO results from an uncoupled remodeling unit with decreased bone formation and increased bone resorption [148]. Multiple mechanisms have been proposed that contribute to this prevalent form of secondary osteoporosis (see Table 1.2).

The GCs alter both the commitment of MSCs to the osteoblast lineage as well as proliferation of committed osteoblasts [222]. It has been shown in vitro that GCs regulate osteoblast differentiation by modifying the expression and action of BMPs as well as Runx2 [222]. GCs also promote an increase in osteoblast and osteocyte apoptosis [223]. GIO is also mediated by a direct inhibitory effect on osteoblasts as well as by decreasing type I collagen expression and destabilizing type I collagen mRNA [224–226].

The GCs inhibit production of IGF-I by osteoblasts, inhibit IGF receptor expression, and decrease the stimulatory effects of TGF-β on osteoblasts [225, 227, 228]. As discussed in Sects. 1.6.5 and 1.6.8, IGF-1 and TGF-β influence bone formation by stimulating osteoblast proliferation and differentiation.

The effect of GCs on increasing bone resorption is seen early in the remodeling sequence where these agents increase expression of RANKL and decrease OPG

Table 1.2 The pathophysiology of glucocorticoid-induced bone loss

Decreased bone formation		
	Preosteoblast	
		↓ Proliferation
		↓ BMP, Runx2
	Osteoblast	
		↑ Apoptosis
		↓ Protein synthesis
		↓ IGF-1, TGF-β
	Osteocyte	
		↓ Viability
		↑ Apoptosis
	Adrenals/gonads	
		↓ Androgens/↓ estrogen
Increased bone resorption		
	↓ OPG, ↑ RANKL	
	GI tract	
		↓ Ca^{2+} absorption
	Kidneys	
		↓ Ca^{2+}/phosphate resorption
		↓ $1,25(OH)_2$ D3 production
	Parathyroid	
		↓ PTH

Abbreviations are as defined in the text

expression, prolonging the life of osteoclasts by limiting apoptosis [229]. GCs reduce intestinal absorption of calcium, increase urinary phosphate and calcium, and reduce production of 1,25-dihydroxyvitamin D leading to secondary hyperparathyroidism [230, 231]. High doses of GCs often suppress gonadotropin secretion thereby reducing levels of androgens and estrogens [232].

This combination of factors leads to a high rate of spontaneous fractures even at levels of BMD that are usually not associated with bone failure [148]. The multiple mechanisms described above provide good evidence supporting the role of GCs in dysfunctional bone remodeling leading to destabilization of bone microarchitecture and increased risk of fracture [226]. An additional known side effect of GC use is loss of muscle mass and strength as well as mypoathy [233]. Muscle pain and weakness may lead to decreased mobility and decreased strength predisposing patients to falls. Another side effect of GC use is osteonecrosis or avascular necrosis, commonly seen in the femur or humerus. Theories on the etiology of this condition include fat emboli, oxidative injury, and osteocyte apoptosis [226].

Up to 50% of people on long-term GC therapy will develop osteoporosis and fracture may quickly ensue [226]. Reid et al. conducted a prospective, longitudinal study on patients beginning high-dose GC therapy (mean dose of prednisone 21 mg/day) and found that they lost a mean of 27% of their lumbar spine BMD during the first year [234]. A large retrospective cohort study in the United Kingdom by Van Staa et al. reported a relative risk of clinical vertebral fracture during oral GC therapy to be 2.6, with a relative risk for hip fracture of 1.6, and overall relative risk for nonvertebral fracture of 1.3 [226, 235]. The overall prevalence of fracture in patients on oral GCs is approximately 28%, the highest proportion of these patients being postmenopausal women [226, 235]. The risk of fracture was shown by Van Staa et al. to be related to the dose and duration of therapy, but is independent of bone mineral density [235]. Low doses of oral GCs (prednisone 5–9 mg) as well as high doses of inhaled steroids may also produce clinically significant osteoporosis [236, 237].

1.8 Cellular Senescence

Cellular senescence refers to the progressive loss in ability of normal cells to divide. This concept was first described in 1961 by Hayflick and Moorhead when they showed that normal human fibroblasts only divide a finite number of times [238]. This concept of limited cell division came to be known as "Hayflick's limit" or replicative senescence [239]. Replicative senescence applies only to cells that are able to divide in vivo, which excludes postmitotic cells [240, 241]. Tissue function may decline with age in part because the ability of cells to replicate and/or repair themselves is lost [240, 242–244].

Various forms of DNA damage may either lead to unregulated cell division (neoplasia) or result in a halt of cell replication by senescence or apoptosis.

Senescent cells are growth arrested in the G_1/S phase of the cell cycle [245]. The G_0 or quiescent phase is excluded. The phenotype of senescent cells is manifested by irreversible growth arrest, resistance to apoptosis, and altered cellular function [240].

It has been suggested that reductions in bone density seen with age may be the result of osteoblast loss, either directly (decreased proliferation and apoptosis) or indirectly (secondary to changes that accompany replicative senescence leading to the loss of a normal osteoblast phenotype) [143, 246–250]. Cultured osteoblasts exhibit a limited proliferative lifespan and an altered phenotype, as evidenced by decreased expression of Runx2, alkaline phosphatase, type I collagen, and osteocalcin [248, 251, 252]. With age, human MSCs display declines in several measures associated with proliferative and osteogenic potential [247, 249, 253–255]. The osteogenic potential of murine MSCs shows a similar decline with increasing donor age [256]. Kassem et al. demonstrated that osteoblast cell strains established from osteoporotic patients had a severely reduced proliferative capacity in vitro [248]. If functional deficits in osteoblasts that occur with cellular senescence play a major role in the uncoupling of bone formation and resorption, then recruitment of osteoblast precursors and osteoblast differentiation become critical components in maintaining the balance between these two opposing processes.

It has also been shown that osteoclasts and osteoblasts may undergo apoptosis [257–261]. The rate of bone formation is largely determined by the number of osteoblasts, which is a product of the number of progenitors and effective lifespan of the mature cell [262]. Jilka et al. showed that PTH serves to increase osteoblast number, bone formation rate, and bone mass in mice with either normal or reduced osteoblastgenesis [262]. This is due to an anti-apoptotic effect of the hormone on osteoblasts [262]. Indeed osteoblast apoptosis is a recognized phenomenon, as seen by GC-induced osteoblast cell death [223].

With senescence, reduced expression of osteoblast markers such as alkaline phosphatase, osteocalcin, and type I collagen has been shown in response to various hormones and growth factors including 1,25-$(OH)_2$ vitamin D3, IGF-I, PTH, and PGE2 [263–270].

A possible marker of cellular senescence in osteoblasts is senescence-associated β-galactosidase (SA β-gal). This marker has been shown to increase with aging of fibroblasts both in vitro and in vivo [244]. Stenderup et al. found that late passage MSCs expressed higher levels of SA β-gal than early passage cells [246]. However, it is unlikely that SA β-gal by itself, truly defines cellular senescence [263, 264].

In summary, potential cellular mechanisms of age-related bone loss include decreases in osteogenic stem cell potential with age, decreased proliferation of osteoblasts, depressed expression of an osteoblast phenotype, apoptosis, or decreased osteoblast responsiveness to extracellular signals [265]. It is still unclear whether the inability of MSCs to differentiate into osteoblasts or the impaired function of senescent osteoblasts makes the greater contribution to age-related bone loss.

1.8.1 Telomere Shortening and Telomerase Dysfunction in Aging Bone

Telomere shortening may be the instrument that cells use to "sense" their replicative history [266]. Telomeres are sequences of repetitive DNA (TTAGGG in vertebrates) that cap the end of chromosomes and prevent genomic instability [240]. With aging, telomere length decreases as end loop structures become uncapped (and more susceptible to degradation), and the number of dysfunctional telomeres increases [267–271]. Telomerases are enzymes present in cells that add short repeat sequences to chromosome ends to prevent shortening. Bodnar et al. showed that telomere shortening is a critical factor limiting the replicative capacity of normal human somatic cells in vitro [272]. Evidence is accumulating for a role of telomere dysfunction in aging. For example, individuals with shorter telomeres have higher mortality rates than those with longer telomeres [273]. Telomere and telomerase status have been shown to affect stem cell behavior in mice [274]. Finally, cells from centenarians have longer telomeres than younger controls [275].

It is hypothesized that telomere shortening contributes to the aging of bone. Osteoblasts and MSCs have been shown to undergo replicative senescence via telomere shortening [276, 277]. Telomerase both extends the lifespan of osteogenic precursors and accelerates the osteogenic differentiation of MSCs in vitro [278]. Conversely, after forced ectopic expression of telomerase in human MSCs, proliferative capacity is extended in vitro and the capacity for bone formation is enhanced when human MSCs are transplanted into mice [271, 276, 277]. These observations provide strong evidence that telomere and/or telomerase function in MSCs is an important component of bone formation and possibly age-related bone loss.

References

1. Srouji S, Livne E. Bone marrow stem cells and biological scaffold for bone repair in aging and disease. Mech Ageing Dev 2005;126:281–7.
2. Bilezikian JP. Osteoporosis in men. J Clin Endocrinol Metab 1999;84:3431–4.
3. Looker AC, Orwoll ES, Johnston CC Jr, et al. Prevalence of low femoral bone density in older U.S. adults from NHANES III. J Bone Miner Res 1997;12:1761–8.
4. McKee MD, Addison WN, Kaartinen MT. Hierarchies of extracellular matrix and mineral organization in bone of the craniofacial complex and skeleton. Cells Tissues Organs 2005;181:176–88.
5. Jilka RL. Biology of the basic multicellular unit and the pathophysiology of osteoporosis. Med Pediatr Oncol 2003;41:182–5.
6. Marcus R, Feldman D, Kelsey J. Osteoporosis. San Diego: Academic Press, 1996.
7. Martin RB, Burr DB, Sharkey NA. Skeletal tissue mechanics. New York: Springer, 1998.
8. Boyde A. The real response of bone to exercise. J Anat 2003;203:173–89.
9. Dempster D. Anatomy and functions of the adult skeleton. In: Favus M, ed. Primer on the metabolic bone diseases and disorders of the mineral metabolism, 6th ed. Washington, DC: The American Society for Bone and Mineral Research, 2006:9.
10. Weiss L. Histology: cell and tissue biology. New York: Elsevier Biomedical, 1983.

11. Silva MJ, Gibson LJ. Modeling the mechanical behavior of vertebral trabecular bone: effects of age-related changes in microstructure. Bone 1997;21:191–9.
12. Parfitt AM, Villanueva AR, Foldes J, Rao DS. Relations between histologic indices of bone formation: implications for the pathogenesis of spinal osteoporosis. J Bone Miner Res 1995;10:466–73.
13. Frost H. Dynamics of bone remodeling. In: Frost H, ed. Bone biodynamics. Boston, MA: Little Brown, 1964:315–33.
14. Manolagas SC. Birth and death of bone cells: basic regulatory mechanisms and implications for the pathogenesis and treatment of osteoporosis. Endocr Rev 2000;21:115–37.
15. Zamberlan N, Radetti G, Paganini C, et al. Evaluation of cortical thickness and bone density by roentgen microdensitometry in growing males and females. Eur J Pediatr 1996;155:377–82.
16. Lu PW, Cowell CT, LLoyd-Jones SA, Briody JN, Howman-Giles R. Volumetric bone mineral density in normal subjects, aged 5-27 years. J Clin Endocrinol Metab 1996;81:1586–90.
17. Seeman E. The structural and biomechanical basis of the gain and loss of bone strength in women and men. Endocrinol Metab Clin North Am 2003;32:25–38.
18. Teitelbaum SL. Bone resorption by osteoclasts. Science 2000;289:1504–8.
19. Boyle WJ, Simonet WS, Lacey DL. Osteoclast differentiation and activation. Nature 2003;423:337–42.
20. Ichinose Y, Tanaka H, Inoue M, Mochizuki S, Tsuda E, Seino Y. Osteoclastogenesis inhibitory factor/osteoprotegerin reduced bone loss induced by mechanical unloading. Calcif Tissue Int 2004;75:338–43.
21. Raisz LG. Pathogenesis of osteoporosis: concepts, conflicts, and prospects. J Clin Invest 2005;115:3318–25.
22. Nuttall ME, Patton AJ, Olivera DL, Nadeau DP, Gowen M. Human trabecular bone cells are able to express both osteoblastic and adipocytic phenotype: implications for osteopenic disorders. J Bone Miner Res 1998;13:371–82.
23. Canalis E. Skeletal growth factors. Philadelphia: Lippincott Williams & Wilkins, 2000.
24. Ogata T, Noda M. Expression of Id, a negative regulator of helix-loop-helix DNA binding proteins, is down-regulated at confluence and enhanced by dexamethasone in a mouse osteoblastic cell line, MC3T3E1. Biochem Biophys Res Commun 1991;180:1194–9.
25. Pittenger MF, Mackay AM, Beck SC, et al. Multilineage potential of adult human mesenchymal stem cells. Science 1999;284:143–7.
26. Lacey DL, Erdmann JM, Teitelbaum SL, Tan HL, Ohara J, Shioi A. Interleukin 4, interferon-gamma, and prostaglandin E impact the osteoclastic cell-forming potential of murine bone marrow macrophages. Endocrinology 1995;136:2367–76.
27. Horwood NJ, Elliott J, Martin TJ, Gillespie MT. IL-12 alone and in synergy with IL-18 inhibits osteoclast formation in vitro. J Immunol 2001;166:4915–21.
28. Mirosavljevic D, Quinn JM, Elliott J, Horwood NJ, Martin TJ, Gillespie MT. T-cells mediate an inhibitory effect of interleukin-4 on osteoclastogenesis. J Bone Miner Res 2003;18:984–93.
29. Gaur T, Lengner CJ, Hovhannisyan H, et al. Canonical WNT signaling promotes osteogenesis by directly stimulating Runx2 gene expression. J Biol Chem 2005;280:33132–40.
30. Lecka-Czernik B, Gubrij I, Moerman EJ, et al. Inhibition of Osf2/Cbfa1 expression and terminal osteoblast differentiation by PPARgamma2. J Cell Biochem 1999;74:357–71.
31. Vaughan T, Pasco JA, Kotowicz MA, Nicholson GC, Morrison NA. Alleles of RUNX2/CBFA1 gene are associated with differences in bone mineral density and risk of fracture. J Bone Miner Res 2002;17:1527–34.
32. Lee B, Thirunavukkarasu K, Zhou L, et al. Missense mutations abolishing DNA binding of the osteoblast-specific transcription factor OSF2/CBFA1 in cleidocranial dysplasia. Nat Genet 1997;16:307–10.
33. Nakashima K, Zhou X, Kunkel G, et al. The novel zinc finger-containing transcription factor osterix is required for osteoblast differentiation and bone formation. Cell 2002;108:17–29.

34. Komori T, Yagi H, Nomura S, et al. Targeted disruption of Cbfa1 results in a complete lack of bone formation owing to maturational arrest of osteoblasts. Cell 1997;89:755–64.
35. Otto F, Thornell AP, Crompton T, et al. Cbfa1, a candidate gene for cleidocranial dysplasia syndrome, is essential for osteoblast differentiation and bone development. Cell 1997;89: 765–71.
36. Mundlos S, Otto F, Mundlos C, et al. Mutations involving the transcription factor CBFA1 cause cleidocranial dysplasia. Cell 1997;89:773–9.
37. Ducy P, Starbuck M, Priemel M, et al. A Cbfa1-dependent genetic pathway controls bone formation beyond embryonic development. Genes Dev 1999;13:1025–36.
38. Sato M, Morii E, Komori T, et al. Transcriptional regulation of osteopontin gene in vivo by PEBP2alphaA/CBFA1 and ETS1 in the skeletal tissues. Oncogene 1998;17:1517–25.
39. Zelzer E, McLean W, Ng YS, et al. Skeletal defects in VEGF(120/120) mice reveal multiple roles for VEGF in skeletogenesis. Development 2002;129:1893–904.
40. Zelzer E, Glotzer DJ, Hartmann C, et al. Tissue specific regulation of VEGF expression during bone development requires Cbfa1/Runx2. Mech Dev 2001;106:97–106.
41. Engsig MT, Chen QJ, Vu TH, et al. Matrix metalloproteinase 9 and vascular endothelial growth factor are essential for osteoclast recruitment into developing long bones [erratum appears in J Cell Biol 2001 Jan 22;152(2):following 417]. J Cell Biol 2000;151: 879–89.
42. Rozman C, Feliu E, Berga L, Reverter JC, Climent C, Ferran MJ. Age-related variations of fat tissue fraction in normal human bone marrow depend both on size and number of adipocytes: a stereological study. Exp Hematol 1989;17:34–7.
43. Chawla A, Lazar MA. Peroxisome proliferator and retinoid signaling pathways co-regulate preadipocyte phenotype and survival. Proc Natl Acad Sci U S A 1994;91:1786–90.
44. Kawaguchi H, Akune T, Yamaguchi M, et al. Distinct effects of PPARgamma insufficiency on bone marrow cells, osteoblasts, and osteoclastic cells. J Bone Miner Metab 2005;23:275–9.
45. Ducy P, Zhang R, Geoffroy V, Ridall AL, Karsenty G. Osf2/Cbfa1: a transcriptional activator of osteoblast differentiation. Cell 1997;89:747–54.
46. Lecka-Czernik B, Moerman EJ, Grant DF, Lehmann JM, Manolagas SC, Jilka RL. Divergent effects of selective peroxisome proliferator-activated receptor-gamma 2 ligands on adipocyte versus osteoblast differentiation. Endocrinology 2002;143:2376–84.
47. Ogawa S, Urano T, Hosoi T, et al. Association of bone mineral density with a polymorphism of the peroxisome proliferator-activated receptor gamma gene: PPARgamma expression in osteoblasts. Biochem Biophys Res Commun 1999;260:122–6.
48. Ohsumi J, Sakakibara S, Yamaguchi J, et al. Troglitazone prevents the inhibitory effects of inflammatory cytokines on insulin-induced adipocyte differentiation in 3T3-L1 cells. Endocrinology 1994;135:2279–82.
49. Ibrahimi A, Teboul L, Gaillard D, et al. Evidence for a common mechanism of action for fatty acids and thiazolidinedione antidiabetic agents on gene expression in preadipose cells. Mol Pharmacol 1994;46:1070–6.
50. Jennermann C, Triantafillou J, Cowan D, Penniink BGA, Connolly KM, Morris DC. Effects of thiazolidinediones on vone turnover in the rat. J Bone Miner Res 1995;10:S241.
51. Mullender MG, Huiskes R. Osteocytes and bone lining cells: which are the best candidates for mechano-sensors in cancellous bone? Bone 1997;20:527–32.
52. Uitterlinden AG, Arp PP, Paeper BW, et al. Polymorphisms in the sclerosteosis/van Buchem disease gene (SOST) region are associated with bone-mineral density in elderly whites. Am J Hum Genet 2004;75:1032–45.
53. Winkler DG, Sutherland MK, Geoghegan JC, et al. Osteocyte control of bone formation via sclerostin, a novel BMP antagonist. EMBO J 2003;22:6267–76.
54. Brunkow ME, Gardner JC, Van Ness J, et al. Bone dysplasia sclerosteosis results from loss of the SOST gene product, a novel cystine knot-containing protein. Am J Hum Genet 2001;68:577–89.
55. Beighton P. Sclerosteosis. J Med Genet 1988;25:200–3.

56. Anderson JJB, Garner SC. Calcium and phosphorus nutrition in health and disease. Boca Raton, FL: CRC Press, 1995.
57. Favus M, Bushinksy D, Lenmann Jr. J. Chapter 13. Regulation of calcium, magnesium and phosphate metabolism. In: Favus M, ed. Primer on the metabolic bone diseases and disorders of mineral metabolism, 6th ed. Washington, DC: ASBMR, 2006:76.
58. Roodman GD. Cell biology of the osteoclast. Exp Hematol 1999;27:1229–41.
59. Ott SM. Sclerostin and Wnt signaling – the pathway to bone strength [comment]. J Clin Endocrinol Metab 2005;90:6741-3.
60. Boyle WJ, Simonet WS, Lacey DL. Osteoclast differentiation and activation. Nature 2003;423:337–42.
61. Troen BR. Molecular mechanisms underlying osteoclast formation and activation. Exp Gerontol 2003;38:605–14.
62. Stejskal D, Bartek J, Pastorkova R, Ruzicka V, Oral I, Horalik D. Osteoprotegerin, RANK, RANKL. Biomed Pap Med Fac Univ Palacky Olomouc Czech Repub 2001;145:61–4.
63. Han KO, Choi JT, Choi HA, et al. The changes in circulating osteoprotegerin after hormone therapy in postmenopausal women and their relationship with oestrogen responsiveness on bone. Clin Endocrinol (Oxf) 2005;62:349–53.
64. Aubin JE, Bonnelye E. Osteoprotegerin and its ligand: a new paradigm for regulation of osteoclastogenesis and bone resorption. Medscape Womens Health 2000;5:5.
65. Zaidi M, Pazianas M, Shankar VS, et al. Osteoclast function and its control. Exp Physiol 1993;78:721-39.
66. Holtrop ME, Cox KA, Eilon G, Simmons HA, Raisz LG. The ultrastructure of osteoclasts in microphthalmic mice. Metab Bone Dis Relat Res 1981;3:123–9.
67. Delaisse JM, Andersen TL, Engsig MT, Henriksen K, Troen T, Blavier L. Matrix metalloproteinases (MMP) and cathepsin K contribute differently to osteoclastic activities. Microsc Res Tech 2003;61:504–13.
68. Baron R, Vignery A, Tran Van P. The significance of lacunar erosion without osteoclasts: studies on the reversal phase of the remodeling sequence. Metab Bone Dis Rel Res 1980;2S:35–40.
69. Glass DA 2nd, Bialek P, Ahn JD, et al. Canonical Wnt signaling in differentiated osteoblasts controls osteoclast differentiation. Dev Cell 2005;8:751–64.
70. Dong XN, Guo XE. Geometric determinants to cement line debonding and osteonal lamellae failure in osteon pushout tests. J Biomech Eng 2004;126:387–90.
71. Burr DB, Schaffler MB, Frederickson RG. Composition of the cement line and its possible mechanical role as a local interface in human compact bone. J Biomech 1988;21: 939–45.
72. Skedros JG, Holmes JL, Vajda EG, Bloebaum RD. Cement lines of secondary osteons in human bone are not mineral-deficient: new data in a historical perspective. Anat Rec A Discov Mol Cell Evol Biol 2005;286:781–803.
73. Reinholt FP, Hultenby K, Oldberg A, Heinegard D. Osteopontin—a possible anchor of osteoclasts to bone. Proc Natl Acad Sci U S A 1990;87:4473–5.
74. Diab T, Condon KW, Burr DB, Vashishth D. Age-related change in the damage morphology of human cortical bone and its role in bone fragility. Bone 2006;38:427–31.
75. Bonewald LF, Mundy GR. Role of transforming growth factor-beta in bone remodeling. Clin Orthop 1990;261–76.
76. Locklin RM, Oreffo RO, Triffitt JT. Effects of TGFbeta and bFGF on the differentiation of human bone marrow stromal fibroblasts. Cell Biol Int 1999;23:185–94.
77. Ueland T. GH/IGF-I and bone resorption in vivo and in vitro. Eur J Endocrinol 2005;152:327–32.
78. Fox SW, Lovibond AC. Current insights into the role of transforming growth factor-beta in bone resorption. Mol Cell Endocrinol 2005;243:19–26.
79. Anderson HC. Matrix vesicles and calcification. Curr Rheumatol Rep 2003;5:222–6.
80. Huiskes R, Ruimerman R, van Lenthe GH, Janssen JD. Effects of mechanical forces on maintenance and adaptation of form in trabecular bone. Nature 2000;405:704–6.

81. Chow JW, Wilson AJ, Chambers TJ, Fox SW. Mechanical loading stimulates bone formation by reactivation of bone lining cells in 13-week-old rats. J Bone Miner Res 1998;13:1760–7.
82. Hauge EM, Qvesel D, Eriksen EF, Mosekilde L, Melsen F. Cancellous bone remodeling occurs in specialized compartments lined by cells expressing osteoblastic markers. J Bone Miner Res 2001;16:1575–82.
83. Garnero P, Sornay-Rendu E, Chapuy MC, Delmas PD. Increased bone turnover in late postmenopausal women is a major determinant of osteoporosis. J Bone Miner Res 1996;11: 337–49.
84. Reid I. Menopause. In: Favus M, ed. Primers of the metabolic bone diseases and disorders of mineral metabolism, 6th ed. Washington, DC: ASBMR, 2006:68.
85. Kumar R. Vitamin D and calcium transport. Kidney Int 1991;40:1177–89.
86. Wasserman RH. Physiological mechanisms of calcium absorption and homeostasis, with emphasis on vitamin D action. In: Bales C, ed. Mineral homeostasis in the elderly. New York: Alan R Liss, 1989:15.
87. Brown AJ, Dusso A, Slatopolsky E. Vitamin D. Am J Physiol 1999;277:F157–75.
88. Reichel H, Koeffler HP, Norman AW. The role of the vitamin D endocrine system in health and disease. N Engl J Med 1989;320:980–91.
89. Larsen ER, Mosekilde L, Foldspang A. Vitamin D and calcium supplementation prevents osteoporotic fractures in elderly community dwelling residents: a pragmatic population-based 3-year intervention study. J Bone Miner Res 2004;19:370–8.
90. Hordon LD, Peacock M. Osteomalacia and osteoporosis in femoral neck fracture. Bone Miner 1990;11:247–59.
91. Mosekilde L. Vitamin D and the elderly. Clin Endocrinol (Oxf) 2005;62:265–81.
92. Garnero P, Munoz F, Borel O, Sornay-Rendu E, Delmas PD. Vitamin D receptor gene polymorphisms are associated with the risk of fractures in postmenopausal women, independently of bone mineral density. J Clin Endocrinol Metab 2005;90:4829–35.
93. Bischoff-Ferrari HA, Dawson-Hughes B, Willett WC, et al. Effect of Vitamin D on falls: a meta-analysis. JAMA 2004;291:1999–2006.
94. Sambrook PN, Chen JS, March LM, et al. Serum parathyroid hormone predicts time to fall independent of vitamin D status in a frail elderly population. J Clin Endocrinol Metab 2004;89:1572–6.
95. Stein MS, Wark JD, Scherer SC, et al. Falls relate to vitamin D and parathyroid hormone in an Australian nursing home and hostel. J Am Geriatr Soc 1999;47:1195–201.
96. Costa EM, Blau HM, Feldman D. 1,25-dihydroxyvitamin D3 receptors and hormonal responses in cloned human skeletal muscle cells. Endocrinology 1986;119:2214–20.
97. Bellido T, Boland R. Effects of 1,25-dihydroxy-vitamin D3 on phosphate accumulation by myoblasts [erratum appears in Horm Metab Res 1991 Jul;23(7):356 Note: Teresita, B corrected to Bellido, T; Ricardo, B corrected to Boland, R]. Horm Metab Res 1991;23:113–6.
98. Pfeifer M, Begerow B, Minne HW, Abrams C, Nachtigall D, Hansen C. Effects of a short-term vitamin D and calcium supplementation on body sway and secondary hyperparathyroidism in elderly women [erratum appears in J Bone Miner Res 2001 Oct;16(10):1935]. J Bone Miner Res 2000;15:1113–8.
99. Avenell A, Gillespie WJ, Gillespie LD, O'Connell DL. Vitamin D and vitamin D analogues for preventing fractures associated with involutional and post-menopausal osteoporosis. [update of Cochrane Database Syst Rev. 2001;(1):CD000227; PMID: 11279685]. Cochrane Database Syst Rev 2005;000227.
100. Jackson RD, LaCroix AZ, Gass M, et al. Calcium plus vitamin D supplementation and the risk of fractures. N Engl J Med 2006;354:669–83.
101. Cummings SR, Browner WS, Bauer D, et al. Endogenous hormones and the risk of hip and vertebral fractures among older women. Study of Osteoporotic Fractures Research Group. N Engl J Med 1998;339:733–8.
102. Bischoff-Ferrari HA, Willett WC, Wong JB, Giovannucci E, Dietrich T, Dawson-Hughes B. Fracture prevention with vitamin D supplementation: a meta-analysis of randomized controlled trials. JAMA 2005;293:2257–64.

103. Bischoff-Ferrari HA, Orav EJ, Dawson-Hughes B. Effect of cholecalciferol plus calcium on falling in ambulatory older men and women: a 3-year randomized controlled trial. Arch Intern Med 2006;166:424–30.
104. Canaff L, Hendy GN. Human calcium-sensing receptor gene. Vitamin D response elements in promoters P1 and P2 confer transcriptional responsiveness to 1,25-dihydroxyvitamin D. J Biol Chem 2002;277:30337–50.
105. Brown EM. PTH secretion in vivo and in vitro. Regulation by calcium and other secretagogues. Miner Electrolyte Metab 1982;8:130–50.
106. Brown EM, MacLeod RJ. Extracellular calcium sensing and extracellular calcium signaling. Physiol Rev 2001;81:239–97.
107. Ooms ME, Lips P, Roos JC, et al. Vitamin D status and sex hormone binding globulin: determinants of bone turnover and bone mineral density in elderly women. J Bone Miner Res 1995;10:1177–84.
108. Agnusdei D, Maioli E, Camporeale A, Zacchei F, Gerardi D, Gennari C. The effect of age on bone and renal responsiveness to parathyroid hormone infusion in man. J Endocrinol Invest 1992;15:69–72.
109. Riggs BL, Melton LJ 3rd. Clinical review 8: Clinical heterogeneity of involutional osteoporosis: implications for preventive therapy. J Clin Endocrinol Metab 1990;70:1229–32.
110. Manolagas SC, Jilka RL. Bone marrow, cytokines, and bone remodeling. Emerging insights into the pathophysiology of osteoporosis. N Engl J Med 1995;332:305–11.
111. Kimble RB, Matayoshi AB, Vannice JL, Kung VT, Williams C, Pacifici R. Simultaneous block of interleukin-1 and tumor necrosis factor is required to completely prevent bone loss in the early postovariectomy period. Endocrinology 1995;136:3054–61.
112. Hughes DE, Dai A, Tiffee JC, Li HH, Mundy GR, Boyce BF. Estrogen promotes apoptosis of murine osteoclasts mediated by TGF-beta. Nat Med 1996;2:1132–6.
113. Gao Y, Qian WP, Dark K, et al. Estrogen prevents bone loss through transforming growth factor beta signaling in T cells. Proc Natl Acad Sci U S A 2004;101:16618–23.
114. Eghbali-Fatourechi G, Khosla S, Sanyal A, Boyle WJ, Lacey DL, Riggs BL. Role of RANK ligand in mediating increased bone resorption in early postmenopausal women. J Clin Invest 2003;111:1221–30.
115. Khosla S, Melton LJ 3rd, Atkinson EJ, O'Fallon WM, Klee GG, Riggs BL. Relationship of serum sex steroid levels and bone turnover markers with bone mineral density in men and women: a key role for bioavailable estrogen. J Clin Endocrinol Metab 1998;83:2266–74.
116. Van Pottelbergh I, Goemaere S, Zmierczak H, Kaufman JM. Perturbed sex steroid status in men with idiopathic osteoporosis and their sons. J Clin Endocrinol Metab 2004;89:4949–53.
117. Khosla S, Melton LJ 3rd, Atkinson EJ, O'Fallon WM. Relationship of serum sex steroid levels to longitudinal changes in bone density in young versus elderly men. J Clin Endocrinol Metab 2001;86:3555–61.
118. Wejda B, Hintze G, Katschinski B, Olbricht T, Benker G. Hip fractures and the thyroid: a case-control study. J Intern Med 1995;237:241–7.
119. Coindre JM, David JP, Riviere L, et al. Bone loss in hypothyroidism with hormone replacement. A histomorphometric study. Arch Intern Med 1986;146:48–53.
120. Britto JM, Fenton AJ, Holloway WR, Nicholson GC. Osteoblasts mediate thyroid hormone stimulation of osteoclastic bone resorption. Endocrinology 1994;134:169–76.
121. Stall GM, Harris S, Sokoll LJ, Dawson-Hughes B. Accelerated bone loss in hypothyroid patients overtreated with L-thyroxine. Ann Intern Med 1990;113:265–9.
122. Faber J, Galloe AM. Changes in bone mass during prolonged subclinical hyperthyroidism due to L-thyroxine treatment: a meta-analysis. Eur J Endocrinol 1994;130:350–6.
123. Abe E, Marians RC, Yu W, et al. TSH is a negative regulator of skeletal remodeling. Cell 2003;115:151–62.
124. Nasu M, Sugimoto T, Chihara M, Hiraumi M, Kurimoto F, Chihara K. Effect of natural menopause on serum levels of IGF-I and IGF-binding proteins: relationship with bone mineral density and lipid metabolism in perimenopausal women. Eur J Endocrinol 1997;136: 608–16.

125. Brixen K, Kassem M, Nielsen HK, Loft AG, Flyvbjerg A, Mosekilde L. Short-term treatment with growth hormone stimulates osteoblastic and osteoclastic activity in osteopenic postmenopausal women: a dose response study. J Bone Miner Res 1995;10: 1865–74.
126. Friedlander AL, Butterfield GE, Moynihan S, et al. One year of insulin-like growth factor I treatment does not affect bone density, body composition, or psychological measures in postmenopausal women. J Clin Endocrinol Metab 2001;86:1496–503.
127. Langlois JA, Rosen CJ, Visser M, et al. Association between insulin-like growth factor I and bone mineral density in older women and men: the Framingham Heart Study. J Clin Endocrinol Metab 1998;83:4257–62.
128. Horowitz MC. Cytokines and estrogen in bone: anti-osteoporotic effects. Science 1993; 260:626–7.
129. Manolagas SC. Role of cytokines in bone resorption. Bone 1995;17:63S–7S.
130. Kitazawa R, Kimble RB, Vannice JL, Kung VT, Pacifici R. Interleukin-1 receptor antagonist and tumor necrosis factor binding protein decrease osteoclast formation and bone resorption in ovariectomized mice. J Clin Invest 1994;94:2397–406.
131. Ershler WB, Harman SM, Keller ET. Immunologic aspects of osteoporosis. Dev Comp Immunol 1997;21:487–99.
132. Kudo O, Sabokbar A, Pocock A, Itonaga I, Fujikawa Y, Athanasou NA. Interleukin-6 and interleukin-11 support human osteoclast formation by a RANKL-independent mechanism. Bone 2003;32:1–7.
133. Takayanagi H, Ogasawara K, Hida S, et al. T-cell-mediated regulation of osteoclastogenesis by signalling cross-talk between RANKL and IFN-gamma. Nature 2000;408:600–5.
134. Effros RB. Replicative senescence of CD8 T cells: effect on human ageing. Exp Gerontol 2004;39:517–24.
135. Pietschmann P, Grisar J, Thien R, et al. Immune phenotype and intracellular cytokine production of peripheral blood mononuclear cells from postmenopausal patients with osteoporotic fractures. Exp Gerontol 2001;36:1749–59.
136. Zaidi M, Fuller K, Bevis PJ, GainesDas RE, Chambers TJ, MacIntyre I. Calcitonin gene-related peptide inhibits osteoclastic bone resorption: a comparative study. Calcif Tissue Int 1987;40:149–54.
137. Zaidi M, Shankar VS, Adebanjo OA, et al. Regulation of extracellular calcium sensing in rat osteoclasts by femtomolar calcitonin concentrations. Am J Physiol 1996;271:F637–44.
138. Fromigue O, Modrowski D, Marie PJ. Growth factors and bone formation in osteoporosis: roles for fibroblast growth factor and transforming growth factor beta. Curr Pharm Des 2004;10:2593–603.
139. Iwaniec UT, Magee KA, Mitova-Caneva NG, Wronski TJ. Bone anabolic effects of subcutaneous treatment with basic fibroblast growth factor alone and in combination with estrogen in osteopenic ovariectomized rats. Bone 2003;33:380–6.
140. Montero A, Okada Y, Tomita M, et al. Disruption of the fibroblast growth factor-2 gene results in decreased bone mass and bone formation. J Clin Invest 2000;105:1085–93.
141. Chen L, Li C, Qiao W, Xu X, Deng C. A Ser(365)→Cys mutation of fibroblast growth factor receptor 3 in mouse downregulates Ihh/PTHrP signals and causes severe achondroplasia. Hum Mol Genet 2001;10:457–65.
142. Kato H, Matsuo R, Komiyama O, et al. Decreased mitogenic and osteogenic responsiveness of calvarial osteoblasts isolated from aged rats to basic fibroblast growth factor. Gerontology 1995;41:20–7.
143. Pfeilschifter J, Diel I, Pilz U, Brunotte K, Naumann A, Ziegler R. Mitogenic responsiveness of human bone cells in vitro to hormones and growth factors decreases with age. J Bone Miner Res 1993;8:707–17.
144. Mayahara H, Ito T, Nagai H, et al. In vivo stimulation of endosteal bone formation by basic fibroblast growth factor in rats. Growth Factors 1993;9:73–80.
145. Yamaguchi A, Komori T, Suda T. Regulation of osteoblast differentiation mediated by bone morphogenetic proteins, hedgehogs, and Cbfa1. Endocr Rev 2000;21:393–411.

146. Gazit D, Zilberman Y, Ebner R, Kahn A. Bone loss (osteopenia) in old male mice results from diminished activity and availability of TGF-beta. J Cell Biochem 1998;70:478–88.
147. Finkelman RD, Bell NH, Strong DD, Demers LM, Baylink DJ. Ovariectomy selectively reduces the concentration of transforming growth factor beta in rat bone: implications for estrogen deficiency-associated bone loss. Proc Natl Acad Sci U S A 1992;89:12190–3.
148. Rosen CJ. 2004. Chapter 11. The epidemiology and pathogenesis of Osteoporosis. In F. Singer (ed.) Diseases of Bone and Mineral Metabolism. http://www.endotext.org/parathyroid/parathyroid11/parathyroidframe11.htm
149. Garnero P, Hausherr E, Chapuy MC, et al. Markers of bone resorption predict hip fracture in elderly women: the EPIDOS Prospective Study. J Bone Miner Res 1996;11:1531–8.
150. Garnero P, Sornay-Rendu E, Claustrat B, Delmas PD. Biochemical markers of bone turnover, endogenous hormones and the risk of fractures in postmenopausal women: the OFELY study. J Bone Miner Res 2000;15:1526–36.
151. Riggs BL, Wahner HW, Seeman E, et al. Changes in bone mineral density of the proximal femur and spine with aging. Differences between the postmenopausal and senile osteoporosis syndromes. J Clin Invest 1982;70:716–23.
152. Cummings SR, Nevitt MC, Browner WS, et al. Risk factors for hip fracture in white women. Study of Osteoporotic Fractures Research Group. N Engl J Med 1995;332:767–73.
153. Ahlborg HG, Johnell O, Turner CH, Rannevik G, Karlsson MK. Bone loss and bone size after menopause. N Engl J Med 2003;349:327–34.
154. Parfitt AM, Mathews CH, Villanueva AR, Kleerekoper M, Frame B, Rao DS. Relationships between surface, volume, and thickness of iliac trabecular bone in aging and in osteoporosis. Implications for the microanatomic and cellular mechanisms of bone loss. J Clin Invest 1983;72:1396–409.
155. McCalden RW, McGeough JA, Barker MB, Court-Brown CM. Age-related changes in the tensile properties of cortical bone. The relative importance of changes in porosity, mineralization, and microstructure. J Bone Joint Surg Am 1993;75:1193–205.
156. Chan GK, Duque G. Age-related bone loss: old bone, new facts. Gerontology 2002;48: 62–71.
157. Keshawarz NM, Recker RR. Expansion of the medullary cavity at the expense of cortex in postmenopausal osteoporosis. Metab Bone Dis Relat Res 1984;5:223–8.
158. Hughes DE, Boyce BF. Apoptosis in bone physiology and disease. Mol Pathol 1997;50: 132–7.
159. Kameda T, Mano H, Yuasa T, et al. Estrogen inhibits bone resorption by directly inducing apoptosis of the bone-resorbing osteoclasts. J Exp Med 1997;186:489–95.
160. Gohel A, McCarthy MB, Gronowicz G. Estrogen prevents glucocorticoid-induced apoptosis in osteoblasts in vivo and in vitro. Endocrinology 1999;140:5339–47.
161. Tomkinson A, Gevers EF, Wit JM, Reeve J, Noble BS. The role of estrogen in the control of rat osteocyte apoptosis. J Bone Miner Res 1998;13:1243–50.
162. Kasten TP, Collin-Osdoby P, Patel N, et al. Potentiation of osteoclast bone-resorption activity by inhibition of nitric oxide synthase. Proc Natl Acad Sci U S A 1994;91:3569–73.
163. Das UN. Nitric oxide as the mediator of the antiosteoporotic actions of estrogen, statins, and essential fatty acids. Exp Biol Med (Maywood) 2002;227:88–93.
164. Cillo JE Jr, Gassner R, Koepsel RR, Buckley MJ. Growth factor and cytokine gene expression in mechanically strained human osteoblast-like cells: implications for distraction osteogenesis. Oral Surg Oral Med Oral Pathol Oral Radiol Endod 2000;90:147–54.
165. Dick IM, Liu J, Glendenning P, Prince RL. Estrogen and androgen regulation of plasma membrane calcium pump activity in immortalized distal tubule kidney cells. Mol Cell Endocrinol 2003;212:11–8.
166. McKane WR, Khosla S, Burritt MF, et al. Mechanism of renal calcium conservation with estrogen replacement therapy in women in early postmenopause –a clinical research center study. J Clin Endocrinol Metab 1995;80:3458–64.
167. Savine R, Sonksen PH. Is the somatopause an indication for growth hormone replacement? J Endocrinol Invest 1999;22:142–9.

168. Lombardi G, Tauchmanova L, Di Somma C, et al. Somatopause: dismetabolic and bone effects. J Endocrinol Invest 2005;28:36–42.
169. Savine R, Sonksen P. Growth hormone—hormone replacement for the somatopause? Horm Res 2000;53:37–41.
170. Anawalt BD, Merriam GR. Neuroendocrine aging in men. Andropause and somatopause. Endocrinol Metab Clin North Am 2001;30:647–69.
171. Giordano R, Lanfranco F, Bo M, et al. Somatopause reflects age-related changes in the neural control of GH/IGF-I axis. J Endocrinol Invest 2005;28:94–8.
172. Ebeling PR, Jones JD, O'Fallon WM, Janes CH, Riggs BL. Short-term effects of recombinant human insulin-like growth factor I on bone turnover in normal women. J Clin Endocrinol Metab 1993;77:1384–7.
173. Grinspoon SK, Baum HB, Peterson S, Klibanski A. Effects of rhIGF-I administration on bone turnover during short-term fasting. J Clin Invest 1995;96:900–6.
174. Johansson AG, Lindh E, Blum WF, Kollerup G, Sorensen OH, Ljunghall S. Effects of growth hormone and insulin-like growth factor I in men with idiopathic osteoporosis. J Clin Endocrinol Metab 1996;81:44–8.
175. Rosen CJ. Growth hormone and aging. Endocrine 2000;12:197–201.
176. Haren MT, Kim MJ, Tariq SH, Wittert GA, Morley JE. Andropause: a quality-of-life issue in older males. Med Clin North Am 2006;90:1005–23.
177. Morales A, Heaton JP, Carson CC 3rd. Andropause: a misnomer for a true clinical entity. J Urol 2000;163:705–12.
178. Harman SM, Metter EJ, Tobin JD, Pearson J, Blackman MR. Baltimore Longitudinal Study of Aging. Longitudinal effects of aging on serum total and free testosterone levels in healthy men. J Clin Endocrinol Metab 2001;86:724–31.
179. Amin S, Zhang Y, Sawin CT, et al. Association of hypogonadism and estradiol levels with bone mineral density in elderly men from the Framingham study. Ann Intern Med 2000;133:951–63.
180. Tenover JS. Effects of testosterone supplementation in the aging male. J Clin Endocrinol Metab 1992;75:1092–8.
181. Snyder PJ, Peachey H, Hannoush P, et al. Effect of testosterone treatment on bone mineral density in men over 65 years of age. J Clin Endocrinol Metab 1999;84:1966–72.
182. Vanderschueren D, Vandenput L, Boonen S, Lindberg MK, Bouillon R, Ohlsson C. Androgens and bone. Endocr Rev 2004;25:389–425.
183. Nair KS, Rizza RA, O'Brien P, et al. DHEA in elderly women and DHEA or testosterone in elderly men. N Engl J Med 2006;355:1647–59.
184. National Institutes of Health, National Institute of Diabetes and Digestive and Kidney Diseases, U.S. Renal Data System, USRDS 2006. Annual data report: atlas of end-stage renal disease in the United States, 2006. Minneapolis, MN usrds@usrds.org
185. Levey AS, Coresh J, Balk E, et al. National Kidney Foundation practice guidelines for chronic kidney disease: evaluation, classification, and stratification [erratum appears in Ann Intern Med. 2003 Oct 7;139(7):605]. Ann Intern Med 2003;139:137–47.
186. Garg AX, Papaioannou A, Ferko N, Campbell G, Clarke JA, Ray JG. Estimating the prevalence of renal insufficiency in seniors requiring long-term care. Kidney Int 2004;65: 649–53.
187. Martin K, Al-Aly ZG E. Chapter 66. Renal osteopdystrophy. In: Favus M, ed. Primer on the metabolic bone dieases and disorder of mineral metabolism, 6th ed. Washington, DC: ASBMR, 2006:359.
188. Hruska KA, Teitelbaum SL. Renal osteodystrophy. N Engl J Med 1995;333:166–74.
189. Arnaud CD. Hyperparathyroidism and renal failure. Kidney Int 1973;4:89–95.
190. Suda T, Udagawa N, Nakamura I, Miyaura C, Takahashi N. Modulation of osteoclast differentiation by local factors. Bone 1995;17:87S–91S.
191. Owen TA, Aronow MS, Barone LM, Bettencourt B, Stein GS, Lian JB. Pleiotropic effects of vitamin D on osteoblast gene expression are related to the proliferative and differentiated state of the bone cell phenotype: dependency upon basal levels of gene expression, duration

of exposure, and bone matrix competency in normal rat osteoblast cultures. Endocrinology 1991;128:1496–504.
192. Fournier A, Oprisiu R, Hottelart C, et al. Renal osteodystrophy in dialysis patients: diagnosis and treatment. Artif Organs 1998;22:530–57.
193. Coburn J, Slatopolsky E. Vitamin D, parathyroid hormone and the renal osteopdystrophies. In: Brenner B, Rector FJ, eds. The kidney, 4th ed. Philadelphia: W.B. Saunders, 1991:2036.
194. Yeh LC, Tsai AD, Lee JC. Osteogenic protein-1 (OP-1, BMP-7) induces osteoblastic cell differentiation of the pluripotent mesenchymal cell line C2C12. J Cell Biochem 2002;87:292–304.
195. Frick K, Bushinksy D. Metabolic acidosis stimulates expression of rank ligand RNA. J Am Soc Nephrol 2002;13:576A.
196. Alem AM, Sherrard DJ, Gillen DL, et al. Increased risk of hip fracture among patients with end-stage renal disease. Kidney Int 2000;58:396–9.
197. Krall EA, Dawson-Hughes B. Walking is related to bone density and rates of bone loss. Am J Med 1994;96:20–6.
198. Chen JS, Cameron ID, Cumming RG, et al. Effect of age-related chronic immobility on markers of bone turnover. J Bone Miner Res 2006;21:324–31.
199. Takata S, Yasui N. Disuse osteoporosis. J Med Invest 2001;48:147–56.
200. Dalsky GP, Stocke KS, Ehsani AA, Slatopolsky E, Lee WC, Birge SJ Jr. Weight-bearing exercise training and lumbar bone mineral content in postmenopausal women. Ann Intern Med 1988;108:824–8.
201. Nishimura Y, Fukuoka H, Kiriyama M, et al. Bone turnover and calcium metabolism during 20 days bed rest in young healthy males and females. Acta Physiol Scand Suppl 1994;616: 27–35.
202. Uhthoff HK, Jaworski ZF. Bone loss in response to long-term immobilisation. J Bone Joint Surg Br 1978;60-B:420–9.
203. Wang B, Zhang S, Wu XY. Effects of microgravity on the gene expression and cellular functions of osteoblasts. Space Med Med Eng (Beijing) 2003;16:227–30.
204. Uebelhart D, Demiaux-Domenech B, Roth M, Chantraine A. Bone metabolism in spinal cord injured individuals and in others who have prolonged immobilisation. A review. Paraplegia 1995;33:669–73.
205. Bikle DD, Sakata T, Halloran BP. The impact of skeletal unloading on bone formation. Gravit Space Biol Bull 2003;16:45–54.
206. Hangartner T. Osteoporosis due to misuse. In: Matkovic V, ed. Physical medicine and rehabilitation clinics of North America: osteoporosis. Philadelphia: W.B. Saunders, 1995:579.
207. Chantraine A, Heynen G, Franchimont P. Bone metabolism, parathyroid hormone, and calcitonin in paraplegia. Calcif Tissue Int 1979;27:199–204.
208. Weiss D. 2006. Osteoporosis and Spinal Cord Injury. http://emedicine.medscape.com/article/322204-print
209. Seattle WA. Northwest Regional Spinal Cord Injury System (NWRSCIS). Common musculoskeletal problems after SCI: contractures, osteoporosis, fractures, and shoulder pain, 2002.
210. Culberson JW. Alcohol use in the elderly: beyond the CAGE. Part 1 of 2: prevalence and patterns of problem drinking. Geriatrics 2006;61:23–7.
211. Substance Abuse and Mental Health Services Administration (Office of Applied Studies). Results from the 2001 National Household Survey on Drug Abuse: Volume 1. Summary of National Findings. Rockville, MD: Department of Health and Human Services, 2002.
212. Moore AA, Hays RD, Greendale GA, Damesyn M, Reuben DB. Drinking habits among older persons: findings from the NHANES I Epidemiologic Followup Study (1982-84). National Health and Nutrition Examination Survey. J Am Geriatr Soc 1999;47:412–6.
213. Turner RT. Skeletal response to alcohol. Alcohol Clin Exp Res 2000;24:1693–701.
214. Sampson HW. Alcohol, osteoporosis, and bone regulating hormones. Alcohol Clin Exp Res 1997;21:400–3.
215. Cheung RC, Gray C, Boyde A, Jones SJ. Effects of ethanol on bone cells in vitro resulting in increased resorption. Bone 1995;16:143–7.

216. Turner RT, Aloia RC, Segel LD, Hannon KS, Bell NH. Chronic alcohol treatment results in disturbed vitamin D metabolism and skeletal abnormalities in rats. Alcohol Clin Exp Res 1988;12:159–62.
217. Kristensson H, Lunden A, Nilsson BE. Fracture incidence and diagnostic roentgen in alcoholics. Acta Orthop Scand 1980;51:205–7.
218. Turner RT, Evans GL, Zhang M, Sibonga JD. Effects of parathyroid hormone on bone formation in a rat model for chronic alcohol abuse. Alcohol Clin Exp Res 2001;25:667–71.
219. Benson BW, Shulman JD. Inclusion of tobacco exposure as a predictive factor for decreased bone mineral content. Nicotine Tob Res 2005;7:719–24.
220. Blum M, Harris SS, Must A, Phillips SM, Rand WM, Dawson-Hughes B. Household tobacco smoke exposure is negatively associated with premenopausal bone mass. Osteoporos Int 2002;13:663–8.
221. Law MR, Hackshaw AK. A meta-analysis of cigarette smoking, bone mineral density and risk of hip fracture: recognition of a major effect. BMJ 1997;315:841–6.
222. Cooper MS, Hewison M, Stewart PM. Glucocorticoid activity, inactivity and the osteoblast. J Endocrinol 1999;163:159–64.
223. Weinstein RS, Jilka RL, Parfitt AM, Manolagas SC. Inhibition of osteoblastogenesis and promotion of apoptosis of osteoblasts and osteocytes by glucocorticoids. Potential mechanisms of their deleterious effects on bone. J Clin Invest 1998;102:274–82.
224. Lukert BP, Raisz LG. Glucocorticoid-induced osteoporosis: pathogenesis and management. Ann Intern Med 1990;112:352–64.
225. Canalis E, Avioli L. Effects of deflazacort on aspects of bone formation in cultures of intact calvariae and osteoblast-enriched cells. J Bone Miner Res 1992;7:1085–92.
226. Sambrook PN. Glucocorticoid-induced osteoporosis. In: Favus M, ed. Primeron the metabolic bone diseases and disorders of mineral metabolism, 6th ed. Washington, DC: ASBMR, 2006:296.
227. Centrella M, McCarthy TL, Canalis E. Glucocorticoid regulation of transforming growth factor beta 1 activity and binding in osteoblast-enriched cultures from fetal rat bone. Mol Cell Biol 1991;11:4490–6.
228. Adler RA, Rosen CJ. Glucocorticoids and osteoporosis. Endocrinol Metab Clin North Am 1994;23:641–54.
229. Hofbauer LC, Gori F, Riggs BL, et al. Stimulation of osteoprotegerin ligand and inhibition of osteoprotegerin production by glucocorticoids in human osteoblastic lineage cells: potential paracrine mechanisms of glucocorticoid-induced osteoporosis. Endocrinology 1999;140:4382–9.
230. Morris HA, Need AG, O'Loughlin PD, Horowitz M, Bridges A, Nordin BE. Malabsorption of calcium in corticosteroid-induced osteoporosis. Calcif Tissue Int 1990;46:305–8.
231. Cosman F, Nieves J, Herbert J, Shen V, Lindsay R. High-dose glucocorticoids in multiple sclerosis patients exert direct effects on the kidney and skeleton. J Bone Miner Res 1994;9:1097–105.
232. MacAdams MR, White RH, Chipps BE. Reduction of serum testosterone levels during chronic glucocorticoid therapy. Ann Intern Med 1986;104:648–51.
233. Askari A, Vignos PJ Jr, Moskowitz RW. Steroid myopathy in connective tissue disease. Am J Med 1976;61:485–92.
234. Reid IR, Heap SW. Determinants of vertebral mineral density in patients receiving long-term glucocorticoid therapy. Arch Intern Med 1990;150:2545–8.
235. Van Staa TP, Leufkens HG, Abenhaim L, Zhang B, Cooper C. Use of oral corticosteroids and risk of fractures. J Bone Miner Res 2000;15:993–1000.
236. Laan RF, van Riel PL, van de Putte LB, van Erning LJ, van't Hof MA, Lemmens JA. Low-dose prednisone induces rapid reversible axial bone loss in patients with rheumatoid arthritis. A randomized, controlled study. Ann Intern Med 1993;119:963–8.
237. Israel E, Banerjee TR, Fitzmaurice GM, Kotlov TV, LaHive K, LeBoff MS. Effects of inhaled glucocorticoids on bone density in premenopausal women. N Engl J Med 2001;345:941–7.

238. Hayflick L, Moorhead PS. The serial cultivation of human diploid cell strains. Exp Cell Res 1961;25:585.
239. de Magalhaes JP. From cells to ageing: a review of models and mechanisms of cellular senescence and their impact on human ageing. Exp Cell Res 2004;300:1–10.
240. Campisi J. From cells to organisms: can we learn about aging from cells in culture? Exp Gerontol 2001;36:607–18.
241. Campisi J. Replicative senescence: an old lives' tale? Cell 1996;84:497–500.
242. Rohme D. Evidence for a relationship between longevity of mammalian species and life spans of normal fibroblasts in vitro and erythrocytes in vivo. Proc Natl Acad Sci U S A 1981;78:5009–13.
243. Martin GM, Sprague CA, Epstein CJ. Replicative life-span of cultivated human cells. Effects of donor's age, tissue, and genotype. Lab Invest 1970;23:86–92.
244. Dimri GP, Lee X, Basile G, et al. A biomarker that identifies senescent human cells in culture and in aging skin in vivo. Proc Natl Acad Sci U S A 1995;92:9363–7.
245. Sherwood SW, Rush D, Ellsworth JL, Schimke RT. Defining cellular senescence in IMR-90 cells: a flow cytometric analysis. Proc Natl Acad Sci U S A 1988;85:9086–90.
246. Stenderup K, Justesen J, Clausen C, Kassem M. Aging is associated with decreased maximal life span and accelerated senescence of bone marrow stromal cells. Bone 2003;33:919–26.
247. D'Ippolito G, Schiller PC, Ricordi C, Roos BA, Howard GA. Age-related osteogenic potential of mesenchymal stromal stem cells from human vertebral bone marrow. J Bone Miner Res 1999;14:1115–22.
248. Kassem M, Ankersen L, Eriksen EF, Clark BF, Rattan SI. Demonstration of cellular aging and senescence in serially passaged long-term cultures of human trabecular osteoblasts. Osteoporos Int 1997;7:514–24.
249. Stenderup K, Justesen J, Eriksen EF, Rattan SI, Kassem M. Number and proliferative capacity of osteogenic stem cells are maintained during aging and in patients with osteoporosis. J Bone Miner Res 2001;16:1120–9.
250. Oreffo RO, Bord S, Triffitt JT. Skeletal progenitor cells and ageing human populations. Clin Sci (Colch) 1998;94:549–55.
251. Kveiborg M, Rattan SI, Clark BF, Eriksen EF, Kassem M. Treatment with 1,25-dihydroxyvitamin D3 reduces impairment of human osteoblast functions during cellular aging in culture. J Cell Physiol 2001;186:298–306.
252. Christiansen M, Kveiborg M, Kassem M, Clark BF, Rattan SI. CBFA1 and topoisomerase I mRNA levels decline during cellular aging of human trabecular osteoblasts. J Gerontol A Biol Sci Med Sci 2000;55:B194–200.
253. Long MW, Ashcraft EK, Normalle D, Mann KG. Age-related phenotypic alterations in populations of purified human bone precursor cells. J Gerontol A Biol Sci Med Sci 1999;54:B54–62.
254. Nishida S, Endo N, Yamagiwa H, Tanizawa T, Takahashi HE. Number of osteoprogenitor cells in human bone marrow markedly decreases after skeletal maturation. J Bone Miner Metab 1999;17:171–7.
255. Erdmann J, Kogler C, Diel I, Ziegler R, Pfeilschifter J. Age-associated changes in the stimulatory effect of transforming growth factor beta on human osteogenic colony formation. Mech Ageing Dev 1999;110:73–85.
256. Bergman RJ, Gazit D, Kahn AJ, Gruber H, McDougall S, Hahn TJ. Age-related changes in osteogenic stem cells in mice. J Bone Miner Res 1996;11:568–77.
257. Hughes DE, Wright KR, Uy HL, et al. Bisphosphonates promote apoptosis in murine osteoclasts in vitro and in vivo. J Bone Miner Res 1995;10:1478–87.
258. Lutton JD, Moonga BS, Dempster DW. Osteoclast demise in the rat: physiological versus degenerative cell death. Exp Physiol 1996;81:251–60.
259. Jilka RL, Weinstein RS, Bellido T, Parfitt AM, Manolagas SC. Osteoblast programmed cell death (apoptosis): modulation by growth factors and cytokines. J Bone Miner Res 1998;13:793–802.

260. Hill PA, Tumber A, Meikle MC. Multiple extracellular signals promote osteoblast survival and apoptosis. Endocrinology 1997;138:3849–58.
261. Kitajima I, Soejima Y, Takasaki I, Beppu H, Tokioka T, Maruyama I. Ceramide-induced nuclear translocation of NF-kappa B is a potential mediator of the apoptotic response to TNF-alpha in murine clonal osteoblasts. Bone 1996;19:263–70.
262. Jilka RL, Weinstein RS, Bellido T, Roberson P, Parfitt AM, Manolagas SC. Increased bone formation by prevention of osteoblast apoptosis with parathyroid hormone. J Clin Invest 1999;104:439–46.
263. Yang NC, Hu ML. The limitations and validities of senescence associated-beta-galactosidase activity as an aging marker for human foreskin fibroblast Hs68 cells. Exp Gerontol 2005;40:813–9.
264. Cristofalo VJ. SA beta Gal staining: biomarker or delusion. Exp Gerontol 2005;40:836–8.
265. Pignolo RJ, Kaplan FS. Interventional spine: An algorithmic approach. In: Slipman CW, Derby R, Simeone FA, Mayer TG, eds. Bone biology. Philadelphia, PA: Elsevier 2008.
266. Chiu CP, Harley CB. Replicative senescence and cell immortality: the role of telomeres and telomerase. Proc Soc Exp Biol Med 1997;214:99–106.
267. Bekaert S, Van Pottelbergh I, De Meyer T, et al. Telomere length versus hormonal and bone mineral status in healthy elderly men. Mech Ageing Dev 2005;126:1115–22.
268. Cristofalo VJ, Lorenzini A, Allen RG, Torres C, Tresini M. Replicative senescence: a critical review. Mech Ageing Dev 2004;125:827–48.
269. Du X, Shen J, Kugan N, et al. Telomere shortening exposes functions for the mouse Werner and Bloom syndrome genes. Mol Cell Biol 2004;24:8437–46.
270. Marrone A, Walne A, Dokal I. Dyskeratosis congenita: telomerase, telomeres and anticipation. Curr Opin Genet Dev 2005;15:249–57.
271. Yudoh K, Matsuno H, Nakazawa F, Katayama R, Kimura T. Reconstituting telomerase activity using the telomerase catalytic subunit prevents the telomere shorting and replicative senescence in human osteoblasts. J Bone Miner Res 2001;16:1453–64.
272. Bodnar AG, Ouellette M, Frolkis M, et al. Extension of life-span by introduction of telomerase into normal human cells. Science 1998;279:349–52.
273. Cawthon RM, Smith KR, O'Brien E, Sivatchenko A, Kerber RA. Association between telomere length in blood and mortality in people aged 60 years or older. Lancet 2003;361:393–5.
274. Flores I, Cayuela ML, Blasco MA. Effects of telomerase and telomere length on epidermal stem cell behavior. Science 2005;309:1253–6.
275. Franceschi C, Mondello C, Bonafe M, Valensin S, Sansoni P, Sorbi S. Long telomeres and well preserved proliferative vigor in cells from centenarians: a contribution to longevity? Aging Clin Exp Res 1999;11:69–72.
276. Simonsen JL, Rosada C, Serakinci N, et al. Telomerase expression extends the proliferative life-span and maintains the osteogenic potential of human bone marrow stromal cells. Nat Biotechnol 2002;20:592–6.
277. Shi S, Gronthos S, Chen S, et al. Bone formation by human postnatal bone marrow stromal stem cells is enhanced by telomerase expression. Nat Biotechnol 2002;20:587–91.
278. Gronthos S, Chen S, Wang CY, Robey PG, Shi S. Telomerase accelerates osteogenesis of bone marrow stromal stem cells by upregulation of CBFA1, osterix, and osteocalcin. J Bone Miner Res 2003;18:716–22.

Chapter 2
Pathologic Fractures

Jesse T. Torbert and Richard D. Lackman

Abstract Pathologic fractures can be caused by any type of bone tumor, but the overwhelming majority of pathologic fractures in the elderly are secondary to metastatic carcinomas. Multiple myeloma is also common in the elderly and has a high incidence of pathologic fractures. Diagnostic laboratory tests and imaging of multiple myeloma and metastatic tumors allow earlier diagnosis and intervention, which lead to decreased morbidity. Chemotherapy and radiation therapy have improved treatment of metastatic disease, but have a variable effect depending on the tumor type. The goals of surgical treatment of impending or pathologic fracture are to provide pain relief and a functionally stable and durable construct that will allow the patient to ambulate shortly after surgery and will persist for the life of the patient. Fixation of metastatic pathologic fractures requires reinforcement or replacement of the compromised bone with a rigid and durable construct. Rehabilitation and prevention of postoperative complications are imperative. The overall effectiveness of treatment in pathologic fractures is improved with a multidisciplinary approach.

Keywords Pathologic fracture • Metastatic • Orthopedic • Tumor • Diagnosis • Treatment

2.1 Introduction

Many pathologic processes, including osteoporosis, weaken bone. Typically, the term pathologic fracture refers to the fracture that occurs in the area of a neoplasm. Pathologic fractures can be caused by any type of bone tumor, but the overwhelming

R.D. Lackman (✉)
Department of Orthopaedic Surgery, Sarcoma Center of Excellence at the Abramson Cancer Center of the University of Pennsylvania, Hospital of the University of Pennsylvania, Philadelphia, PA 19104, USA
e-mail: rilack@pahosp.com

R.J. Pignolo et al. (eds.), *Fractures in the Elderly*, Aging Medicine,
DOI 10.1007/978-1-60327-467-8_2, © Springer Science+Business Media, LLC 2011

majority of pathologic fractures in the elderly are secondary to metastatic carcinomas. Multiple myeloma is also common in the elderly and has a high incidence of pathologic fractures.

2.2 Metastatic Tumors of Bone

The most common primary malignancies that metastasize to bone are breast, lung, kidney, prostate, and thyroid carcinomas, which account for approximately 700,000 new primary cases in the U.S. annually. Metastatic bone disease can have very detrimental effects on quality of life. The prognosis for patients with metastases to bone largely depends on the aggressiveness of the primary tumor, with lung cancer patients having the shortest length of survival. Unlike primary bone tumors, the early diagnosis and treatment of secondary tumors will not result in a cure. However, much of the significant morbidity related to bone metastases and pathologic fracture can be lessened with early intervention. The evaluation and management of patients with metastatic bone disease is best done with a multidisciplinary approach including medical oncologist, radiologist, pathologist, orthopedic surgeon, physical therapist, and social worker.

2.2.1 Location

Skeletal metastases are often multifocal; however, renal and thyroid carcinomas are notorious for producing solitary lesions. By far the most common location for osseous metastases is the axial skeleton, followed by the proximal femur and proximal humerus. Metastatic spine tumors are 40 times more frequent than all primary bone tumors combined [1]. In autopsy series, vertebral body metastases were found in over one-third of patients who died of cancer [2]. The anterior elements of the spine are 20 times more likely to be involved than the posterior elements [3].

2.2.2 Presentation

Patients with metastatic bone disease can have varied presentations. Lesions may vary from extremely painful and disabling to asymptomatic. Most metastases present with a bone lesion detected on bone imaging after patients complain of localized musculoskeletal pain. Bone metastases rarely present with an associated soft-tissue mass, and the presence of such a mass should increase the suspicion of a primary sarcoma. Fractures after a minor or insignificant injury should always raise the suspicion of an underlying lesion, especially in patients with a previously diagnosed malignancy. Most symptomatic patients with metastatic bone disease present with pain that is mechanical in nature, worse at night, and unresponsive to anti-inflammatory medications and narcotics. Neurological complaints may be the presenting symptoms especially in cases of spinal metastases with associated nerve root or spinal cord compression. It is also common for patients with pelvic metastases to present with leg pain, which mimics sciatica. As such, it is important to include imaging of the pelvis in the work-up of patients with metastatic bone disease and leg pain because radiographs and magnetic resonance imaging (MRI) of the lumbar spine may miss these lesions. Thorough clinical examination is mandatory in all cases to evaluate not only the presenting lesion, but also any other metastatic foci that may be less symptomatic. In patients with previous bony metastasis, regular follow-up evaluation is needed to assess painful sites and screen for impending fractures.

2.2.3 Diagnostic Laboratory Tests

The laboratory work-up in a patient with a metastatic bone tumor can be involved if the primary tumor has not already been diagnosed. A complete blood count (CBC) with a differential is important when working up any suspected malignancy. Elevated erythrocyte sedimentation rates (ESR) and C-reactive protein (CRP) levels signal that an inflammatory process is involved, but cannot consistently differentiate an infectious process from a malignancy. Carcinoembryonic antigen (CEA) is a marker of adenocarcinomas from various primary sites such as colonic, rectal, pancreatic, gastric, and breast. Prostate-specific antigen (PSA) levels can help diagnose prostate cancer. A thyroid panel can help eliminate the suspicion of a rare thyroid primary. Lactate dehydrogenase (LDH) isoenzymes 2 and 3 can suggest a diagnosis of lymphoma. To evaluate for liver cancer, alpha fetal protein (AFP) levels are often obtained in patients with hepatitis C or those that are heavy drinkers. A chemistry panel can be used to assess kidney function and allows calcium and phosphate levels to be followed to detect and avoid the development of malignant hypercalcemia. Urinary N-telopeptides serve as an indicator for bone collagen breakdown, which parallels tumor burden, and can provide a baseline to evaluate treatment progress.

2.2.4 Imaging

High quality, plain anteroposterior and lateral radiographs that show the involved bone, including one joint proximally and distally, are the standard for initial assessment of metastatic bone disease. One should look for lytic, blastic, or mixed lesions. Metastases from lung, renal, and thyroid tumors tend to be entirely lytic (Fig. 2.1). Breast metastases may be lytic or may show a mixed lytic–blastic

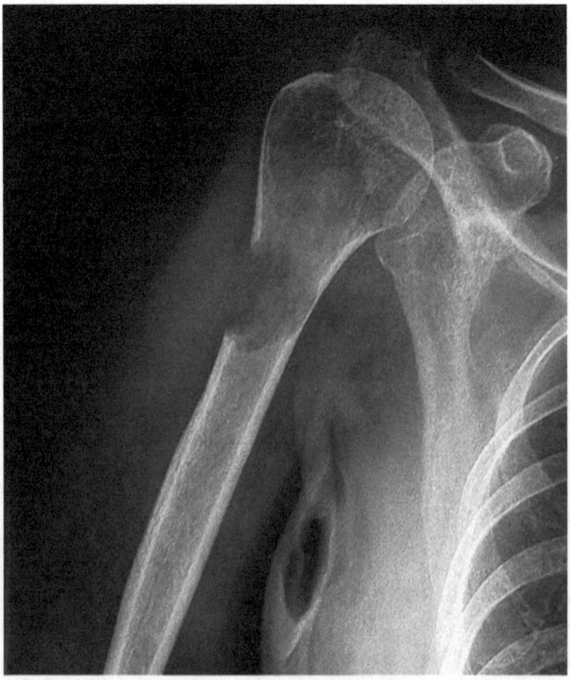

Fig. 2.1 This is an AP radiograph of a right humerus lytic lesion in a patient with metastatic carcinoma. These images are courtesy of UPenn Orthopaedic Trauma Service

appearance. The majority of prostate bone metastases are blastic (Fig. 2.2) though lytic lesions do occur. Pelvic radiographs should include an anteroposterior view and obturator and iliac oblique Judet views of the pelvis. A significant amount of bone must be destroyed before a lesion will appear lytic on radiographs. Therefore, a patient with a malignancy and bone pain often requires further evaluation despite normal-appearing plain radiographs.

Computed tomography (CT) is the study of choice when looking for bone detail and cortical destruction, but is not as sensitive at assessing marrow replacement. MRI on the other hand is very sensitive to early marrow replacement and can locate metastases prior to their appearance on radiographs and CT, but is not as helpful for bony anatomy.

Total body radionuclide bone scan is useful in searching for other skeletal sites of tumor involvement. It is a fairly sensitive technique for the detection of bone metastases and can detect these lesions earlier than plain films; however, one disadvantage is low specificity. Bone scans demonstrate areas of osteoblastic activity, and the radionuclide accumulates at sites of fracture, infection, degenerative disease, bone metastases, and benign tumors such as hemangioma and fibrous dysplasia. False-negative bone scans are often due to destructive activity that exceeds reactive or blastic activity, as in multiple myeloma and in tumors which are confined to the medullary cavity and do not affect the cortex.

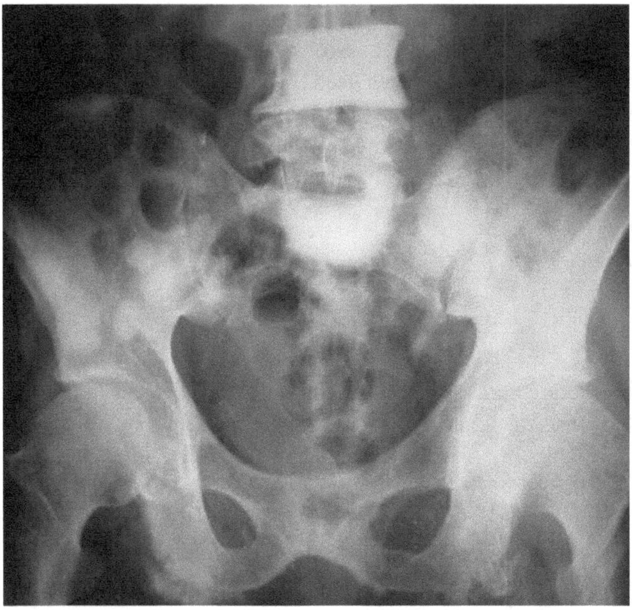

Fig. 2.2 This is an AP radiograph of the pelvis in a patient with metastatic prostate cancer with multiple blastic lesions in the pelvis and fourth lumbar vertebra

2.2.5 Management Options

2.2.5.1 Medical/Radiation Therapy

Patients with cancer are often in a hypercoagulable state. Prophylaxis against deep vein thrombosis (DVT) with pharmacologic agents and/or sequential compression devices (SCD's) is provided for patients who are non-ambulatory and at risk. Bisphosphonates inhibit osteoclastic activity, suppressing bone resorption, and are commonly used to treat destructive bony lesions from metastatic disease. One common bisphosphonate used in cancer patients is pamidronate, which in conjunction with systemic chemotherapy, has been shown to decrease or delay pathologic fractures due to bone metastases in breast cancer [4] and multiple myeloma patients [5]. Zolendronate is also commonly used is many protocols.

Chemotherapy and radiotherapy should be used as indicated to stop or slow the neoplastic progression. Postoperatively, chemotherapy and radiotherapy are often delayed between 7 and 14 days after surgery in order to allow unimpeded would healing.

Prostate, lymphoid, and breast neoplasms are the most sensitive to radiation therapy. Lung and thyroid cancers are intermediately responsive; gastrointestinal, melanoma, and renal tumors are typically radiotherapy-resistant lesions. Treatment for metastatic lesions in the extremities can range from a single 8 Gy dose to a

40 Gy dose divided over 15 daily fractions. Large single doses are usually utilized for treating pain related to metastatic lesions, while smaller fractional dosing allows a higher cumulative dose and is often used for definitive treatment or when attempting to decrease the size of metastatic lesions. Metastatic bone lesions with a low risk of fracture may be initially treated with radiation, which may negate the need for subsequent surgical intervention.

2.2.5.2 Surgery

Indications

A pathologic fracture can be devastating in an elderly cancer patient and is a clear indication for surgical intervention, with the patient's medical condition and expected survival playing a role in the decision to proceed to surgery. The treatment of metastatic bone lesions in the absence of fracture is not so well-defined. Because pathologic fractures are extremely detrimental, prophylactic surgical treatment of impending fractures has been shown to improve outcomes [6]. In 1989, Mirels [7] developed a scoring system designed to predict the risk of pathologic fracture due to bone metastases in the extremities.

The Mirels classification is based on the degree of pain, lesion size, lytic versus blastic nature, and anatomic location as shown in Table 2.1. Mirels recommended prophylactic fixation for a total score ≥9. The variability in quality of surrounding bone, behavior of metastases from different tumor types, response of these metastases to treatment including radiation, and patient activity level can also have an effect on the probability of fracture. While this scoring system is helpful, we feel that the most reliable predictor of impending fracture is mechanical pain. Mechanical pain is a physiologic indicator that the involved bone cannot withstand the physical stresses placed upon it, and is therefore at risk of fracture. As a result, all metastatic lesions in the extremities that exhibit mechanical pain should be considered for prophylactic fixation.

One important caveat to any surgeon considering operative intervention for a suspected bone metastasis is to recognize the possibility of an unrelated primary bone tumor in a patient with a previously diagnosed malignancy. As a general rule, the first time a tumor presents with metastasis to bone, histological confirmation

Table 2.1 The scoring system proposed by Mirels [7] (reprinted with permission)

Score	1	2	3
Pain	Mild	Moderate	Mechanical pain
Lesional size/diameter of bone involved	<1/3	1/3–2/3	>2/3
Lesion type (blastic versus lytic)	Blastic	Mixed	Lytic
Anatomic site	Upper limb	Lower limb	Peritrochanteric (proximal femur)

with a biopsy or intra-operative frozen section should precede definitive surgical intervention. When the diagnosis is confirmed, immediate internal fixation is reasonable. If concern for a potential primary bone sarcoma persists, definitive surgery should be postponed. Passing an intramedullary nail through a primary bone sarcoma will result in distal seeding of the medullary canal and will frequently necessitate amputation.

Treatment Options

The goals of surgery for impending or pathologic fracture in the setting of metastatic disease are to provide pain relief and a functionally stable and durable construct that will allow the patient to ambulate shortly after surgery and will persist for the life of the patient. This is quite a challenge in some cases given the large amount of bone loss, the degree of osteoporosis in the elderly, and the decreased ability of bone to heal in the local setting of tumor. Therefore, techniques used in patients with pathological fractures differ from those used in young patients with traumatic fractures in which fixation is placed as a temporary stabilizing measure while fracture healing occurs. The idea in the fixation of metastatic pathologic fractures is to reinforce or replace the compromised bone with a rigid and durable construct. This typically requires plates or intramedullary rods with the addition of methylmethacrylate, or bone cement, to fill the bone defects. If the fracture is near a joint, and stable and durable fixation cannot be achieved by the described methods, joint arthroplasty may provide a more durable construct and may require less operative time and blood loss. Occasionally, segmental replacement prostheses may be used (Fig. 2.3), which not only replace the joint surface and nearby bone but also replace varying lengths of diaphyseal bone with metal. These are typically used in malignant primary tumors of bone where large segments of bone must be resected; although they may also play a role in metastatic bone disease. Surgical alternatives, although not all-inclusive, for fixation or reconstruction of impending or pathologic fractures in the extremities were proposed by Lackman et al. [8] and are presented in Table 2.2.

Postoperative Care

The postoperative physical therapy largely depends on the type of construct used and the intra-operative observations made by the surgeon regarding the quality of bone, screw purchase, and overall stability of the construct. The goal is to achieve mobility and independence in order to improve the quality of life and to decrease cardiopulmonary complications that are associated with immobility in the elderly patient.

Adequate pain control is necessary for participation in physical therapy. DVT prophylaxis is very important in cancer patients that are immobilized. Bisphosphonates, radiation therapy, and chemotherapy should be used as indicated, keeping in mind that radiation and chemotherapy decrease wound healing and may be delayed.

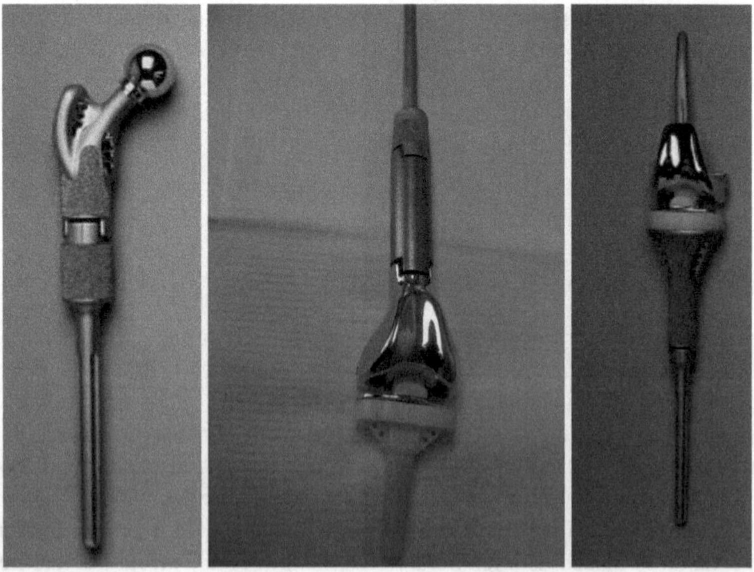

Fig. 2.3 These are images of tumor replacement prostheses. The left image is a proximal femur replacement prosthesis. The middle image shows a distal femoral replacement prosthesis which includes the knee replacement. The image on the right is a proximal tibial replacement prosthesis and includes the knee replacement. These images are courtesy of UPenn Orthopaedic Trauma Service

Table 2.2 Surgical alternatives for fixation or reconstruction of impending or pathologic fractures in bones of the extremities [8] (reprinted with permission)

Region	Surgical approach
Clavicle and scapula	No surgical intervention needed (radiotherapy sufficient)
Proximal humerus	Plate and cement or intramedullary rod ± cement or segmental replacement endoprosthesis
Humeral shaft	Intramedullary rod ± cement
Distal humerus	Plate and cement or segmental replacement endoprosthesis
Proximal radius	No surgical intervention needed (radiotherapy sufficient)
Radial and ulnar shaft	Plate/rod ± cement if radiotherapy fails
Distal radius	Plate and cement
Femoral head and neck	Endoprosthesis (total or hemiarthroplasty)
Intertrochanteric	Compression hip screw ± cement or intramedullary rod ± cement or segmental replacement endoprosthesis
Subtrochanteric	Intramedullary rod ± cement
Femoral shaft	Intramedullary rod ± cement
Distal femoral metaphysis	Plate and cement or retrograde intramedullary rod ± cement or segmental replacement prosthesis
Proximal tibial metaphysis	Plate and cement or segmental replacement prosthesis
Tibial shaft	Intramedullary rod ± cement
Distal tibia	Plate and cement

2.3 Multiple Myeloma

Multiple myeloma is a B-cell lymphoproliferative disease that is characterized by involvement of the skeleton at multiple sites. Multiple myeloma causes 1% of all cancer deaths in the Western countries. It is more common in men and those with African descent. The peak incidence occurs between 50 and 60 years of age. Most myeloma patients will present with multiple lesions; however, a small percentage will present with a solitary lesion and a negative bone marrow aspirate. Those with a solitary myeloma have a much better prognosis.

2.3.1 Presentation

The clinical features of multiple myeloma arise from the effects of organs infiltrated with tumor cells and the production of excessive immunoglobulin (Ig). Hypercalcemia resulting from bone resorption can give rise to confusion, weakness, lethargy, constipation, and polyuria. Decreased production of normal Ig predisposes the patient to recurrent infections. Renal insufficiency occurs in half of multiple myeloma patients, and is often an ominous manifestation. Chronic renal failure may develop insidiously or acute renal failure may present with oliguria. Infiltration of bones causes pain, pathologic fractures, spinal cord compressions, and hypercalcemia. Patients often present with bone pain and pathologic fracture, which is a major source of morbidity. One study followed 165 multiple myeloma patients for an average of 3.2 years and found approximately two pathologic fractures, mostly vertebral and rib fracture, per patient [9].

2.3.2 Diagnostic Laboratory Tests

The diagnosis of myeloma can be confirmed by the identification of monoclonal proteins in the serum or urine via serum protein electrophoresis (SPEP) or urine protein electrophoresis (UPEP). Monoclonal proteins are more often absent or undetectable in solitary myeloma compared to multiple myeloma. A chemistry panel can be used to assess kidney function and allows calcium and phosphate levels to be followed to detect and avoid the development of malignant hypercalcemia. Formal diagnostic criteria have been put forth by the Mayo Clinic and the International Myeloma Working Group for the diagnosis of symptomatic multiple myeloma [10–12].

2.3.3 Imaging

Multiple punched-out lesions on a lateral skull radiograph are a classic finding for multiple myeloma. A skeletal survey often reveals other lytic bone lesions. These often appear as medullary lytic lesions with sharp margins, but little periosteal

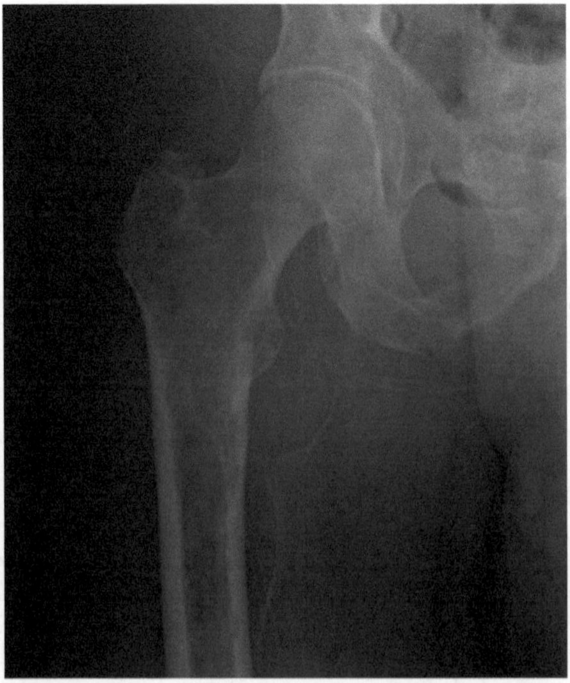

Fig. 2.4 This is an AP radiograph of the right hip in an elderly male with multiple myeloma. Multiple, medullary punched-out, lytic lesions, a classic finding, are present. There is little periosteal reaction. The most inferior lesions have sharp margins, another classic finding. This image is courtesy of UPenn Orthopaedic Oncology Service

reaction (Fig. 2.4). Bone scans are often negative secondary to the lack of bone reaction. MRI scans, especially of the spine, are useful.

2.3.4 Management Options

2.3.4.1 Medical Therapy

Chemotherapy and radiation have been the mainstays of treatment. Radiation will often result in less bone pain and decreased need for surgical treatment. Bisphosphonates have been shown to reduce pain, pathologic fractures, and increase survival [13].

2.3.4.2 Surgery

Surgical Treatment Options

Surgical intervention is typically reserved for decompression of neural structures in the case of spinal involvement and stabilization of lower extremity pathologic fractures. Upper extremity fractures may respond well to radiation therapy. Surgery may be the best treatment for recurrent lesions or those that do not respond to radiotherapy. The goals are the same as those for metastatic carcinoma lesions: to provide a functionally stable and durable construct that will allow the patient to ambulate shortly after surgery and will persist for the life of the patient. Again, this can be accomplished with internal fixation and the addition of bone cement for bone defects or joint/bone replacing prostheses.

Postoperative

The postoperative care of multiple myeloma patients is similar to those with metastatic bone metastases. The goal is to achieve mobility and independence in order to improve the quality of life, while decreasing cardiopulmonary complications that are associated with immobility in the elderly patient. Pain control and DVT prophylaxis are necessary. In addition, bisphosphonates are often continued postoperatively due to their demonstrated effects on pain, fractures, and survival.

References

1. Harrington KD. Metastatic disease of the spine. In: Harrington KD, ed. Orthopaedic management of metastatic bone disease. St. Louis: Mosby, 1988:309–383.
2. Wong DA, Fornasier VL, MacNab I. Spinal metastases: the obvious, the occult, and the impostors. Spine 1990;15:1–4.
3. Brihaye J, Ectors P, Lemort M. The management of spinal epidural metastases. Adv Tech Stand Neurosurg 1988;16:121–176.
4. Hortobagyi GN, Theriault RL, Lipton A. Long-term prevention of skeletal complications of metastatic breast cancer with pamidronate. Protocol 19 Aredia Breast Cancer Study Group. J Clin Oncol 1998;16:2038–2044.
5. Berenson JR, Lichtenstein A, Porter L. Efficacy of pamidronate in reducing skeletal events in patients with advanced multiple myeloma. Myeloma Aredia Study Group. N Engl J Med 1996;334:488–493.
6. Ward WG, Holsenbeck S, Dorey FJ. Metastatic disease of the femur: surgical treatment. Clin Orthop Relat Res 2003;(415 Suppl):S230–S244.
7. Mirels H. Metastatic disease in long bones. A proposed scoring system for diagnosing impending pathologic fractures. Clin Orthop Relat Res 1989;(249):256–264.
8. Lackman RD, Torbert JT, Hosalkar HS. Treatment of metastases to the extremities and pelvis. Oper Tech Orthop 2004;14:288–295.
9. Melton LJ, Kyle RA, Achenbach SJ. Fracture risk with multiple myeloma: a population-based study. J Bone Miner Res 2005;20:487–493.
10. Smith A, Wisloff F, Samson D. Guidelines on the diagnosis and management of multiple myeloma 2005. Br J Haematol 2006;132:410–451.
11. International Myeloma Working Group. Criteria for the classification of monoclonal gammopathies, multiple myeloma and related disorders: a report of the International Myeloma Working Group. Br J Haematol 2003;121:749–757.
12. Rajkumar SV, Dispenzieri A, Kyle RA. Monoclonal gammopathy of undetermined significance, Waldenstrom macroglobulinemia, AL amyloidosis, and related plasma cell disorders: diagnosis and treatment. Mayo Clin Proc 2006;81:693–703.
13. Berenson JR, Rajdev L, Broder M. Bone complications in multiple myeloma. Cancer Biol Ther 2006;5:1082–1085.

Chapter 3
Falls

Amy M. Corcoran and Bruce Kinosian

Abstract Falls and fall-related injuries contribute substantially to morbidity and mortality in older adults each year. It is important to understand the additive nature of risk factors associated with falls, to annually screen for falls and associated contributing factors, and to target interventions to the identified risk factors. Since each older adult's risk profile and capacities (both biological and social) will vary, each will require an individualized treatment plan to reduce the chance of future falls.

Keywords Falls • Accidents • Fracture • Older adults • Elderly

3.1 Introduction

Falls affect approximately 30% of all persons older than 65 years old each year [1, 2]. Over 13,000 older adults (>65 years old) died from falls or fall-related injuries in 2003. All-cause mortality rate is 24% at 12 months for a hip fracture in an older adult [3]. Understanding how to assess for fall risks both before and after an injurious fall can help tailor interventions to prevent future injury [4]. Thus proper screening before, and appropriate assessment after a fall are prerequisites to keeping an older adult independent for a longer period of time. This chapter outlines prevention strategies, risk assessment, clinical evaluation and testing in older adults who have fallen or are at risk of falling.

Older adults fall frequently – up to one-third of elders living in the community [5]. The definition of a fall is the unintentional change in the position of the body in which it comes to rest on the ground or strikes an object [6]. Falls are considered one of the more common "geriatric syndromes," along with urinary incontinence, pressure ulcers, delirium, and functional decline. All of these geriatric syndromes

A.M. Corcoran (✉)
Department of Medicine, Division of Geriatrics, University of Pennsylvania, Penn-Ralston Center, 3615 Chestnut Street, Philadelphia, PA 19104, USA
e-mail: amym.corcoran@uphs.upenn.edu

R.J. Pignolo et al. (eds.), *Fractures in the Elderly*, Aging Medicine,
DOI 10.1007/978-1-60327-467-8_3, © Springer Science+Business Media, LLC 2011

have in common multiple contributing factors/risks (i.e., older age, baseline cognitive impairment, baseline functional impairment, and impaired mobility), in addition to being associated with increased morbidity [7]. The key concept of a geriatric syndrome is that multiple deficits, and impaired capacity to adjust to those deficits, lead to a common, clinically observed condition. In the case of falls, just as in other geriatric syndromes, these deficits are additive, so that the greater the number of deficits, the greater the risk that the syndrome (i.e., a fall) will occur. Below we provide an overview of the risk factors associated with falls, fall prevention strategies, as well as post-fall assessment and care.

3.2 Epidemiology

Heath care providers are caring for older adults who fall and suffer fall-related injuries in a variety of settings. About 35–40% of older community dwellers fall annually [5], in contrast, the fall rate in nursing facilities and hospitals is three times this rate amounting to about 1.5 falls per institution bed annually [8, 9]. Falls often lead to injuries, with 20–30% of older adults suffering moderate to severe injuries such as hip fractures or head traumas that ultimately reduce mobility and independence [10]. Injuries are a leading cause of death in older adults, ranking sixth among those aged 65–74 years old [11]. Up to 25% of those who sustain hip fractures and survive remain institutionalized at 1 year, while another 25% do not survive the first year post-fracture [12]. In the United States, falls are also an expensive part of health care, with fall-related injuries accounting for 6% of all medical expenditures in those over 65 years old [8, 9]. In hospitalized patients, 30–48% of falls result in injury, with 5–10% considered serious injuries [13–17].

Almost 13,000 people older than 65 died from fall-related injuries in 2002, while in 2003 approximately 1.8 million elderly were treated in emergency departments for nonfatal fall-related injuries, and of these, more than 421,000 were hospitalized [1, 18]. Subsequent to a fall, fear of future falling can lead to a significant curtailment in activity, resulting in additional functional decline [19].

3.3 Risk Factors and Screening

Identification of risk factors associated with falls is essential to formulating interventions to prevent them. Risk factors may be divided into intrinsic or extrinsic factors as outlined in Table 3.1. In addition to numerous individual meta-analyses, the American Geriatrics Society, British Geriatrics Society and American Academy of Orthopaedic Surgeons Panel on Falls Prevention jointly performed a univariate meta-analysis of the most common risk factors for falls in older adults. Of the 16 studies examined, the following were found to be the most common risk factors: muscle weakness, history of falls, gait deficit, balance deficit, use of assistive device, visual deficit, arthritis, impaired activities of daily living (ADLs), depression,

Table 3.1 Risk factors and causes for falling in older adults [5, 20]

Intrinsic	Extrinsic
Functional and cognitive impairment	Polypharmacy (≥3 medications)
Postural hypotension	Restraints
Musculoskeletal or neuromotor dysfunction	Poor footwear or problem with assistive device
Chronic medical problems	Environmental factors:
Sensory problems	Unsecured area rugs or uneven floors
Visual	Poor lighting
Auditory	Absent grab bars where needed
Vestibular	Poor accessibility to food, phone, etc.
Neuropathic	Inappropriate clothing

cognitive impairment, and age greater than 80 years old [5]. Some of these are markers for other risk factors (e.g., use of an assistive device, age > 80, ADL impairment, and history of falls), while other factors have direct links to the observed risk (e.g., muscle weakness, gait, balance, and visual deficits).

The Saint Louis Veterans Administration Geriatric Research Education and Clinical Center (GRECC) developed a helpful pneumonic to allow rapid recall of the major causes of falls for screening purposes, "SAFE AND SOUND." "SAFE" is an acronym for Strength problems, Alcohol, Food-associated hypotension, and Environmental Factors. "AND" stands for Atherosclerotic Disease (syncope), No freedom, and Drugs. "SOUND" stands for Sight problems, Orthostasis, Unsteady balance, Nocturia, and Delirium [21].

Since a past fall is highly predictive of future falls, one of the main screening recommendations suggested by the 2001 Joint Guidelines [5] is that, as part of the routine care of older persons, health professionals should ask the patient or caregiver about falls at least once a year. The more falls an older adult has over the course of a year, the greater the risk of having a hip fracture [21, 22]. It is not correct to assume that prior falls without injury indicate a reduced risk of future injury. Given the all-cause mortality rate of 24% at 12 months post-hip fracture [3], screening for risk factors and careful post-fall assessment is necessary in all older adults.

3.4 Fall Assessment

3.4.1 Post-fall Assessment and Evaluation

3.4.1.1 First Fall

After the first fall, evaluation of lower extremity strength, balance, and gait dysfunction should be performed [5, 9, 23]. These may be assessed in any variety of

Table 3.2 Comprehensive multidisciplinary post-fall assessment [9, 23]

Factor	Assessment
Gait, balance or mobility problems	"Get Up and Go"
	Physical therapy evaluation
	Assessment of cognitive function and gaits associated with them (i.e., Parkinson's disease)
	Assessment of lower extremities for arthritis
Postural hypotension/syncope	Check orthostatic blood pressures
	Review medications
	Review causes for syncope
Cognitive impairment/psychological problems	Screen using a standardized cognitive status examination (i.e., Mini-Mental State Examination, Mini-Cognitive testing)
	Screen for depression (i.e., Geriatric Depression Scale short-form)
	Screen for fear of falling
Urinary incontinence	Ask about difficulties urinating and frequency
Polypharmacy (see Table 3.5)	Review all medication
Sensory deficits	Visual assessment with referral to an ophthalmologist
	Auditory assessment
	Neuropathy assessment
Acute illness	Evaluate for changes in medical condition
	Evaluate for delirium
Environmental hazards (see Table 3.1)	Home safety evaluation

ways, the most common one being the "Get Up and Go Test" which has the patient rise from a chair without using their arms, walk 10 feet, turn and return to the chair [24, 25]. Normal performance time is less than 10 s. Those who exhibit any unsteadiness or take longer than 20 s should undergo further evaluation as deemed appropriate (Table 3.2). Possible prevention strategies should be individualized.

3.4.1.2 Recurrent Falls

If multiple falls have occurred, a more thorough evaluation is warranted, focusing on elements common to the multiple falls. A thorough assessment should include: a general medical and falls history, medication review, vision evaluation, gait and balance testing, inspection of lower limb joints, as well as a complete neurological and cardiovascular exam [5, 23]. It is critical to obtain a good history of circumstances surrounding the fall(s) and any associated symptoms. If the patient is cognitively impaired, history will require identifying reliable reporters of the events, if available. A complete evaluation includes a valid reconciliation of medications taken, a history of alcohol or illicit drug use, assessment of acute and chronic medical problems, as well as orthostatic blood pressure measurements, inspection of footwear, and assessment of functional and cognitive status. Basic laboratory studies are often used to screen for reversible causes of weakness and unsteady gait, which include a complete blood count, chemistries, thyroid-stimulating hormone, vitamin B12 level, urinalysis, and other laboratory tests dictated by history and examination findings. If the patient's history suggests syncope, an electrocardiogram, carotid dopplers, echocardiogram, or ambulatory cardiac monitoring may be indicated. Table 3.2 provides an overview by contributing factor on how to evaluate an older adult after a fall.

3.5 Fall Prevention

Prevention of a fall is what all providers and patients strive for. When looking at the different prevention strategies, we can describe them as primary, secondary, and tertiary. If a "fall" is the event, then preventing a "fall" would be considered a primary prevention. A secondary prevention would be one that reduces injury from the event, or "fall."

3.5.1 Primary Prevention

Primary preventive interventions are intended to prevent falls, and thus prevent the resultant fractures or other injuries. These preventive interventions are the ones that primary medical providers should be advising and educating older adults about early in the geriatric assessment process.

3.5.1.1 Exercise

Exercise has long been deemed important in primary prevention [26], with walking, balance training, and muscle strengthening each having been demonstrated to reduce falls and subsequent fractures [27–30]. Table 3.3 provides simple exercises that can be done in the patient's home with the assistance of a stable chair. Any provider can quickly explain these exercises to the patient or caregiver in a short amount of time. Tai Chi has also been studied extensively and shown to be helpful in preventing falls, principally by improving balance. One study that compared Tai Chi three times per week to stretching showed that the risk of multiple falls over a 6-month time period was 55% lower in the Tai Chi group [32]. There was also significant improvement in measures of functional balance, physical performance, and reduced fear of falling [32]. Tai Chi classes have spread widely, and are now often offered at community senior centers.

Screening and intervention for those who have a history of falls are elements of secondary prevention. Simply asking the patient on an annual basis if they have ever fallen has been shown to be a useful screen. However, more focused assessment

Table 3.3 Simple balance and strengthening exercises [31]

Balance	Plantar flexion – stand behind the chair and rise to toes 8–15 times
	Knee flexion – extending/flexing knee while standing behind the chair and using the chair for stability
	Hip flexion
	While standing behind the chair, raise leg and flex hip
	Bend forward over the chair for stability and lift one leg backward
	Bend forward over the chair for stability and lift one leg to the side (abducting the leg)
Strengthen upper extremity	Sitting in an armless chair with feet on the ground and arms at the side, then raise arms to shoulder level, hold for 1 s and then relax with arms down to side. Repeat 8–15 times. Eventually add weights, starting with one pound and then gradually adding more
	Biceps curls – alternating arms with 8–15 repetitions and starting with light weights
Strengthen lower extremity	Plantar flexion – see above
	Quadriceps strengthening exercises with knee extension exercises. Sit in stable chair with arms at side and feet on floor, then lift feet until straight in front or level with hips/knees, holding for 1–2 s. Repeat 8–15 times. Rest and then repeat

based on a risk-factor targeted history (see Sect. 3.3) and on physical examination is necessary to prescribe subsequent interventions.

3.5.1.2 Importance of Vitamin D

Screening for vitamin D deficiency is important, both because its prevalence is high among the fall-prone elderly and because vitamin D supplementation has been shown to be an effective intervention. Supplementation reduces both fall risk as well as fracture risk by having a positive effect on functional performance, reaction time, and balance [33]. It has been shown to reduce the risk of falls in both ambulatory and institutionalized older individuals with stable health by 22% in a recent meta-analysis [34]. The benefit was most clearly established in women using active vitamin D, with the number needed to treat for fracture prevention found to be 15 (i.e. 15 people need to be treated for 1 year in order to prevent one fracture) [34]. Previously, the effect of vitamin D on factures was attributed to bone mineral density changes, but now felt to be directly related to improvement in neuromuscular or neuroprotective function [33]. Initial recommended daily doses for the elderly population should probably be at least 1,000 International Units (IU) per day. Replacement doses in deficient individuals are much higher, requiring laboratory testing to initially evaluate and then monitor replacement. Recent studies have suggested that optimal levels of Vitamin D (25-OH) for functional performance are in the 90–100 nmol/L range (36–40 ng/mL) [35], which are substantially above the usually reported "normal" laboratory values.

3.5.1.3 Sarcopenia and Nutrition

Screening for those at risk of sarcopenia, or those who have sarcopenia, identifies another target for intervention. Sarcopenia is a condition associated with frailty. Sarcopenia is defined as low muscle mass secondary to lack of specific nutrients, lack of adequate macronutrients (protein and calories), and/or lack of trophic factors (often mediated via exercise). A brief clinical evaluation can be useful in classifying individuals at-risk of nutritionally associated complications, including falls and fractures. Of these, the Mini-Nutritional Assessment (MNA) has had the most extensive validation in acute and long-term care settings [36]. A reduced version of the full MNA has recently been developed and validated that uses six items: decreased food intake due to loss of appetite, digestive problems, chewing, or swallowing difficulties; weight loss; mobility; neuropsychological problems; acute illnesses; and the person's body mass index [36]. The MNA-SF (short form) has a sensitivity of 0.96 for identifying those clinically judged to be "undernourished." The recommended use of the MNA-SF is as the first step in a two-step process – those who score above 12 on the MNA-SF should be evaluated with the full MNA [37]. Using this approach, there is a 14% false-positive rate for the MNA-SF, but only a 3.4% false-negative rate. To emphasize the importance of the relationship between cognitive function and nutritional risk, both clinical guidelines [38] and the MNA use the Folstein Mini-Mental Status Examination for cognitive assessment, the Katz ADL screen for assessment of self-care function, and the Geriatric Depression Scale (short-form) for depression screening.

A different stream of research developed from the surgical specialties, and focused on the targeted use of forced feeding (enteral or parenteral nutrition). The conceptual breakthrough was to define protein–energy malnutrition as another nutrient deficiency, using the standard definition for a vitamin. That is, a vitamin is a substance, the absence of which is associated with a clinical syndrome, and the provision of which eliminates the clinical condition. "Clinically relevant" malnutrition was defined as a condition associated with adverse clinical events, which did not occur with the provision of adequate protein and energy. A number of predictive equations were developed to relate assessment variables with clinical complications. None of the equations did better, however, than a clinical technique termed "Subjective Global Assessment (SGA)" of nutritional status [39]. The method is designed to assign *risk* of malnutrition-associated complications, not to identify a specific state of malnutrition. The underlying assumption is that the fluctuations of nutrients, rather than the stock of nutrients, is principally related to the risk of complications. This was supported by refeeding studies in anorexic patients where organ function (heart, skeletal muscle, immune cells) normalizes within 10–14 days, well before substantial lean body mass is accumulated [40].

Loss of weight, and the pattern of weight loss, is assigned primary importance in the above paradigm. If an individual loses substantial weight, but then starts to regain some weight, they are assigned less risk than an individual who is still losing weight. Change in dietary intake is the primary cause of fluctuations in nutrient consumption. When making assessments, the duration of the dietary change and the current diet type should be noted. These are (1) suboptimal solid diet, (2) full liquid diet, (3) hypocaloric liquids, and (4) starvation. Daily nutrient intake can also be mitigated by the presence of significant gastrointestinal symptoms (e.g., nausea, vomiting, diarrhea, and anorexia). Patients with changes in their nutrient consumption often present as weak and are easily fatigued. These nutrient changes can also result in physical changes such as skin breakdown, infections, loss of subcutaneous fat, and muscle wasting. Weight loss history is adjusted if it is accompanied by ankle and sacral edema. This is because the edema may be masking the total weight loss experienced by the patient. To find detectable edema, fluid retention must be in excess of 3–4 L.

SGA uses a three-level classification system that is based on the patient's pattern of weight change [39]. The assessment relies on information regarding the patient's current weight and their weight 6 months prior to admission. The weight 2 weeks prior is used to determine the most recent direction of weight change. Depending upon the pattern of change, a patient is classified as being: (a) low risk for malnutrition-associated complications (less than 5% weight loss, or more than 5% total loss, but recent weight gain and increased appetite), (b) moderate risk for malnutrition-associated complications (those with 5–10% weight loss without recent stabilization or gain, poor dietary intake, and slight loss of subcutaneous tissue); or (c) at severe risk of malnutrition-associated complications (ongoing weight loss of more than 10% with severe subcutaneous tissue loss and muscle wasting).

The central, common element of all the methods is the amount and pattern of weight loss. The surgical equations use various serum protein measures and a measure of weight loss; SGA uses weight loss and has slightly improved specificity with the addition of an albumin level. The subjective components in SGA incorporate the other elements of the MNA – functional level, mobility, cognitive state, and appetite. Having a prior weight and a current weight is crucial. A good historian may give the correct estimate of change for purposes of SGA classification, but for many patients obtaining reliable historical data may be difficult. However, those who have had recent contact with the medical system, or reside in institutional settings (e.g., nursing homes) may well have a prior weight available, which should be obtained. All patients should be weighed on admission or at first evaluation.

3.5.2 Secondary Prevention

The aim of secondary prevention is to prevent injury from a fall, or the prevention of future falls. There are several classes of devices which are employed in secondary prevention – those that alert others when a person at risk of falling is rising to a sitting or standing position, those that identify individuals when they have fallen (to reduce their down time), and those that buffer the faller in order to reduce injury.

3.5.2.1 Technological Devices

There are many devices, which attach directly to the patient that are used to alert staff members in facilities that a fall may be imminent. Nursing home facilities often use bed or chair alarms attached to the resident that trigger with standing or sitting up. Often, a low bed with surrounding mats can also be utilized to help decrease the chance of injury. Other types of fall detectors include: user activated alarms and pendants, automatic wearable fall detectors (watches), video-monitoring-based fall detectors, and floor-vibration-based fall detectors [41–43]. Independently living older adults may also be offered technology to monitor for falls and even fall risks. There are diagnostic technology systems that consist of a personal wearable device that can monitor pulse-ox, blood glucose, heart rate, respiratory rate and other information, with the integration of a home telecare system and camera [44, 45].

3.5.2.2 Hip Protectors

Among other devices to protect the faller is the hip protector. The hip protector is relatively inexpensive (approximately $100 for a pair), however patient adherence is often a problem. A recent meta-analysis of randomized control trials of hip protectors in men and women showed that hip protectors may be effective in long-term care settings (where compliance with use is easier to enforce) [46]. However, there was little evidence of effectiveness in community populations when analyzed by intention-to-treat. Community studies found that fractures in the treatment arm tended to occur when individuals were not wearing their hip protectors [46]. Overall, there is substantial variation in hip protector styles and effectiveness in the long-term care setting, and little evidence to support using them in community dwellers if they are not likely to be worn. In addition to adherence issues, limitations include: skin irritation, abrasion, and local discomfort [46–50].

3.5.2.3 Post-fall Interventions

Post-fall interventions vary depending on the given situation. Both single interventions (i.e., balance training) and multifactorial interventions have been studied. Table 3.4 provides an overview of the recommendations for good single-intervention strategies. Medication review is a single-intervention strategy applicable to potential fallers in all settings. Medication links to fall risk in older adults are listed in Table 3.5.

Table 3.4 Overview of single intervention fall prevention strategies [5, 9, 35, 51]

Exercise
Tai Chi
Walking
Balance and strength training
Environment
Home safety evaluation
Medication review/audit
Have patient or caregiver/family bring all medications in for review
Discontinue all unnecessary medications
Assistive devices
Review need for and ensure proper use of device
Bone and muscle strengthening strategies
Calcium (1,500 mg/day)
Vitamin D (≥1,000 IU/day)
Identifying and treating underlying osteoporosis (i.e., bisphosphonates)
Footwear
Assess for appropriate footwear with skid-proof soles
Evaluate for need of shoe lift and/or orthotics
Elimination of restraints
Remove bedrails
Remove unnecessary lines (i.e., foley or IV)
Hip protectors
May be helpful for those older adults who will wear them

3.5.2.4 Community-based Older Adults

Recommendations for community dwellers include: appropriate use of assistive devices, review and modification of medications, exercise programs with strength and balance training, treatment of postural hypotension, corrections of environmental hazards, and treatment of cardiac disorders. Medications should be evaluated whether or not they are new to the patient regimen, and their side-effect profiles should be reviewed with respect to contributions to potential fall risk. Special attention should be paid to those medications that have been linked to falls, which include: antipsychotics, sedatives/hypnotics, neuroleptics, antidepressants, and benzodiazepines [52–57]. In general, older adults tend be at higher risk of developing side effects from medications due to pathophysiological changes associated with aging. For example, the slower reaction times found among the elderly, which impair balance, are further exacerbated with use of benzodiazepines, making balance even more tenuous.

The set of interventions for community dwelling fallers should vary directly with the number of risk factors identified. As with other geriatric syndromes, there is no single "cause" of falls to identify from a list of differential diagnostic possibilities. Thus, there is no single intervention to be prescribed for all fallers.

Table 3.5 Medications linked to fall risk in older adults [23, 52–57]

Types of medications	Examples
Sedatives/hypnotics	Benzodiazepines (i.e., lorazepam, diazepam, alprazolam)
	Barbiturates (i.e., phenobarbitol)
	Opioids (i.e., morphine, codeine)
	Antihistamines (i.e., diphenhydramine)
Anticholinergics	Atropine, scopolamine
	Glycopyrrolate
	Benztropine, trihexphenidyl
Neuroleptics/antipsychotics	Haloperidol, risperidone
Antidepressants	Tricyclic antidepressants (i.e., nortriptyline)
	Selective serotonin-reuptake inhibitors (i.e., paroxetine, fluoxetine, sertraline)
Anti-arrhythmics	Digoxin
Diuretics	Loop diuretics (i.e., furosemide)
	Thiazides (i.e., hydrochlorothiazide)
Antihypertensives	Beta-blockers (i.e., metoprolol)

3.5.2.5 Facility-based Older Adults

In the long-term care setting, comprehensive assessment, staff education, gait training, proper use of assistive devices, as well as review and modification of medications have been shown to be important [9]. As in other settings, each patient should have an individualized treatment plan depending on their assessment and evaluation of their current clinical situation.

3.5.2.6 Inpatient-Based Older Adult

In the hospital setting, a multifactorial approach is best used to target risk factors. Evaluation should emphasize medication review, orthostatic blood pressure monitoring, screening for and addressing underlying causes for delirium, balance and gait assessment, care of bowel or bladder incontinence, and physical therapy assessment of muscle strength [13].

Limiting psychotropic medications is important in the hospitalized older adult. One study showed that patients who received fewer psychotropic medications had a lower in-hospital fall rate (0.28 versus 0.64 falls per 100 patient-days; $P = 0.001$) [58]. Providing a restraint free environment (e.g., by the use of hi-lo beds instead of side rails) has also been shown to reduce falls and subsequent injury.

Bastow et al. [59, 60] used nutritional supplementation in moderately and severely malnourished women post hip fracture in the early 1980s, showing lower mortality and quicker rehabilitative recovery. This is still likely to be one of the most effective interventions to reducing fall risk after hip fracture.

3.5.3 Tertiary Prevention

Tertiary prevention focuses on rehabilitation from a fall with injury (see Chap. 15).

References

1. Centers for Disease Control and Prevention (CDC). Fatalities and injuries from falls among older adults – United States, 1993-2003 and 2001-2005. MMWR Morb Mortal Wkly Rep 2006;55:1221–4.
2. Hausdorff JM, Rios DA, Edelberg HK. Gait variability and fall risk in community-living older adults: a 1-year prospective study. Arch Phys Med Rehabil 2001;82:1050–6.
3. Huddleston JM, Whitford KJ. Medical care of elderly patients with hip fractures. Mayo Clin Proc 2001;76:295–8.
4. Administration on Aging. http://www.aoa.gov/prof/Statistics/future_growth/future_growth.asp. Accessed July 2007.
5. American Geriatrics Society, British Geriatrics Society, and American Academy of Orthopaedic Surgeons Panel on Falls Prevention. Guidelines for the prevention of falls in older persons. J Am Geriatr Soc 2001;49:664–72.
6. Kiel DP. The evaluation of falls in the emergency department. Clin Geriatr Med 1993;9:591–9.
7. Inouye SK, Studenski S, Tinetti ME, Kuchel GA. Geriatric syndromes: clinical, research, and policy implications of a core geriatric concept. J Am Geriatr Soc 2007;55:780–91.
8. Cumming RG, Kelsey JL, Nevitt MC. Methodologic issues in the study of frequent and recurrent health problems. Falls in the elderly. Ann Epidemiol 1990;1:49–56.
9. Tinetti ME. Clinical practice. Preventing falls in elderly persons. N Engl J Med 2003; 348:42–9.
10. Sterling DA, O'Connor JA, Bonadies J. Geriatric falls: injury severity is high and disproportionate to mechanism. J Trauma 2001;50:116–9.
11. Dellinger AM, Stevens JA. The injury problem among older adults: mortality, morbidity and costs. J Safety Res 2006;37:519–22.
12. Magaziner J, Hawkes W, Hebel JR, et al. Recovery from hip fracture in eight areas of function. J Gerontol A Biol Sci Med Sci 2000;55:M498–507.
13. Amador LF, Loera JA. Preventing postoperative falls in the older adult. J Am Coll Surg 2007;204:447–53.
14. Hitcho EB, Krauss MJ, Birge S, et al. Characteristics and circumstances of falls in a hospital setting: a prospective analysis. J Gen Intern Med 2004;19:732–9.
15. Ash KL, MacLeod P, Clark L. A case-control study of falls in the hospital setting. J Gerontol Nurs 1998;24:7–15.
16. Krauss MJ, Evanoff B, Hitcho E, et al. A case-control study of patient, medication, and care-related risk factors for inpatient falls. J Gen Intern Med 2005;20:116–22.
17. Uden G, Nilsson B. Hip fracture frequent in hospital. Acta Orthop Scand 1986;57:428–30.
18. Centers for Disease Control and Prevention. National Center for Injury Prevention and Control. Available at http://www.cdc.gov/injury/index.html. Last accessed on November 10, 2010.
19. Scheffer AC, Schuurmans MJ, van Dijk N, van der Hooft T, de Rooij SE. Fear of falling: measurement strategy, prevalence, risk factors and consequences among older persons. Age Ageing 2008;37(1):19–24.
20. Rubenstein LZ, Josephson KR. Falls and their prevention in elderly people: what does the evidence show? Med Clin North Am 2006;90:807–24.
21. Morley JE. Falls – where do we stand? Mo Med 2007;104:63–7.

22. Cumming RG, Klineberg RJ. Fall frequency and characteristics and the risk of hip fractures. J Am Geriatr Soc 1994;42:774–8.
23. King MB. Falls. In: Hazzard WR, Blass JP, Halter JB, Ouslander JG, Tinetti ME, eds. Principles of Geriatric Medicine and Gerontology. 5th edn. New York: McGraw-Hill, 2003:1517–29.
24. Wall JC, Bell C, Campbell S, Davis J. The Timed Get-up-and-Go test revisited: measurement of the component tasks. J Rehabil Res Dev 2000;37:109–13.
25. Podsiadlo D, Richardson S. The timed "Up & Go": a test of basic functional mobility for frail elderly persons. J Am Geriatr Soc 1991;39:142–8.
26. Centers for Disease Control and Prevention (CDC). Strength training among adults aged >/=65 years – United States, 2001. MMWR Morb Mortal Wkly Rep 2004;53:25–8.
27. Carter ND, Kannus P, Khan KM. Exercise in the prevention of falls in older people: a systematic literature review examining the rationale and the evidence. Sports Med 2001;31:427–38.
28. American College of Sports Medicine Position Stand. Exercise and physical activity for older adults. Med Sci Sports Exerc 1998;30:992–1008.
29. Butler RN, Davis R, Lewis CB, Nelson ME, Strauss E. Physical fitness: benefits of exercise for the older patient. 2. Geriatrics 1998;53:46.
30. Gregg EW, Pereira MA, Caspersen CJ. Physical activity, falls, and fractures among older adults: a review of the epidemiologic evidence. J Am Geriatr Soc 2000;48:883–93.
31. Komara FA. The slippery slope: reducing fall risk in older adults. Prim Care 2005;32: 683–97.
32. Li F, Harmer P, Fisher KJ, et al. Tai Chi and fall reductions in older adults: a randomized controlled trial. J Gerontol A Biol Sci Med Sci 2005;60:187–94.
33. Dhesi JK, Jackson SH, Bearne LM, et al. Vitamin D supplementation improves neuromuscular function in older people who fall. Age Ageing 2004;33:589–95.
34. Bischoff-Ferrari HA, Dawson-Hughes B, Willett WC, et al. Effect of Vitamin D on falls: a meta-analysis. JAMA 2004;291:1999–2006.
35. Bischoff-Ferrari HA, Giovannucci E, Willett WC, Dietrich T, Dawson-Hughes B. Estimation of optimal serum concentrations of 25-hydroxyvitamin D for multiple health outcomes. Am J Clin Nutr 2006;84:18–28.
36. Vellas B, Guigoz Y, Garry PJ, et al. The Mini Nutritional Assessment (MNA) and its use in grading the nutritional state of elderly patients. Nutrition 1999;15:116–22.
37. The Mini Nutritional Assessment (MNA) 2007. Available at http://www.mna-elderly.com/MNA_proceedings.pdf. Last accessed on November 10, 2010.
38. Thomas DR, Ashmen W, Morley JE, Evans WJ. Nutritional management in long-term care: development of a clinical guideline. Council for Nutritional Strategies in Long-Term Care. J Gerontol A Biol Sci Med Sci 2000;55:M725–34.
39. Detsky AS, Smalley PS, Chang J. The rational clinical examination. Is this patient malnourished? JAMA 1994;271:54–8.
40. Lopes J, Russell DM, Whitwell J, Jeejeebhoy KN. Skeletal muscle function in malnutrition. Am J Clin Nutr 1982;36:602–10.
41. Brownsell S, Hawley MS. Automatic fall detectors and the fear of falling. J Telemed Telecare 2004;10:262–6.
42. Cheek P, Nikpour L, Nowlin HD. Aging well with smart technology. Nurs Adm Q 2005; 29:329–38.
43. Tideiksaar R, Feiner CF, Maby J. Falls prevention: the efficacy of a bed alarm system in an acute-care setting. Mt Sinai J Med 1993;60:522–7.
44. Chun H, Kang J, Kim KJ, Park KS, Kim HC. IT-based diagnostic instrumentation systems for personalized healthcare services. Stud Health Technol Inform 2005;117:180–90.
45. Demiris G, Rantz M, Aud M, et al. Older adults' attitudes towards and perceptions of "smart home" technologies: a pilot study. Med Inform Internet Med 2004;29:87–94.
46. Sawka AM, Boulos P, Beattie K, et al. Do hip protectors decrease the risk of hip fracture in institutional and community-dwelling elderly? A systematic review and meta-analysis of randomized controlled trials. Osteoporos Int 2005;16:1461–74.

47. Howland J, Peterson E, Kivell E. Hip protectors efficacy and barriers to adoption to prevent fall-related injuries in older adults: findings and recommendations from an international workgroup. J Saf Res 2006;37:421–4.
48. Sugioka Y, Koike T, World Health Organization. Absolute risk for fracture and WHO guidelines. Fall and fracture in elderly people: risk factors and strategies for prevention. Clin Calcium 2007;17:1059–65.
49. Holzer G, Holzer LA. Hip protectors and prevention of hip fractures in older persons. Geriatrics 2007;62:15–20.
50. Kannus P, Uusi-Rasi K, Palvanen M, Parkkari J. Non-pharmacological means to prevent fractures among older adults. Ann Med 2005;37:303–10.
51. Chang JT, Morton SC, Rubenstein LZ, et al. Interventions for the prevention of falls in older adults: systematic review and meta-analysis of randomised clinical trials. BMJ 2004;328: 680.
52. Leipzig RM, Cumming RG, Tinetti ME. Drugs and falls in older people: a systematic review and meta-analysis: I. Psychotropic drugs. J Am Geriatr Soc 1999;47:30–9.
53. Leipzig RM, Cumming RG, Tinetti ME. Drugs and falls in older people: a systematic review and meta-analysis: II. Cardiac and analgesic drugs. J Am Geriatr Soc 1999;47:40–50.
54. Arfken CL, Wilson JG, Aronson SM. Retrospective review of selective serotonin reuptake inhibitors and falling in older nursing home residents. Int Psychogeriatr 2001;13:85–91.
55. Ensrud KE, Blackwell T, Mangione CM, et al. Central nervous system active medications and risk for fractures in older women. Arch Intern Med 2003;163:949–57.
56. Hien le TT, Cumming RG, Cameron ID, et al. Atypical antipsychotic medications and risk of falls in residents of aged care facilities. J Am Geriatr Soc 2005;53:1290–5.
57. Landi F, Onder G, Cesari M, et al. Psychotropic medications and risk for falls among community-dwelling frail older people: an observational study. J Gerontol A Biol Sci Med Sci 2005;60:622–6.
58. Peterson JF, Kuperman GJ, Shek C, Patel M, Avorn J, Bates DW. Guided prescription of psychotropic medications for geriatric inpatients. Arch Intern Med 2005;165:802–7.
59. Bastow MD, Rawlings J, Allison SP. Benefits of supplementary tube feeding after fractured neck of femur: a randomised controlled trial. 1983. Nutrition 1995;11:323–6.
60. Bastow MD, Rawlings J, Allison SP. Benefits of supplementary tube feeding after fractured neck of femur: a randomised controlled trial. Br Med J (Clin Res Ed) 1983;287:1589–92.

Part II
Perioperative Management

Chapter 4
Preoperative Assessment of Risk

Joan Weinryb

Abstract Preoperative risk assessment for geriatric patients must include an acknowledgment of the hazards of iatrogenic events associated with hospitalization of elderly persons. These include adverse drug events, bowel and bladder dysfunction, delirium, falls, malnutrition, nosocomial infections, and pressure sores. Evaluation includes individual assessment of risk for each adverse outcome and strategies for avoiding each.

The consultant should provide:

- Systematic medication regimen review
- Recommendations for avoidance or timely elimination of tubes and gadgets
- Recommendations that diminish over-restriction of nutrition and over- or under-utilization of fluids
- Identification and modification of pressure ulcer-related risk factors
- Recommendations for, access to toilets, use of laxatives, avoidance of medications with side-effect profiles associated with bowel and bladder function disturbance, and avoidance or early removal of urinary catheters
- Recommendations for postoperative pain management
- Minimization of restraints, including high beds and bedrails, avoidance of medications associated with falls or mental status changes in the elderly
- Recommendations for liberal and appropriate use of physical, occupational and speech therapy modalities, assistive devices, and interim care sites

Preoperative assessment has a threefold purpose. One is to reduce personal risk and improve outcome, both by determining the interface between the procedure and individual's characteristics and by designating appropriate perioperative strategies to decrease the likelihood of morbidity and mortality. Another is to eliminate unnecessary testing that leads to unneeded procedures that may add morbidity and

J. Weinryb (✉)
Division of Geriatric Medicine, University of Pennsylvania Health System, Philadelphia, PA, USA
e-mail: weinrybj@mail.med.upenn.edu

R.J. Pignolo et al. (eds.), *Fractures in the Elderly*, Aging Medicine,
DOI 10.1007/978-1-60327-467-8_4,

mortality of their own (e.g., cardiac stress testing on low risk individuals or those who are facing low risk procedures, that could lead to cardiac catheterization and contrast-induced renal failure). The third is to eliminate unnecessary interventions that contribute to financial waste.

In some instances, there is already a substantial literature. Designation for whom perioperative beta blockade reduces perioperative cardiac events is fairly well established. Benefits of DVT prophylaxis have been amply demonstrated, though which medication in which circumstance remains an active research topic. Procedure type and medication management to avoid bleeding complications is fairly well described.

Areas more specific to geriatric patients like preoperative functional capacity and strategies for avoiding delirium are still in evolution. As the proportion of the population who are elderly increases, it is increasingly important to optimize preoperative evaluation and perioperative management to reduce mortality, morbidity, and unnecessary cost.

Keywords Risk stratification • Risk index • Functional status • Preoperative testing

4.1 Introduction

In our aging society, the elderly proportion of our population is expanding most rapidly. More than half of all surgical procedures occurs in older patients [1]. The likelihood of many ophthalmologic, orthopedic, and cardiovascular surgical procedures increases with advancing age. The previous view, common as late as 1980, of avoiding surgery at all costs in persons older than 65 years has changed with the increasing life expectancy of older persons and declining surgical mortality. Still, a disproportionate number of older patients suffer from postoperative complications. Three quarters of perioperative mortality occurs in persons over age 65 [2]. The major causes of postoperative death include cardiovascular, pulmonary, and infectious events.

Age as an independent predictor of operative risk remains controversial. Advancing age brings increasing rates of medical illnesses including pulmonary, cardiac, renal, and endocrine diseases that do have a clear influence on surgical morbidity and mortality. At least 90% of those over the age of 70 years have at least one comorbidity [2].

Research has led to the concept of reduced physiologic reserves related to aging that influence recovery. Surgical mortality rates have been declining from 20% in the 1960s to about 5%, despite the aging of our society and the increasing likelihood that persons older than 65 years will undergo surgery. The trend extends to the extremes of age as a small study of surgical outcomes among centenarians demonstrated [3]. Expanding knowledge of what influences outcome has enabled improved identification and modification of risk factors leading to poor outcome.

It is clear that while aging affects normal physiology, the aging process differs from person to person and, for each individual, aging does not even affect each organ system uniformly. A perioperative complication in an elderly person is more likely to lead to further complications. Failure of one organ is more likely to lead to failure in multiple organs. Preoperative risk assessment involves assessing the general factors relating to all persons in an age group, type of risks, risks relating to the procedure, and patient-specific factors of health and functional status. Geriatricians give both a general idea of risk versus benefit and assess for strategies to minimize morbidity due to postoperative complications likely to occur in the aged without preemptive management. Preoperative assessment and perioperative management are inextricably intertwined.

Common parlance terms preoperative evaluation as the "Pre-Op Clearance."

Clearance is a misnomer. Preoperative evaluation can assess status and underlying risk and define strategies for limiting potentially avoidable complications. Assessments can identify the multiple comorbid conditions common in elderly persons, characterize functional capacity, and add what is known about the risk inherent in the particular procedure. The goal is to help to determine what care can minimize the risk of one or more organ systems failing, leading to complications, morbidity and disability, or death. Risk, once identified, allows patient and practitioner more understanding of the benefit of the proposed procedure. Risk may be modified by medications, preventive treatments, and collaboration with specialists.

4.2 Risk Factors

Risk is divided into procedure-specific factors and patient-specific factors. The former may help determine the necessity for assessing for the latter. Some classes of risk are more related to procedure-specific factors; e.g., pulmonary complications relative to site of surgery. Assessment of burden of illness helps estimate perioperative mortality.

The most familiar patient-specific factor to both requesting surgeon and consultant is preoperative cardiac risk. For geriatric patients, this is only "the tip of the iceberg." To optimize the management of geriatric patients, the assessment must encompass a broader range of concerns. The assessment includes the individual's pre-existing comorbidities, and the effects of the physiological process of aging, both generally and specifically to that patient. Additionally, the risk and necessity of each procedure, as well as the elective or emergent nature of the surgery, must be evaluated.

There are a number of challenges in interpreting statistical studies of the effects of surgical management on older persons. Older people are a heterogeneous population. They include those who are frail and have multiple comorbidities, as well as those of the same chronological age who have a minimal burden of medical problems. Chronological age does not necessarily parallel physiologic age. Additionally, though there are studies detailing the deterioration of physiologic function with "normal aging," the reserve function of various organ systems is not known for any particular individual until the system is challenged. Older people may be well compensated when unstressed, but unable to tolerate, in one or more organ groups, any additional burden. Older people may be well compensated because of complex medication regimens that must be modified for surgery. Older people are more likely to develop fluid and electrolyte disturbances. They suffer more frequently from drug toxicities and interactions. Their medical histories may be long, with missing or unobtainable data. Some are unable to supply adequate or correct detail about themselves to allow accurate assessment.

The challenge for the geriatric preoperative consultant is to be familiar with the general risk stratifications, to understand the effects of various comorbidities, to eliminate modifiable sources of risk, and to advocate proactively for care that maximizes the likelihood of positive outcome in geriatric patients. For the geriatrician, preoperative assessment and perioperative management are intertwined. Components of risk stratification, preoperative testing recommendations, and functional assessment lead to recommendations for preoperative optimization and perioperative management.

4.3 Risk Stratification

The ACC/AHA has organized the approach to the risk stratification of procedures [4].

High risk procedures are those considered to have >5% mortality. These include emergency surgery, aortic surgery, surgery for peripheral vascular disease, and surgery that involves prolonged anesthesia time and large fluid shift or blood loss.

Intermediate risk, with risk of 1–5%, includes orthopedic procedures outlined in subsequent chapters, urologic surgeries, uncomplicated head and neck, abdominal and thoracic surgeries.

Low risk, with risk <1%, includes dermatologic, endoscopic procedures, cataract surgery and breast surgery. It is noteworthy that emergent surgeries have a 5- to 20-fold increase in mortality for those who are 80 years and above compared to electively scheduled surgeries.

Risk stratification is only the first step in preparing the elderly patient for surgery. It is a framework useful in guiding preoperative evaluation and testing. It is not the result of the testing.

4.4 Preoperative Cardiac Evaluation

Much has been written about the estimation of cardiac risk prior to noncardiac surgery. Cardiac risk indices mainly identify markers of coronary artery disease and ventricular dysfunction. Once identified, determination can be made of whether the risk of surgery outweighs the benefit to the particular patient and which evaluations and treatments should be initiated to decrease the risk. The use of reliable indexes of risk has the added benefit of limiting the extent of invasive preoperative testing.

Noteworthy is the Goldman Cardiac Risk Index [5]. Published in 1977, it assigns points to nine clinical risk factors. Age > 70 years automatically adds 5 points. The sum of the points places the patient in a certain "Class" of cardiac risk. Class I confers the lowest risk (<1%) whereas Class IV the highest risk (78%). Detsky modified the Cardiac Risk Index in 1986 by adding two more variables, pulmonary edema and angina [6].

The Revised Goldman Cardiac Risk Index (RCRI), published in 1999, was simplified to six independent predictors of major cardiac complications (cardiac death, nonfatal MI, nonfatal cardiac arrest) [7]. The RCRI is thought to have the best predictive value.

One of the problems noted for all these indices is that very few patients with aortic stenosis, increasingly common with aging, were included in the studies determining the usefulness of the indices. Moderate to severe aortic stenosis significantly increases risk for cardiac complications (hypotension, myocardial infaction, heart failure, and arrhythmia). When aortic valvular disease is determined to be present, the appropriate recommendation is for valve replacement before intermediate- or major-risk elective surgery in patients who have criteria for valve replacement [8]. For emergency procedures, or if the patient has refused valve replacement, aggressive intraoperative hemodynamic monitoring can be recommended to ensure maintenance of adequate preload. Preoperative evaluation allows the consultant to make recommendations about the advisability of valvular surgery prior to the planned procedure or to arrange an opportunity for the anesthesiologist to determine beforehand what appropriate intraoperative hemodynamic monitoring, including invasive modalities, will be optimal.

Multiple randomized and nonrandomized trials over the past decade have lead to the conclusion that beta blockers confer a mortality benefit for patients undergoing intermediate to high risk noncardiac surgical procedures [9, 10]. These medications are thought to minimize the risk of intraoperative cardiac ischemia by decreasing cardiac oxygen demand and inhibiting the large sympathetic surge associated with surgery. In 2005, a large meta-analysis of randomized controlled trials of preoperative beta blocker use for noncardiac surgery found that the data were too inconclusive to make a sweeping recommendation for beta blocker use [10]. The POISE trial and the subsequent 2008 meta-analysis, does not support initiation of prophylactic perioperative beta blockers in the majority of patients undergoing noncardiac surgery [11, 12]. Beta blockers for low risk patients undergoing low risk procedures do more harm than good. The 2009 ACC/AHA Guideline updates recommend beta-blocker therapy to be continued in patients already taking them, and although weakly recommended, to be initiated in those undergoing vascular surgery who have evidence of ischemia in preoperative cardiac testing. Patients whose preoperative testing shows CAD, or those with multiple intermediate risk factors who are undergoing either vascular surgery or intermediate/high risk nonvascular surgery, are felt to benefit if heart rate is tightly controlled. Patients undergoing low risk surgery who have not been taking beta blockers, patients with low cardiac risk undergoing vascular surgery, and patients with no or one intermediate risk factor undergoing intermediate to high risk surgeries are not candidates for beta blockers.

The geriatrician can advise choice of a beta-1 selective agent. Atenolol (long acting) is considered to be more effective than metoprolol (short acting). Assessment for renal insufficiency may bring about a recommendation for metoprolol instead. Optimally, the medication is started 30 days prior to elective surgery and titrated to a heart rate of 50–60 bpm. If it is not possible to start so far in advance, intravenous beta blockers can be given prior to surgery and intraoperatively (e.g., 5–10 mg IV atenolol every 6 h), continuing with oral medication continued postoperatively for at least a month.

4.5 Preoperative Pulmonary Evaluation

Normal aging and chronic pulmonary diseases confer increased risk of developing perioperative complications such as aspiration, pneumonia, hypoventilation, hypoxia, and bronchospasm [13–15]. Postoperative pulmonary complication rates for patients over age 65 are 11.3%, compared with younger patients' rate of 1.5%. The incidence among men is 7.8%, compared with 5.7% among women. Pulmonary complications account for 20% of perioperative deaths in the elderly.

The site of surgery is an important risk factor for developing postoperative pulmonary complications [14]. The closer to the diaphragm, the higher the risk. Pulmonary complications prolong hospital stays. For abdominal surgical patients, this is by an average of 10 days over the 6-day mean length of stay for abdominal surgery. Highest pulmonary complication risk is associated with thoracic and upper abdominal surgeries (cholecystectomy), neck surgery, and abdominal aortic aneurysm repairs. Procedures lasting more than 4 h also confer greater risk of complications [14]. Orthopedic procedures generally do not confer a relatively greater risk of pulmonary complications due to surgical sites in proximity to the diaphragm or from prolonged procedures.

Aging leads to diminished pulmonary reserve. Normal aging also leads to loss of elasticity of the pharyngeal support structures, potentiating an increased risk of aspiration. The chest wall becomes stiffer with age, the thorax becomes enlarged and the diaphragm flattens, increasing residual volume. Keeping alveoli open thus requires more energy, especially in a supine position. Older people are at higher risk of ventilation–perfusion mismatch and increased A-a gradients, regardless of surgical procedure.

Common lung diseases including chronic bronchitis and emphysema, add even greater risk for postoperative complications. In fact, COPD has been shown to be an independent major risk factor for the development of perioperative pulmonary complications. Cigarette smoking, even in the absence of COPD, can increase surgical risk. It appears that the number of pack-years correlates with the amount of increased risk [16]. All patients, regardless of their age should be advised to stop smoking more than 8 weeks prior to their surgery (smoking cessation <4 weeks prior to surgery is associated with greater risk). If surgery is elective and the procedure is one with increased likelihood of pulmonary complication, the consultant may advise postponement until smoking cessation has been accomplished [16].

COPD is a major surgical risk factor, conferring three to five times greater risk of perioperative pulmonary complications. Abnormalities on pulmonary auscultation are even more predictive than chest X-ray or spirometry. Risk indices for predicting postoperative pneumonia after noncardiac surgery include factors of age, location of surgery, functional status, weight loss, transfusion history, laboratory abnormalities have shown validity [14, 17]. Preoperative spirometry and arterial blood gases are mainly reserved for patients undergoing thoracic or upper abdominal procedures or who have significant underlying lung disease. Pulmonary function testing is mainly helpful for those undergoing lobectomy or pneumonectomy to predict adequacy of postoperative lung function. The consultant may advise expectant management with bronchodilators for COPD patients, pre- and postoperatively. Early mobilization to an upright position, so as to allow full diaphragmatic excursion, and supervised incentive spirometry benefit most older patients and may be suggested as priorities. Chest physiotherapy and mucolytics may also be recommended. The consultant may advise treatment of any COPD exacerbation with steroids without significant increase in infection or interference with wound healing.

Asthmatics do not necessarily have increased pulmonary risk. Management to keep the peak expiratory flow rate at 80% of the individual's best decreases their risk of complications. Asthmatics should be advised to use their medications to this end.

4.6 Infection and Perioperative Antibiotics

Perioperative antibiotic management involves not only knowledge of standard of care "prophylaxis," but the recognition of perioperative signs of infection which may be absent, diminished or different in the elderly.

4.7 Thromoembolic Risk

Older persons are more likely to have underlying venous insufficiency and immobility. Thromboembolic complications, DVT, and pulmonary embolus, increase with age and type of surgery. Additional risk factors include a history of thromboembolism, stroke, malignancy, and hypercoagulable states. Hip fracture, lower extremity orthopedic surgery or spinal cord injuries confer risk. Meta-analyses have indicated incidence of DVT without prophylaxis after orthopedic surgery to lie in the range of 50–60% [18]. Fatal pulmonary embolism has been calculated to occur in almost 4–14% of hip fracture patients who have not received prophylaxis against thromboembolism. Limb immobility associated with stroke is also associated with high rates of thromboembolism. Guidelines for appropriate DVT/PE prophylaxis, tailored for specific procedures, recommended and amended by experts, should be consulted and followed [19]. Further information about anticoagulation in the elderly can be found elsewhere in this volume.

4.8 Gastrointestinal Risks and Obesity

The gastrointestinal system is affected by aging [20]. Gastric acid production decreases, and gastric motility lessens. Hepatic blood flow decreases, and intestinal peristalsis may be slower and more prone to disruption by medications, immobility, and dehydration.

Medications that require acid for activation or absorption may be affected. Medications that are activated by liver metabolism may have reduced effect and those that are inactivated by the liver may have increased effect at the same dose as used for a younger person. Older persons may have vitamin B12 or vitamin D deficiency on the basis of reduced absorptive capacity.

Older persons often have reduced perception of thirst and may not maintain their hydration status without urging. Reduced saliva flow, sense of smell and taste may affect appetite. Dental and swallowing problems may cause nutrition and hydration problems perioperatively. Constipation, common in the elderly, may be exacerbated by limited fiber intake, anesthetic and analgesic medications, immobility, and lack of timely access to toilet facilities.

Obesity has become increasingly common in the elderly. Obesity alone does not appear to increase perioperative cardiac or pulmonary risk; however, it can interfere with mobilization postoperatively and add to the risk of operative wound infection. Highly obese patients who underwent primary hip replacement were 2.3 times more likely to stay in the hospital more than 5 days, and 2.6 times more likely to be discharged to a skilled nursing facility (SNF) [21]. Some procedures require modification to avoid complications associated with obesity. Surgeons have found, for example, that left colectomy, as opposed to right colectomy, in obese persons often results in intraabdominal collections. Therefore prophylactic drains are more commonly inserted. Many older persons lack the vision and manual dexterity to manage drains alone, even if they have the cognitive ability to understand the directions. Discharge planning must take this into account.

4.9 Nutritional Risks

Nutrition is a factor that influences perioperative risk. Up to 20% of older persons are malnourished at the time of their hospitalization. Up to 50% of nursing home residents are malnourished. Both weight loss and visceral protein depletion may occur.

Total cholesterol of <160 mg/dl is associated with increased mortality in the elderly [22]. Serum albumin <3.5 confers a fourfold increase in the risk of complications and a sixfold increase in perioperative deaths among elderly persons [23]. Dental issues may inhibit the ability to take nutrition. Social isolation, mood disorders, memory loss, and functional incapacities may have interfered with obtaining, preparing, and ingesting a diet that allows maintenance of a normal nutritional status.

Older persons are more likely to suffer from occult vitamin deficiencies. Reduced intake, decreased absorption, increased demand, and decreased ability of the body to convert ingested vitamins to their active forms all contribute to deficiencies. Vitamin deficiency can be a sign of underlying metabolic problems or diseases. Vitamin deficiency can affect vitamin–coenzyme interactions affecting many aspects of metabolic activity from immune function to wound healing and the production of new erythrocytes. It has been found that B12 and Vitamin D subclinical deficiency are relatively common. Vitamin D appears to play a role in muscle strength, as well as in bone health. Malnutrition due to suppression of the ability to utilize nutrients by inflammatory cytokines related to chronic inflammation may also be present. Diseases such as Alzheimer's are associated with high production of interleukin-1 and tumor necrosis factor-alpha in the peripheral blood. Swallowing issues are often worsened by the stress of surgery, medications, dry mouth due to NPO status, lack of assistance with denture insertion, and poor positioning when food is offered. Decreased thirst sensation and sense of smell may diminish older person's acceptance of meals with suboptimal palatability.

Malnutrition increases likelihood of perioperative complications. Factors influenced include not only wound healing, but also energy to be mobilized upright and ability to fend off nosocomial infection. Physical findings include muscle wasting or decrease in strength, and posterior column symptoms. The skin color, tongue color, and presence of papillar atrophy can signal vitamin, protein or iron deficiency states. The consultant evaluates for co-morbid conditions leading to malabsorption such as sprue, previous gastrointestinal surgeries, as well as for other underlying maladies which may have led to malnutrition. The consultant can help avoid vitamin toxicites from the use of inappropriate or excess supplementation. An example of this may be the recommendation of nonspecific zinc administration to all persons with wounds. Though it is clear that zinc deficiency affects wound healing, it is also clear that excess zinc can affect the copper metabolism involved in producing erythrocytes and may lead to anemia [24]. Additionally, it can lead to mouth sores and perception of bad taste, increasing eating problems. Assessment is necessary so that the consultant may be able to recommend supplements and other nutrient strategies to minimize the likelihood of malnutrition interfering with recovery. (S)he may involve the speech therapist and dietician in the perioperative management of the patient, and can be on hand to ensure that prolonged periods without nutrients that can occur with surgery and are much less well tolerated by aged persons, do not occur.

4.10 Renal and Urological Complications

Kidney function declines at about 1% per year after age 35. In one NIH study, moderate renal function impairment increased from 18% in those aged 65–74 years to 96% in those 85 years or older [25]. Many elderly kidneys are affected by hypertension, atherosclerosis, and diabetes mellitus. As aging occurs, total body fat increases; declining muscle mass results in decreased creatinine production. Though the serum creatinine may appear normal, calculated creatinine clearance often reveals significant decreases in glomerular filtration. At the same time, total body water decreases. The impact of these changes is to render the elderly person more sensitive to the effects of intravenous infusions and medications. Since the aging kidney is less able to conserve sodium and water, dehydration and derangement of serum electrolytes may occur because of the type or volume of the intravenous solutions chosen. Additionally, medications that are lipophilic are dissolved in a greater volume of distribution and have increased half-lives. Medications that are hydrophilic have a smaller volume of distribution and a greater effect at the same dose given to a younger person. Therefore, the dictum in geriatric pharmacology: "start low, go slow."

Glomerular filtration rate influences pharmocokinetics in the elderly. Currently, many laboratories are automatically supplying the MDRD GFR calculator, and calculating GFR for all measurements of renal function. The National Kidney Foundation has indicated that this may not be reliable in persons over 70 years. Other calculators include the Cockroft and Gault method, which has the advantage of including modification for the patient's weight and the Jeliffe method, which is felt to be more reliable in persons with unstable renal function, since it corrects for rising creatinine. Aging, liver disease and muscle mass which is unusually high (athletes) or low (malnourished), as well as dietary creatinine intake (high with creatine supplements, low in vegetarians) can affect the accuracy of calculated creatinine. Calculated creatinine clearance, based on a single blood sample and not requiring a 24-h urine collection is much more convenient and more likely to occur. Though there is controversy about the reliability of various equations designed to allow calculation of creatinine clearance, the use of 24-h urine collection for the estimation of GFR has not been shown to be more reliable than serum creatinine-based equations [26]. Since both pharmacodynamics, the study of the relationship between serum concentration and therapeutic effect and pharmacokinetics, are altered in the elderly, it is important for the consultant to quantify the level of renal impairment. Information about appropriate medication doses, modified for renal function, as well as intravenous fluid management to avoid electrolyte imbalances, dehydration or fluid overload will decrease nosocomial morbidity.

Older persons are more likely to develop urologic complications during hospitalization. Infection is more common and associated with both indwelling and condom catheters [27]. Dehydration, retention, and constipation also increase the risk of urinary tract infection. Rates of urinary retention are increased in the elderly, sometimes as a result of underlying anatomic issues. Elderly men with enlarged prostates, able to urinate when standing, may be unable to empty their bladders when immobilized in bed. Retention may be associated with particular medications, especially those with anticholinergic side effects. Indwelling catheterization of longer than 48 h dramatically increases the risk of retention. Rates of urinary incontinence increase, both as a result of medications and due to functional impairment engendered by the surgery, hospital equipment or other environmental factors. Risk factors for retention, incontinence and infection require preoperative assessment and intervention.

4.11 Perioperative Management of Diabetes Mellitus

Diabetes mellitus is increasingly common with aging. Normal blood glucose assists healing, decreases infection, and minimizes morbidity and mortality. If preoperative assessment reveals a HbA1c > 9% or fasting glucose > 180 mg/dl or postprandial glucose > 230 mg/dl, a case may be made for postponing elective surgery until better control is achieved. Diabetics require screening for heart, kidney, and autonomic and peripheral nervous system problems which will affect their management.

Long acting oral medications cannot be used until reliable PO nutrition is restored. Metformin should be held in the perioperative period. For patients receiving insulin previously, the custom has been to give one half the usual dose of long- or intermediate-acting insulin injected in the morning of surgery and then to use "sliding scale" insulin. This method is also used for patients who usually receive oral agents and for those in whom there has been no previous treatment for hyperglycemia. Unpredictable absorption because of changes in tissue perfusion, and depletion of the insulin reservoir due to delay or prolongation of surgery, can cause deterioration in glucose control. Insulin drips, providing easily variable dosing, and long duration insulins like insulin glargine are preferable. The goal is blood glucose levels of 110–180 mg/dl and normal fluid and electrolyte balance.

4.12 Neurological Risk

Preoperative assessment of neurologic status is important in several ways. Older persons may have previous brain insults for which they are well compensated, but that, with the stress of surgery, may appear as a new neurologic deficit. Delirium, which may occur in up to 50% of elderly (>70) surgical patients, contributes to increased morbidity, mortality, prolonged hospital stays, and increased likelihood of institutionalization [28]. Hypoactive delirium often goes unrecognized. Delirium often results in accidental injury. It adds to the likelihood of physical or chemical restraints. The effects of delirium may last for months or years. Older persons with cognitive deficits, underlying vascular disease of the brain, and sensory deficits are especially at risk. Perioperative dehydration, polypharmacy, and medical gadgetry all increase the risk of perioperative delirium. (An in depth approach to delirium is found elsewhere in this volume.) Perioperative strokes can occur with and without atrial fibrillation.

It is important to assess baseline cognitive/neurological function by physical examination and cognitive assessments. Dementia increases surgical mortality up to 52% when compared to nondemented general surgery patients [29]. In addition, psychological factors have been found to be important predictors of surgical outcome. Depression may present as apathy or self neglect. It may interfere with the ability to recover from surgery or may be a marker for as yet undiagnosed dementia. Proper assessment and treatment may be required preoperatively.

Two frequently used methods of cognitive function assessment are the Folstein Minimental Score, a screening tool to determine the presence of cognitive impairment, and the Confusion Assessment Method (CAM), a standardized assessment to quickly identify delirium. The long version of the CAM is a comprehensive instrument, while the short version includes four features that distinguish delirium from other types of cognitive impairment and can be done quickly and easily at the bedside [30]. Myriads of other tools exist with various purposes and varying levels of validation. It is important for each consultant to be comfortable with validated, easily administered tools for evaluation of cognitive and functional status and for the evaluation of delirium.

Geriatricians can advise and monitor postoperative elimination of tubes and gadgets as soon as possible, early mobilization, return of sensory aids such as hearing aides and glasses, appropriate treatment of pain, and careful scrutiny of medications help to reduce delirium.

Withholding of medications while NPO can affect ability to cope with the stress of surgery. For example, unmedicated, patients with Parkinson's disease may develop worsening tremor and rigidity, motor abilities, dysphagia, and hypoxia. Patients with bipolar disorder may destabilize if medications are withheld. The consultant can make sure that usual regimens are restored as soon as possible or suggest alternative management.

Deprivation of nutrition, with resultant ketosis, can lead to decreased levels of brain function, including alertness, understanding, and cooperation with postoperative mobilization and instructions. The consultant can ensure that intravenous administration includes glucose, that some route for nutrients is utilized, and that oral nutrition is restored in a timely fashion.

4.13 Assessment of Functional Status

Functional status evaluation remains the sine qua non of geriatric preoperative evaluation. In general medical evaluations, functional assessment has been used to refer to exercise capacity and is associated with perioperative cardiac risk. Assessment of metabolic equivalent levels for usual activities, or directly measuring by exercise stress testing can help define operative prognosis. One common rule of thumb is that if a person can walk up a flight of stairs carrying a bag of groceries, or run to catch a bus, (s)he has at least a metabolic equivalent of 4 METS and can be considered as having adequate functional capacity. Conversely, inability to exercise to a heart rate of at least 100 bpm is associated with increased risk for both cardiac and pulmonary complications with surgery [31].

For geriatric patients, assessment of ability to complete the basic and the instrumental activities of daily living also carries important prognostic information. Deficits in Basic Activities of Daily Living (BADL) (i.e., washing, dressing, toileting, transferring and feeding) independently predict perioperative complications in patients over 70 years [32]. Patients with low ADL scores, especially men, are almost 10 times more likely to die in the year following surgery. Level of preoperative dependence in Instrumental Activities (IADL) (i.e., medication management, housework, shopping, financial management, ability to use the telephone, and to travel unaided) helps determine appropriate discharge planning. BADL and IADL assessment may also provide a forum for discussion with patient and family of the goals of care appropriate for the particular patient. A surgical procedure that may be appropriate for an older person with good functional status may be undesirable in a person with impaired functional status due to cognitive or physical disability, because the gains and the risks are altered by the individual's functional status. Previous studies of family experience with relatives dying in hospital indicate that families feel pressured to accept invasive interventions [33]. We may extrapolate from this to older persons faced with a surgical procedure. The consultant can lay out the positives and negatives, with the prognostic information available that will allow the patient and family to make informed decisions.

Multiple studies have shown that, though normal aging and common disease processes do affect function of major organs, older people have increasingly positive surgical outcome, surviving even such procedures as cardiac valve replacement and adding years of quality time to their lives. The normal aging process does affect functional reserve, but that does not necessarily translate into adverse outcomes, even when concomitant chronic diseases are superimposed on the normal aging process. Risk assessment and modification through perioperative management can minimize the likelihood of poor outcome.

4.14 Unnecessary Preoperative Testing

Extensive preoperative testing, based on expert opinion, prior to even minor surgical procedures evolved in an effort to do the best for patients and to avoid litigation. More recently, research has sought to better define what is actually beneficial.

Often, preoperative testing which is not indicated is undertaken. Cardiac indexes that assess the risk inherent in the procedure, as well as the individual patient's risk are helpful in limiting unnecessary and invasive testing. Pulmonary specialty guidelines, recommending chest X-ray only for findings that would require intervention prior to the planned procedure and PFTs only for lung surgery are helping to make clear what is in the patient's best interest [34].

There is still a dearth of evidence-based studies. Some recommendations remain by consensus. Chest X-rays are recommended for those over age 50 who have cardiopulmonary disease, and are to undergo high risk surgeries or ones that involve thoracic, upper abdominal, aortic, esophageal, or neck sites [35]. EKGs are recommended for those undergoing intermediate or high risk procedures. Often, they are done for any patient older than 55 years. It is often difficult for the individual physician to refrain from testing for which there is neither evidence nor expert opinion, but which has become a matter of custom. Common examples include EKGs for patients awaiting colonoscopy. Many coagulation tests (e.g., PT/PTT) are done for patients without hematological histories or physical findings indicating bleeding problems who are not scheduled for procedures in areas of high bleeding risk. Such areas include tissue prone to bleeding (oral, nasal, tonsillar, gynecologic, prostatic, urogenital sites) or sites where homeostatic control is difficult during procedures (e.g., liver or kidney biopsies, knee arthroscopy, and brain surgeries).

References

1. Souders J, Rooke A. Perioperative care for geriatric patients. Ann Longterm Care. 2005;13:17–29.
2. Thomas DR, Ritchie CS. Preoperative assessment of older adults. J Am Geriatr Soc. 1995;43:811–21.
3. Warner MA, Saletel RA, et al. Outcomes of anesthesia and surgery in people 100 years of age and older. J Am Geriatr Soc. 1998;46:988–93.
4. Fleisher LA, Beckman JA, et al. ACC/AHA 2007 guidelines on perioperative cardiovascular evaluation and care for noncardiac surgery: a report of the American College of Cardiology/American Heart Association Task Force on Practice Guidelines. Circulation. 2007;116:e418–99.
5. Goldman L, Caldera DL, et al. Multifactorial index of cardiac risk in noncardiac surgical procedures. N Engl J Med. 1977;297:845–50.
6. Detsky AS, Abrams HB, et al. Predicting cardiac complications in patients undergoing non-cardiac surgery. J Gen Intern Med. 1986;1(4):211–9.
7. Lee TH, Marcantonio ER, Mangione CM, et al. Derivation and prospective evaluation of a simple index for prediction of cardiac risk of major noncardiac surgery. Circulation. 1999;100:1043–9.
8. Kertai MD. Aortic stenosis: risk factor for perioperative complications in patients undergoing non-cardiac surgery. Am J Med. 2004;116:8–13.
9. Mangano DT, Layug EL, et al. The effect of atenolol on mortality and cardiovascular morbidity after non-cardiac surgery. N Eng J Med. 1996;341:1789–94.
10. Lindenauer PK, Pekow P, et al. Perioperative beta blocker therapy and mortality after major non-cardiac surgery. N Engl J Med. 2005;353:349–61.
11. POISE Study Group, Devereaux PJ, Yang H, et al. Effects of extended-release metoprolol succinate in patients undergoing non-cardiac surgery (POISE trial): a randomised controlled trial. Lancet. 2008;371:1839.
12. Bangalore S, Wetterslev J, Pranesh S, et al. Perioperative beta blockers in patients having non-cardiac surgery: a meta-analysis. Lancet. 2008; 372:1962.

13. Smetana G. A 68 year old man with COPD contemplating colon cancer surgery. JAMA. 2007;287:2121–30.
14. Smetana GW. Current concepts: preoperative pulmonary evaluation. N Engl J Med. 1999;340:937–44.
15. Arozullah AM, Khuri SF, et al. Development and validation of a multifactorial risk index for predicting postoperative pneumonia after major non-cardiac surgery. Ann Intern Med. 2001;135:847–57.
16. Nakagawa M, Tanaka H. Relationship between the duration of the preoperative smoke-free period and the incidence of postoperative pulmonary complications after pulmonary surgery. Chest. 2001;120:705–10.
17. Palda V. Pre-opportunity knocks a different way to think about the preoperative evaluation. Am Fam Physician 2000;62:308–311.
18. Clagett GP, Anderson FA, et al. Prevention of thromboembolism. Chest. 1998;114: 531S–560S.
19. Geerts Wh, Pineo GF, et al. Prevention of venous thromboembolism: Seventh ACCP Conference on Antithrombotic and Thrombolytic Therapy. Chest. 2004;126(3 Suppl): 338S–400S.
20. Beyth RJ. Medication use. In: Duthie E, Katz P, et al (eds) Practice of geriatrics, 4th edn. WB Saunders, Philadelphia, 2007, pp 38–48.
21. Turgeon Th, et al. Influence of obesity on outcome following primary hip replacement surgery, paper session, 73rd Annual Meeting. American Academy of Orthopedic Surgeons, Chicago, IL, 2006.
22. Ersan T. Perioperative management of the Geriatric Patient, emedicine from WEB MD, updated 5/1/2005. Accessed 10/2007. Ersan T, et al., Perioperative Management of the Geriatric Patient. http://www.emedicine.com/med/TOPIC3175.HTM
23. Gibbs J, Cull W, et al. Preoperative serum albumin level as a predictor of operative mortality and morbidity: results from the national VA Surgical Risk Study. Arch Surg. 1999;134: 36–42.
24. Hoffman R, Benz E, et al. Hoffman. Hematology: basic principles and practice, 4th edition. Elsevier Publishing, Churchill Livingston, 2005.
25. National Kidney Foundation. http://www.kidney.org/professionals/tools/
26. Giannella SV, et al. Magnitude of underestimation of impaired kidney function in older adults with normal serum creatinine. J Am Ger Soc. 2007;55(6):816–23.
27. Thomas DR, Ritchie CS. Preoperative assessment of older adults. J Am Geriatr Soc. 1995;43:811–21.
28. Milisen K, Forman M, et al. A nurse-led interdisciplinary intervention program for delirium in elderly hip-fracture patients. J Am Geriatr Soc. 2001;49:523–32.
29. Dasgupta M, Dumbrell AC. Preoperative risk assessment for delirium after non- cardiac surgery: a systematic review. J Am Geriatr Soc. 2006;54:1578–89.
30. Inouye S, Viscoli C, et al. A predictive for delirium in hospitalized elderly medical patients based on admission characteristics. Ann Int Med. 1993;119:474–81.
31. Eagle KA et al. ACC/AHA Guideline Update for perioperative cardiovascular evaluation for noncardiac surgery. J Am Coll Cardiol. 2002;39:542–553.
32. Browner WS, Li j, et al. In hospital and long term mortality in male veterans following noncardiac surgery. JAMA. 1992;268:228–32.
33. Dy SM, et al. A systematic review of satisfaction with care at the end of life. J Am Geriatr Soc. 2008;56:124–129.
34. Qaseem A, et al. Risk assessment for and strategies to reduce perioperative pulmonary complications in patients undergoing non-cardiothoracic surgery: guideline from ACP. Ann Int Med. 2006;144:575–80.
35. Schein O, et al, The value of routine preoperative medical testing before cataract surgery. N Engl J Med. 2000;342:168–75.

Further Reading

Cohn S, Smetana G. Update in perioperative medicine. Ann Intern Med. 2007;147:263–70.

American Society of Anesthesiologists. ASA Physical Status Classification System. http://www.asahq.org/clinical/physicalstatus.htm.

Arora VM, et al, Quality indicators for hospitalization and surgery in vulnerable elders. J Am Geriatr Soc. 2007;55(s2):S347–58.

Chapter 5
Anticoagulation

Kathleen Walsh and John Bruza

Abstract Anticoagulation in the elderly can be very challenging. UFH, LMWH, and warfarin are effective first line agents for VTE prophylaxis in hip fracture patients. However, the use aspirin as a single agent after major orthopedic surgery is controversial, but more strongly favored by orthopedic surgeons. Differences in the approach taken by orthopaedic surgeons as compared to medical specialists have been discussed, and need to be further evaluated. There is often a greater fear of bleeding in the elderly due to age-associated risk, coexisting diseases, and polypharmacy that is appreciated by both orthopaedic surgeons and medical specialists alike. Intermittent compression devices may provide an added beneficial effect to other interventions, and carry no risk of bleeding.

Keywords Deep vein thrombosis • Pulmonary embolism • Anticoagulation • Heparin • Aspirin • Warfarin • Low molecular weight heparins • Heparin-induced thrombocytopenia • Intermittent pneumatic compression devices • Inferior vena caval filters

5.1 Introduction

Hip fracture surgery is usually performed on older patients and carries a high risk for developing venous thromboembolism (VTE). VTE risk is increased depending on the surgery type, increased age, previous VTE, obesity, varicose veins, venous stasis, cardiac dysfunction, nephrotic syndrome, malignancy, presence of a coagulation inhibitor deficiency state, and prolonged immobility. Aging itself is a risk factor for VTE [1]. Without prophylaxis after hip fracture surgery, about 50% of patients will

---

J. Bruza (✉)
Division of Geriatric Medicine, University of Pennsylvania School of Medicine,
3615 Chestnut Street, Philadelphia, PA 19104-2676, USA
e-mail: jcjohnso@mail.med.upenn.edu

R.J. Pignolo et al. (eds.), *Fractures in the Elderly*, Aging Medicine,
DOI 10.1007/978-1-60327-467-8_5,

develop a deep vein thrombosis (DVT) and 1.4–7.5% will develop a fatal pulmonary embolism (PE) within 3 months [2]. Therefore many, including these authors, recommend that routine thromboprophylaxis be provided to all patients undergoing hip fracture surgery given the high morbidity associated with VTE. The choices among pharmacologic and nonpharmacologic prophylaxis are many and clinical practices vary widely. This chapter will review the latest evidence-based guidelines to prevent VTE in the perioperative period for older adults.

Compared with elective hip and knee arthroplasty, fewer trials have been performed to study patients undergoing hip fracture surgery. For this reason, some of our recommendations for hip fracture patients are extrapolated from clinical trials for elective arthroplasty (Table 5.1).

The high risk for VTE associated with orthopedic surgery is related to many factors contributing to a hypercoagulable state. The supine position on the operating table and the positioning of the extremity during surgery increase the stasis of venous blood flow. As a consequence of the surgical procedure vein wall endothelium becomes damaged, promoting changes in the coagulation cascade in response to tissue factor release from the intimal injury and increasing the risk of thrombosis [3]. The type of anesthesia may also influence the likelihood of VTE, with spinal anesthesia possibly reducing the incidence by affecting sympathetic blockade and actually increasing blood flow to the lower extremities [4]. The time delay between the injury and surgery may also affect the incidence of thrombosis [3].

5.2 Pharmacologic Methods of Prophylaxis

5.2.1 Aspirin

Aspirin is an antiplatelet agent that helps to prevent blood from clotting by inhibiting cyclooxygenase and reducing the synthesis of prostaglandin and thromboxane A2. Aspirin promotes vasodilation and inhibits platelet aggregation [4].

A portion of the Pulmonary Embolism Prevention (PEP) trial randomized over 13,000 patients undergoing hip fracture surgery (mean age 79 years old) to aspirin 160 mg daily or placebo. There was a 43% reduction in PE and 29% reduction in DVT in the group that received aspirin. Though this study concluded that low dose of aspirin reduces the risk of PE and symptomatic DVT, there were confounding factors. For example, additional thromboprophylactic measures such as unfractionated heparin (UFH), low molecular weight heparin (LMWH), and graded compression stockings were used in 18%, 26%, and 30% of patients, respectively. There was a small but significant increase in gastrointestinal bleeding, wound-related bleeding, and a drop in mean perioperative hemoglobin concentration. The mean transfusion volume was greater with aspirin among those receiving transfusion for any reason [5]. In the subgroup analysis of patients who also received prophylaxis with a LMWH, there was no statistically significant difference in the rate of VTE between aspirin and placebo [2].

Table 5.1 Summary of therapeutic anticoagulation options for elderly hip fracture patients

Intervention (References)	Dosing	Advantages	Disadvantages
Fondaparinux [11, 24–26]	2.5 mg SQ daily	Once daily dosing	No antidote
		No risk for HIT	Contraindication in creatinine clearance < 30 mL/min
		Lab monitoring not required	Expensive
LMWH: enoxaparin [13, 19–21]	30 mg SQ q12 or 40 mg SQ daily	Antidote: protamine	Injection site hematomas
		Lab monitoring not required	Dose adjustment needed for creatinine clearance < 30 mL/min and obesity
			HIT – but lower risk than UFH
UFH [11–15]	5,000 units SQ TID	Antidote: protamine	Injection site hematomas HIT
Warfarin [2, 9, 10]	Target INR 2.0–3.0	Antidote: vitamin K No need to adjust for renal impairment or obesity	Frequent blood monitoring Difficulty maintaining therapeutic levels
Aspirin [2, 5–8]	160 mg daily 100 mg BID		Conflicting results of efficacy in preventing VTE and risk of GI bleeding
Intermittent compression devices [30, 31]		Additive effect to other treatments	Not effective in preventing VTE when used alone
		No risk for bleeding	Uncomfortable
		No risk for HIT	May be perceived as a restraint in delirious patient and increase risk for falls
			Use with caution in arterial insufficiency

HIT heparin-induced thrombocytopenia

A double-blinded, randomized, controlled trial was used to study the relative efficacy and safety of a low molecular weight heparinoid (Orgaran) compared with aspirin for the prevention of postoperative VTE in patients undergoing hip fracture surgery. Orgaran is a mixture of sulfated glycosaminoglycans, including heparan sulfate, dermatan sulfate and chondroitin sulfate. Two-hundred and fifty-one patients (average age of 76 years) received aspirin 100 mg twice daily or Orgaran. Patients were excluded from the trial if they had a history of bleeding disorders, recent gastrointestinal bleeding, peptic ulcer disease, or severe renal dysfunction. Venography (the gold standard) was used to detect DVT. About 28% of the Orgaran group and 44% of the aspirin group developed VTE. Seventy-six percent of all the thromboses detected were on the operated leg. There was more major bleeding in the aspirin group (though not statistically significant). Bleeding was classified as major if overt and led to transfusion of >2 units of blood, decrease in hemoglobin > 2 g/dL, or if retroperitoneal, intra-articular or intracranial in origin The study concluded that low molecular weight heparinoid is significantly more effective than and at least as safe as aspirin as a prophylactic agent for postoperative VTE after hip fracture. It also confirms that the incidence of all VTE is high when aspirin is used as the only means of prophylaxis in these patients [6].

The American College of Chest Physicians (ACCP) Evidence Based Guidelines do not recommend aspirin to be used alone as VTE prophylaxis [2] and conclude that aspirin is inferior to warfarin, heparins, and fondaparinux. However, the American Academy of Orthopaedic Surgeons Clinical Guideline on Prevention of Symptomatic Pulmonary Embolism in Patients Undergoing Total Hip or Knee Arthroplasty views aspirin as a viable alternative to other types of chemoprophylaxis in patients at standard risk of both PE and major bleeding [7]. A pooled analysis of 14 randomized controlled trials (RCTs) cited by the ACCP guidelines determined that VTE rates with aspirin were not significantly different from rates for vitamin K antagonists, low molecular weight heparins, and pentasaccharides, with operative site bleeding relative risks lowest for aspirin [8].

5.2.2 Vitamin K Antagonists (Warfarin)

Limited evidence suggests that prophylaxis with warfarin is effective and safe in hip fracture surgery patients. In 1976, Morris published a prospective, randomized control trial, on the prophylactic value of warfarin sodium in 160 elderly hip fracture patients [9]. Patients were randomized to received warfarin or placebo within 24 h of admission to the hospital. There was a significantly lower incidence of DVT in the warfarin group. No treated patient died from PE. There was a decrease in mortality in the treatment group, though it was not statistically significant [9].

In 1989, Powers published a randomized placebo-controlled trial of warfarin, aspirin or placebo in postoperative hip surgery patients [10]. Those in the warfarin group received 10 mg as soon as possible after surgery. Patients in the aspirin group received 650 mg twice daily postoperatively. Impedence plethysmography and ^{125}I-fibrinogen scanning were performed on all patients (both of which are no longer utilized). If positive, the patient underwent a venogram. The warfarin group (target INR 2.0–2.7) had a statistically significant decrease in development of DVT and/or PE. There was little difference between aspirin and placebo. There was no significant difference in terms of bleeding or number of required transfusions between the three groups [10]. Desirable traits of warfarin include the ease of reversibility, if necessary, with vitamin K and unrestricted use with morbid obesity and renal impairment. A potential drawback to warfarin management is the need for frequent blood draws and difficulty in maintaining therapeutic levels. Target INR range should be 2.0–3.0, as per ACCP guidelines [2].

5.2.3 *Heparins*

Unfractionated heparin (UFH) is an inexpensive anticoagulant that is administered subcutaneously and is effective in preventing postoperative DVT and PE. Heparins consist of heterogenous mixtures of glycosaminoglycan molecules that are derived from animal tissues and potentiate the antifactor Xa and antifactor IIa activity of antithrombin [11]. The advantages of UFH include immediate onset of action and immediate protamine sulfate reversal if necessary [12]. A recent Cochrane review of VTE prophylaxis after hip fracture surgery found a significant reduction in incidence of any DVT when heparin (LMWH or UFH) is compared with placebo or control groups, and without increasing hematoma rates [13].

A recent meta-analysis compared twice-daily dosing of UFH 5,000 units to three-times-daily dosing in hospitalized medical patients [14]. The authors found that three-times-daily heparin significantly decreased the incidence of the combined outcome of proximal DVT or PE and showed a trend toward decreasing the incidence of PE. Though the three-times-daily regimen is likely superior to twice-daily for preventing VTE in hospitalized medical patients, the bleeding rates may be increased with this approach [14].

Low molecular weight heparins (LMWH) have a lower and more uniform average molecular weight (compared to UFH). Because of this, LMWH has a longer half-life and more predictable pharmacokinetics [11]. These agents produce less heparin-induced thrombocytopenia (HIT) than UFH [15]. Dose adjustment is required in patients with renal failure and obesity [12].

A prospective, randomized, double-blind trial compared LMWH (Fragmin) given perioperatively (for 6 days) to placebo in 68 hip fracture surgery patients. A 50% reduction in incidence of DVT was demonstrated [16]. This study excluded patients in nursing homes. Transfusion requirements were higher in the Fragmin group, but there were no differences in major bleeding complications, injection hematomas, or signs of hemodynamic insufficiency [16].

There is insufficient data to determine the superiority of UFH over LMWH, or vice versa [13]. Monreal et al. performed a small, randomized, double-blinded clinical trial using UFH 5,000 units every 8 h versus a LMWH (dalteparin) 5,000 units subcutaneously daily [17]. The results showed significantly lower incidence of DVT and PE in the UFH group when compared to the LMWH group, and without increased bleeding [17].

A randomized, prospective trial compared LMW heparinoid (Lomoparan) with warfarin for efficacy in preventing DVT in patients who had hip fracture surgery. Both drugs were begun preoperatively. In one group, Lomoparan was given 750 units subcutaneously every 12 h for 9 days postoperatively and warfarin was added on the seventh day. The other group received only warfarin. Seven percent of the Lomoparan group and 21% of the warfarin group developed a DVT. There were no differences in intraoperative blood loss or in transfusion requirement between the groups. Major bleeding was similar in both groups secondary to wound hematoma, cerebrovascular bleeding and GI bleeding. The authors concluded that LWM heparinoid is a safe, convenient antithrombotic agent for prevention of VTE after hip fracture surgery. This study excluded patients with GI bleeding within 3 months of surgery, renal dysfunction, abnormal liver function tests, and intracranial hemorrhage within the past 12 months [18].

Enoxaparin has been compared to UFH in elective total hip replacement patients. Senaran et al. compared enoxaparin 40 mg daily (initiated 12 h preoperatively) with heparin 5,000 units every 8 h (initiated 8 h preoperatively) in 100 total hip replacement patients. These patients underwent lower extremity duplex ultrasonography prior to discharge from the hospital. Two patients in the heparin group developed DVT and two patients in the enoxaparin group had late DVT during the postoperative period of 6 weeks. Seven patients in each group had minor and major bleeding episodes. The authors concluded that enoxaparin is as safe and effective as standard heparin in total hip replacement surgery [19].

Thaler et al. studied the efficacy of enoxaparin in the prevention of clinically apparent VTE in hip fracture patients. Nearly 900 of these patients were operated on and received enoxaparin 60 mg (in divided doses of 20 and 40 mg) for the first 5 days and then 40 mg daily for 5 weeks. The majority of patients in this trial had spinal anesthesia. Patients were examined daily for symptomatic DVT, PE, and bleeding during hospitalization. After discharge, they were examined once a week for at least 5 weeks postoperatively. If signs or symptoms of a DVT occurred, contrast venography was performed. Patients with suspected PE underwent spiral computed tomographic scanning. Five patients had confirmed DVT and two patients developed PE. Major bleeding occurred in 42 patients (4.7%) defined as including intracerebral bleeding, subdural hematomas, wound hematomas requiring surgical intervention, and transfusion of more than two units of packed red blood cells. There were no cases of heparin-induced thrombocytopenia. The authors concluded that thromboprophylaxis with enoxaparin is safe and appropriate in hip fracture patients [20].

A randomized, double-blinded trial of total hip replacement patients assessed the efficacy of continued enoxaparin for 5 weeks upon discharge. All these patients received enoxaparin 40 mg daily while in the hospital and had a negative venogram study on the day of discharge. Once discharged, patients received enoxaparin 40 mg daily or placebo. The primary endpoint was occurrence of DVT or PE. By day 21, three patients in the enoxaparin group and seven patients in the placebo group had developed DVTs. There was more (minor) bleeding in the enoxaparin group, namely bruising at the injection site. No major bleeding was noted. This study supports continued prophylaxis with enoxaparin for 35 days after surgery to reduce the rate of DVT in total hip replacement patients [21].

Taken together, the above results indicate that UFH dosed 5,000 units three times daily or LMWH are both effective first line agents for VTE prophylaxis in hip fracture patients.

5.2.4 Fondaparinux

Fondaparinux is a relatively new synthetic pentasaccharide that causes selective inhibition of activated factor X (factor Xa) by binding (almost exclusively) to antithrombin with a higher affinity than UFH or LMWH. Once the antithrombin in the plasma is saturated, the excess fondaparinux is excreted through the kidneys. Its half-life of 17–21 h allows for once-daily dosing. Fondaparinux has no known effect on platelets or platelet factor 4 [11]. A potential drawback of fondaparinux is that there is no antidote, although high doses of factor VIIa have had some potential benefits in reversing its anticoagulation effect in healthy volunteers [22, 23]. Fondaparinux is contraindicated in patients with severe renal impairment (creatinine clearance < 30 mL/min) [12].

Eriksson et al. studied 1,711 patients (average age 77 years old) undergoing surgery for femur fractures and randomized them to fondaparinux 2.5 mg once daily or enoxaparin 40 mg once daily. The primary outcome was VTE up to postoperative day 11. The incidence of VTE was 8.3% in the fondaparinux group versus 19.1% in the enoxaparin group. There were no significant differences between the two groups in the incidence of death or bleeding [24]. A United Kingdom study found fondaparinux to be more cost effective to the healthcare system than enoxaparin up to 5 years following orthopedic surgery [25]. There were fewer VTE events (initial and recurrent) and VTE-related deaths in the fondaparinux group, with the greatest clinical benefit seen in hip fracture patients [25].

A double-blinded, multi-center, randomized, placebo-controlled, trial (PENTHIFRA Plus) consisting of 656 patients (average 79 years) undergoing hip fracture surgery evaluated the use of fondaparinux 2.5 mg daily for 3 weeks postoperatively [26]. All patients received fondaparinux initially for 1 week after surgery but were then randomized to further fondaparinux or placebo for the next 3 weeks. Fondaparinux significantly reduced the incidence of VTE compared with placebo from 35 to 1.4%. There was no fatal bleeding and no thrombocytopenia noted [26]. ACCP guidelines authors recommend routine use of fondaparinux (Grade 1A) for patients undergoing hip fracture surgery [2].

5.3 Timing and Duration of Prophylaxis

The appropriate timing and duration of anticoagulation in hip fracture patients is unclear, although initiation of prophylaxis as soon as possible after injury is likely to be the most prudent strategy [27]. Studies suggest that the risk of VTE in hip fracture patients starts from the time of the injury, not from the time of surgical repair. The ACCP guidelines recommend weighing risks and benefits for the particular agent used in terms of the timing of initiation of prophylaxis [2]. The North American Fragmin Trial showed that extended out-of-hospital treatment (up to 35 days) in postelective hip surgery resulted in significantly lower frequencies of DVT compared with in-hospital warfarin therapy followed by out-of-hospital placebo [1]. The PENTHIFRA Plus trial demonstrated extended prophylaxis with fondaparinux for 3 weeks after hip fracture surgery reduced the risk of VTE by 96% [26].

Despite adequate thromboprophylaxis, VTE does occur in postoperative hip fracture patients. After surgery, the affected limb is swollen and tender and the diagnosis of DVT may be difficult. Lieberman et al. found that 6.1% of elderly patients, despite receiving conventional thromboprophylaxis with enoxaparin and graduated compression stockings, developed a proximal DVT following hip surgery [3]. In addition, patients who develop VTE have a prolonged rehabilitation process and increased risk of mortality. Thus medical, ethical, and economic issues mandate the screening of all patients for DVT in the postoperative period. Although further studies are needed to determine the optimal time for screening [3], ACCP guidelines do not support screening for asymptomatic DVT. Prehospital discharge screening with venous doppler ultrasonography is very costly and has the potential to falsely diagnose DVT [2].

Suggested recommendations for duration of anticoagulation therapy is 3–5 weeks postdischarge, and preferably until the patient is fully ambulatory. Screening for asymptomatic DVT is not recommended during this period.

5.4 Risks of Anticoagulation

One of the major risks of anticoagulation is bleeding. A recent prospective study was conducted to address surgeons' concerns about the use of LMWH, namely surgical and injection site complications, hematoma formation, and drainage [28]. Two-hundred and ninety patients who underwent total hip and total knee arthroplasty were given 10-day course of enoxaparin, starting the morning after surgery. When compared to a cohort of short duration warfarin, the total hip arthroplasty patients receiving enoxaparin had a higher incidence of complications, including bleeding at the surgical site and sanguineous wound drainage requiring prolonged hospitalization. Prolonged wound drainage was a minor complication requiring discontinuation of enoxaparin, antibiotics, or suture needed to close a drain site

[28]. Ximelagatran, an oral prodrug of the direct thrombin inhibitor melagatran, was found to produce less heparin-induced thrombocytopenia and injection sight hematomas or discomfort in phase III trials. However, despite these advantages, ximelagatran has no available reversing agent, and the FDA denied its approval because of liver function abnormalities [11].

5.4.1 Heparin-Induced Thrombocytopenia

One of the major risks with heparin is the possibility of developing heparin-induced thrombocytopenia (HIT). HIT is an immune-mediated disorder characterized by the formation of heparin-dependent IgG antibodies acting against the heparin–platelet factor 4 complex and causing platelet aggregation. Patients with HIT are at risk to develop venous or arterial thrombosis. Thrombocytopenia typically appears five or more days after the start of heparin therapy. HIT is seen less often with LMWH than UFH. The fondaparinux molecule may be too small to bind to platelet factor 4. It does not cross react with HIT antibodies from patients with HIT [12]. In a randomized, double-blinded, controlled trial of 665 elective hip surgery patients receiving VTE prophylaxis with either UFH heparin or LMWH, heparin-dependent IgG antibodies were measured in those whose platelet counts dropped below 150,000 after 5 days of treatment with one of the study drugs [29]. HIT was found in 2.7% of patients who received UFH and in none the LMWH group. In eight out of nine patients with HIT, a thrombotic event occurred [29].

5.5 Nonpharmacologic Methods of Prophylaxis

Mechanical methods of prophylaxis include graduated elastic compression stockings and intermittent pneumatic compression devices. These devices increase venous outflow and reduce stasis within the veins of the legs. They also increase the plasma fibrinolytic activity by stimulating the release of plasminogen activator from the blood vessel walls [30]. These devices are safe and inexpensive [31]. The fact that there is no increased risk of bleeding or incidence of heparin-induced thrombocytopenia makes these methods very attractive. To date, no mechanical prophylaxis option alone has been shown to reduce the risk of death or PE [2].

Graduated elastic compression stockings are made of various materials, including rubber or synthetics. They are available in a variety of lengths (calf to thigh), sizes, and ranges of compression, with the greatest pressure at the ankle [32]. The effectiveness of these stockings is dependent upon their appropriate fit. The use of elastic stockings is an option in certain patient groups, including those who are high risk for bleeding, but there has been no randomized trial testing the efficacy of stockings alone as DVT prophylaxis after hip fracture [13]. However, elastic stockings used in combination with pharmacologic agents may increase the efficacy of thromboembolic prophylaxis [15].

Intermittent pneumatic compression devices augment the ability of the calf muscles to work as a venous pump. Compression devices are available in a variety of lengths including foot pumps, foot–calf pumps, calf pumps, and calf–thigh pumps [31]. These devices provide intermittent pressure (inflating and deflating) at predetermined periods of time. A 3-year, prospective, randomized clinical trial demonstrated that pneumatic compression devices are effective in reducing the frequency of thromboembolic events after hip trauma when compared to no prophylaxis. There was a statistically significant difference in the prevention of isolated DVT, but only a trend was apparent in the prevention of PE [30].

Mechanical methods of prophylaxis are recommended primarily for patients who are at high risk of bleeding, but more commonly as an adjunct to pharmacologic therapies. A low overall rate of DVT was seen in a prospective cohort study of 200 hip fracture patients over age 60 who wore bilateral calf compression devices immediately postrepair in addition to chemical prophylaxis (aspirin or warfarin per surgeons' preference). Mechanical prophylaxis, in addition to some form of chemoprophylaxis, may be a safe, and efficacious means of preventing DVT in posthip surgery patients [31]. In a randomized control trial, femoral neck fracture patients were given aspirin 325 mg twice daily or foot-pumps [4]. Both groups wore elastic stockings. The foot-pumps were worn for at least 18 h a day and removed for ambulation. There was no significant difference between the two groups in development of DVT during postoperative days 7–10 (5.7% in the foot-pump group and 9.5% in the aspirin group). Of note, this study excluded those with prior history of VTE, gastritis, or peptic ulcer disease [4].

A recent Cochrane Review included five clinical trials (487 patients) of mechanical prophylaxis and concluded that although the rate of DVT was reduced with these devices, the existing studies were small and flawed [13]. In addition, some patients find these mechanical devices difficult to tolerate [33]. In a study that randomized 100 patients with total hip replacement to foot-pumps versus LMWH, 12 found them uncomfortable and 37 reported difficulty with sleeping [34]. Possible reasons for noncompliance of the compression devices include blisters, intolerance of the foot-pumps, and foot sores [13].

It is imperative that these devices are fitted properly to each individual and should not interrupt the activity of ambulation. Graduated compression stockings should be used with caution in patients with arterial insufficiency [2]. Caution should also be taken in the elderly delirious patient since they may perceive these devices as a restraint, which may potentially increase the risk for falls.

In summation, compression stockings and intermittent pneumatic compression devices can be additive to pharmacologic prophylaxis strategies in reducing VTE risk for hip fracture patients but they must be properly fitted and assessed for tolerability.

5.5.1 Inferior Vena Caval Filters

Inferior vena caval (IVC) filters can be an effective intervention to prevent fatal PE in certain patients. IVC filters should be considered when there is a clear documented contraindication to anticoagulation therapy. A decision to place an IVC filter encompasses several factors including the patient's clinical condition, the types of filters available within the institution, and the expertise of the physician placing the filter. Unlike anticoagulant therapy, an IVC filter offers no beneficial effect on the prevention of incident DVT, DVT extension or recurrence [15].

Vaughn et al. studied mid-60-year-old patients who were about to undergo a total hip or knee replacement. IVC filters were inserted prophylactically into those patients deemed at exceptionally high risk for a fatal PE because of previous thromboemboli. Other patients had an IVC filter placed postoperatively because of failed prophylaxis with warfarin or complications from anticoagulation. Only one person in this group of 66 patients had a fatal PE postoperatively. Although long-term follow-up was not reported, IVC filters may be beneficial in patients at high risk for PE, and in those who have a contraindication to, or a complication from therapeutic anticoagulation [35].

A recent retrospective cohort study reviewed 95 cases of patients (mean age 71.2 years) who underwent 127 joint arthroplasties and had received an IVC filter. Twenty of these patients had suffered a fracture of some type, 17 of whom received an IVC filter preoperatively for confirmed DVT and prior history of PE and the remaining filters were inserted for postoperative PE and DVT, prior history of DVT or PE, or contraindication to anticoagulation [36]. All but two patients with a filter were also anticoagulated with warfarin (goal INR 1.5–1.7). None of the patients who received an IVC filter developed a fatal PE. Two patients had recurrent nonfatal PE despite filter placement. Five patients developed symptomatic DVT after filter placement. Although the incidence of postthrombotic syndrome may be increased, IVC filters did seem to be effective in preventing fatal PE in the total joint arthroplasty population [36].

Death directly attributed to the insertion of an IVC filter is rare; however, there are numerous complications associated with the use of these filters [36]. By causing flow disturbances, thrombosis can occur within the filter itself, leading to the development of collateral veins, vena caval obstruction, lower extremity venous stasis, and the formation of PE (as thrombus moves above the filter). Bleeding, hematoma or infection can occur at the puncture site. The filter can migrate. Clots can arise from proximal sites such as renal veins, right atrium, and upper extremities [36]. The indications and long-term outcomes for the use of retrievable IVC filters are unclear and the role for concomitant anticoagulation for patients with IVC filters is not clearly defined (37).

Still, there may be a role for IVC filter placement in patients with major bleeding or clear contraindication to anticoagulation therapy. Whenever possible, however, pharmacologic anticoagulation is the preferred approach to VTE prophylaxis (35).

Differences in the approach taken by orthopaedic surgeons as compared to medical specialists have been discussed [38, 39], and need to be further evaluated.

References

1. Hull RD, Pineo GF, Francis C, et al. Low-molecular-weight heparin prophylaxis using dalteparin extended out-of-hospital vs in-hospital warfarin/out-of-hospital placebo in hip arthroplasty patients: a double-blind, randomized comparison. North American Fragmin Trial Investigators (see comment). Arch Intern Med. 2000 Jul;160(14):2208–15.
2. Geerts WH, Pineo GF, Heit JA, et al. Prevention of venous thromboembolism: the seventh ACCP conference on antithrombotic and thrombolytic therapy (see comment). Chest. 2004 Sep;126(3 Suppl):338S–400S.
3. Lieberman DV, Lieberman D. Proximal deep vein thrombosis after hip fracture surgery in elderly patients despite thromboprophylaxis. Am J Phys Med Rehabil. 2002 Oct;81(10):745–50.
4. Kennedy JG, Soffe KE, Rogers BW, et al. Deep vein thrombosis prophylaxis in hip fractures: a comparison of the arteriovenous impulse system and aspirin. J Trauma. 2000 Feb;48(2):268–72.
5. Prevention of pulmonary embolism and deep vein thrombosis with low dose aspirin. Pulmonary embolism prevention (PEP) trial (see comment). Lancet. 2000 Apr;355(9212): 1295–302.
6. Gent M, Hirsh J, Ginsberg JS, et al. Low-molecular-weight heparinoid orgaran is more effective than aspirin in the prevention of venous thromboembolism after surgery for hip fracture. Circulation. 1996 Jan;93(1):80–4.
7. American Academy of Orthopaedic Surgeons. Clinical guideline on prevention of pulmonary embolism in patients undergoing total hip or knee arthroplasty. 2007 http://www.aaos.org/research/guidelines/PE_guideline.pdf Last accessed 4-3-10.
8. Brown GA. Venous thromboembolism prophylaxis after major orthopaedic surgery: a pooled analysis of randomized controlled trials. J Arthroplasty. 2009;24: 77–83.
9. Morris GK, Mitchell JR. Prevention and diagnosis of venous thrombosis in patients with hip fractures. A survey of current practice. Lancet. 1976 Oct;2(7991):867–9.
10. Powers PJ, Gent M, Jay RM, et al. A randomized trial of less intense postoperative warfarin or aspirin therapy in the prevention of venous thromboembolism after surgery for fractured hip. Arch Intern Med. 1989 Apr;149(4):771–4.
11. Andersen JC. Advances in anticoagulation therapy: the role of selective inhibitors of factor Xa and thrombin in thromboprophylaxis after major orthopedic surgery. Semin Thromb Hemost. 2004 Dec;30(6):609–18.
12. Ketz J. Enoxaparin clinical pearl. Pharmacotherapy Update The Cleveland Clinic Center for Continuing Education. 2003;VI(1). Available at http://www.clevelandclinicmeded.com/medicalpubs/pharmacy/janfeb2003/enoxaparin.htm. Last accessed on November 10, 2010.
13. Handoll HH, Sherrington C. Mobilisation strategies after hip fracture surgery in adults. Update of Cochrane Database Syst Rev. 2004;(4):CD001704; PMID: 15495015. Cochrane Database Syst Rev. 2007;(1):001704.
14. King CS, Holley AB, Jackson JL, et al. Twice vs three times daily heparin dosing for thromboembolism prophylaxis in the general medical population: a metaanalysis. Chest. 2007 Feb;131(2):507–16.
15. Pini M, Spyropoulos AC. Prevention of venous thromboembolism. Semin Thromb Hemost. 2006 Nov;32(8):755–66.
16. Jorgensen PS, Knudsen JB, Broeng L, et al. The thromboprophylactic effect of a low-molecular-weight heparin (fragmin) in hip fracture surgery. A placebo-controlled study. Clin Orthop. 1992 May;(278):95–100.

17. Monreal M, Lafoz E, Navarro A, et al. A prospective double-blind trial of a low molecular weight heparin once daily compared with conventional low-dose heparin three times daily to prevent pulmonary embolism and venous thrombosis in patients with hip fracture (see comment). J Trauma. 1989 Jun;29(6):873–5.
18. Gerhart TN, Yett HS, Robertson LK, et al. Low-molecular-weight heparinoid compared with warfarin for prophylaxis of deep-vein thrombosis in patients who are operated on for fracture of the hip. A prospective, randomized trial. J Bone Joint Surg Am. 1991 Apr;73(4):494–502.
19. Senaran H, Acarolu E, Ozdemir HM, et al. Enoxaparin and heparin comparison of deep vein thrombosis prophylaxis in total hip replacement patients. Arch Orthop Trauma Surg. 2006 Jan;126(1):1–5.
20. Thaler HW, Roller RE, Greiner N, et al. Thromboprophylaxis with 60 mg enoxaparin is safe in hip trauma surgery. J Trauma. 2001 Sep;51(3):518–21.
21. Planes A, Vochelle N, Darmon JY, et al. Efficacy and safety of postdischarge administration of enoxaparin in the prevention of deep venous thrombosis after total hip replacement. A prospective randomised double-blind placebo-controlled trial. Drugs. 1996;52(Suppl 7):47–54.
22. Bijsterveld NR, Moons AH, Boekholdt SM, et al. Ability of recombinant factor VIIa to reverse the anticoagulant effect of the pentasaccharide fondaparinux in healthy volunteers. Circulation. 2002 Nov;106(20):2550–4.
23. Bijsterveld NR, Vink R, van Aken BE, et al. Recombinant factor VIIa reverses the anticoagulant effect of the long-acting pentasaccharide idraparinux in healthy volunteers. Br J Haematol. 2004 Mar;124(5):653–8.
24. Eriksson BI, Bauer KA, Lassen MR, et al. Fondaparinux compared with enoxaparin for the prevention of venous thromboembolism after hip-fracture surgery (see comment). N Engl J Med. 2001 Nov;345(18):1298–304.
25. Gordois A, Posnett J, Borris L, et al. The cost-effectiveness of fondaparinux compared with enoxaparin as prophylaxis against thromboembolism following major orthopedic surgery. J Thromb Haemost. 2003 Oct;1(10):2167–74.
26. Eriksson BI, Lassen MR, PENTasaccharide in HIp-FRActure Surgery Plus, Investigators. Duration of prophylaxis against venous thromboembolism with fondaparinux after hip fracture surgery: a multicenter, randomized, placebo-controlled, double-blind study (see comment). Arch Intern Med. 2003 Jun;163(11):1337–42.
27. Grant PJ, Jaffer AK. When should prophylactic anticoagulation begin after a hip fracture? Cleve Clin J Med. 2006 788, 790–2; Sep;73(9):785–6.
28. Burnett RS, Clohisy JC, Wright RW, et al. Failure of the American college of chest physicians-1A protocol for lovenox in clinical outcomes for thromboembolic prophylaxis. J Arthroplasty. 2007 Apr;22(3):317–24.
29. Warkentin TE, Levine MN, Hirsh J, et al. Heparin-induced thrombocytopenia in patients treated with low-molecular-weight heparin or unfractionated heparin (see comment). N Engl J Med. 1995 May;332(20):1330–5.
30. Fisher CG, Blachut PA, Salvian AJ, et al. Effectiveness of pneumatic leg compression devices for the prevention of thromboembolic disease in orthopaedic trauma patients: a prospective, randomized study of compression alone versus no prophylaxis. J Orthop Trauma. 1995 Feb;9(1):1–7.
31. Westrich GH, Rana AJ, Terry MA, et al. Thromboembolic disease prophylaxis in patients with hip fracture: a multimodal approach. J Orthop Trauma. 2005 Apr;19(4):234–40.
32. Rice KL, Walsh ME. Minimizing venous thromboembolic complications in the orthopaedic patient. Orthop Nurs. 2001 Nov–Dec;20(6):21–7.
33. Merli GJ. Prevention of thrombosis with warfarin, aspirin, and mechanical methods. Clin Cornerstone. 2005;7(4):49–56.
34. Pitto RP, Hamer H, Heiss-Dunlop W, et al. Mechanical prophylaxis of deep-vein thrombosis after total hip replacement a randomised clinical trial. J Bone Joint Surg Br. 2004 Jul;86(5):639–42.
35. Vaughn BK, Knezevich S, Lombardi AV Jr, et al. Use of the Greenfield filter to prevent fatal pulmonary embolism associated with total hip and knee arthroplasty. J Bone Joint Surg Am. 1989 Dec;71(10):1542–8.

36. Austin MS, Parvizi J, Grossman S, et al. The inferior vena cava filter is effective in preventing fatal pulmonary embolus after hip and knee arthroplasties. J Arthroplasty. 2007 Apr;22(3):343–8.
37. Jaff MR, Goldhaber SZ, Tapson VF. High utilization rate of vena cava filters in deep vein thrombosis. Thromb Haemost. 2005 Jun;93(6):1117–9.
38. Johanson NA, Lachiewicz PF, et al. AAOS Clinical Practice Guideline Summary. Prevention of symptomatic pulmonary embolism in patients undergoing total hip or knee arthroplasty. J Am Acad Orthop Surg. 2009 March;17:183–96.
39. Eikelboom JW, Karthikeyan G, et al. American Association of Orthopedic Surgeons and American College of Chest Physicians guidelines for venous thromboembolism prevention in hip and knee arthroplasty differ: what are the implications for clinicians and patients? Chest 2009 Feb;135:513–20.

Chapter 6
Prevention and Management of Perioperative Delirium

Jerry C. Johnson

Abstract Delirium, arguably the most important perioperative morbidity in patients undergoing hip fracture surgery, is underdiagnosed, and undertreated in patients with fractures. However, delirium can be diagnosed with high sensitivity and specificity and effective means of reducing the severity of delirium and the improving outcomes are known. A comprehensive history and examination are necessary with a focus on the presence of acute alteration in awareness and attention. The cardinal features of delirium are acute onset of cognitive disturbances or attention deficits, and fluctuating course. Multidisciplinary teams with expertise in geriatrics have shown the most success in controlled studies of delirium postoperative prevention and treatment. Managing delirium is largely a matter of reducing and eliminating risk factors. Screening for cognitive impairment, medications known to increase the risk of delirium, and acute metabolic disturbances and acute infections is key. Treatment should include correction of acute problems and maintenance doses of analgesics. Eliminating physical restraints, mobilization, and minimizing room changes are important. Psychotropics are most helpful in persons with clear psychotic symptoms, and when used, they initially be given on a maintenance schedule.

Keywords Delirium • Fractures • Perioperative • Prevention • Management

6.1 Background

6.1.1 Significance of Delirium in Elderly Patients with Fractures

The high rate of delirium and its morbidity and sequelae make it the single most important postoperative morbidity after hip fracture surgery [1], and since most of

J.C. Johnson (✉)
Division of Geriatric Medicine, Department of Medicine, University of Pennsylvania School of Medicine, 3615 Chestnut Street, Philadelphia, PA 19104-2676, USA
e-mail: jcjohnso@mail.med.upenn.edu

R.J. Pignolo et al. (eds.), *Fractures in the Elderly*, Aging Medicine,
DOI 10.1007/978-1-60327-467-8_6,

the delirium literature pertains to hip fracture procedures, the orthopedic surgery evidence upon which this chapter rests derives for the most part from studies of that population. Although the prevalence of delirium in persons undergoing elective hip surgery may be 10–20% [2], the prevalence of delirium in most hip fracture studies approximates 40% [3] and can be as high as 70% after emergency procedures [4]. Delirium can lead to dehydration, malnutrition, inability to cooperate with therapy, increased rates of infection, and other complications, resulting in prolonged hospitalization, increased mortality, and increased likelihood of discharge to a nursing home [3, 5–8]. Delirium is often unrecognized in its early stages [9], its predisposing and precipitating factors are often underappreciated [3, 5, 9–11], and even patients with established delirium often remain unevaluated and under treated. Multiple reasons may contribute to these failures: (1) ambivalence about the most appropriate diagnostic term in the medical literature, (2) changes in the diagnostic criteria espoused by various neurologic and psychiatric organizations, (3) uncertainty as to how to efficiently apply the criteria for delirium in a clinical setting, (4) failure on the part of practicing physicians to appreciate the significance of delirium, and (5) uncertainty about the most effective management.

Physicians often substitute non-specific or descriptive terms such as "change in mental status" or "sundowning" for a diagnosis of delirium [9, 12–14]. Formal criteria for delirium, established by the American Psychiatric Association, reflect the current thinking on the definition of this syndrome. Using these criteria, it is appropriate to use the term "acute confusional state" synonymously with delirium. However, terms such as "change in mental status" or "confusion" without the "acute" prefix have little value diagnostically. Confusion, defined as a loss of one's capacity to think with usual clarity and coherence, is caused by several different psychiatric syndromes that require distinct diagnostic and treatment approaches. It is imperative, therefore, that the clinician not elevate "confusion," which is a symptom, to the level of a diagnosis. Nor is "sundowning," another descriptive term, an appropriate diagnosis.

Many of the predisposing and precipitating factors of delirium can be prevented or reduced. Mostly persons undergoing hip fracture surgery who develop delirium postoperatively have early symptoms, highlighting the importance of screening so that optimal prevention strategies can be started [15]. Persons with more severe manifestations of delirium have much worse outcomes than those with mild or moderate delirium, but even persons with subsyndromal presentations who do not meet the full criteria of delirium are at increased risk of complications [16]. Therefore, it is critical to identify risk factors and reduce them, when possible, from the moment of admission to the hospital. However, physicians have failed to recognize delirium and cognitive impairment in the elderly 25–50% of the time [4]. Armstrong et al. examined the association of the misdiagnosis of delirium with other features in 221 patients studied over a 5-year period [17] and found a 46% misdiagnosis rate. Male patients most often had no diagnosis while women patients were mislabeled as depressed. The medical housestaff were more accurate in identifying delirium than the surgical housestaff, and patients were misdiagnosed in the critical care units more frequently than on the ward.

Physicians vary in their approaches to managing delirium, often obtaining inappropriate tests or administering mediations that are likely to precipitate delirium or to use doses of medication that are too high [12]. Clinicians must first recognize delirium and conduct an appropriate history and medical examination with an emphasis on the neuropsychiatric evaluation, then establish a structured program of risk factor reduction, treat persons with established delirium, and monitor persons throughout the hospital stay. This chapter presents an approach to evaluation, risk factor assessment, diagnosis, and management of delirium in patients with fractures.

6.1.2 Recognizing Delirium

Delirium, a syndrome of disturbed consciousness, attention, cognition, or perception, which develops acutely and fluctuates during the course of the day, is a clinical diagnosis. Psychiatrists and neurologists have used variable terms to label delirium and variable criteria to define it. For example, the third, fourth, and fourth revised editions of the diagnostic and statistical manual of the American Psychiatric Association used different criteria for delirium [18]. The core criteria reflect some combination of three critical elements of delirium: acute onset, cognitive or attention deficits, and fluctuating course.

Some patients posthip fracture enter the hospital with delirium, but in most the onset of delirium occurs postoperatively. The hyperactive, agitated, delirious patient has received the most attention from clinicians because these patients are the most difficult to manage, but physicians should not reserve consideration for delirium to patients who are hyperactive. Hyperactive behavior includes motor restlessness, combativeness, yelling, and screaming. However, many elderly delirious patients are hypoactive, manifesting a passive demeanor, slow speech, and, in extreme cases, stupor and coma. Hyper- and hypoactivity are not mutually exclusive. Over the course of the illness, many patients manifest both behaviors [16, 19, 20]. In most studies about 20–40% are hypoactive, 40 are hyperactive, and others are mixed. However, whether the presentation is hypoactive or hyperactive, the cardinal features described in the definition of delirium must be met.

An attention deficit, defined as the inability to maintain, shift, and focus attention, is the fundamental characteristic of delirium [21]. As a result of inattention, patients demonstrate impaired registration of new information, leading to memory deficits and to disorganized thinking manifested by incoherent or rambling speech. Disorientation to time and place follows, but disorientation to person is rarely seen. Impairment in recent memory is more common than remote memory, although both are evident in the full syndrome. Thinking is illogical and incoherent. Judgment is lost, and insight is poor. Many patients describe persecutory delusions, suspiciousness, bizarre thoughts and images, and loose associations.

Perceptual abnormalities may include distortions, illusions, or frank hallucinations. Distortions are alterations in the form or quality of a sensory experience. Illusions are misinterpretations of external sensory stimulation. Visual illusions are most common, followed in frequency by auditory and tactile illusions. Hallucinations are usually visual. When present, hallucinations may cause the delirious patient to react vigorously in a dangerous and harmful manner, for example, by fleeing, attacking, or committing suicide.

Fluctuation in symptoms ranging from severe perceptual disturbances to lucid, coherent intervals may be seen over minutes to hours. Because of the fluctuating symptoms, some patients may appear normal when first seen, only to decompensate later. Other patients may be impaired initially but become lucid when seen later. These patterns are not suggestive of any particular cause of delirium. Clinicians have also described a disturbed sleep–wake cycle in which patients are intermittently awake at night and sleep during the day.

Delirium should not be mistaken for dementia, a chronic syndrome in which most patients have been symptomatic for a year or longer, and certainly for more than 6 months [9, 22]. The delirious patient with no history of dementia manifests new cognitive deficits, whereas delirious patients with a prior evidence of dementia manifest a definite worsening of cognitive symptoms. However, delirium and dementia are not mutually exclusive; delirium is often superimposed on an underlying dementia.

6.1.3 Causes of Delirium

Rather than a single illness, most patients with delirium have two or more coexisting problems. Alcohol withdrawal, although associated with the classic hyperactive delirious patient, occurs much less frequently in the elderly than do other causes of delirium [10, 11, 23]. Although delirium in patients with fractures in seen most often postoperatively, concomitant acute medical problems in these patients may also result in delirium on admission. Studies on the elderly comparing delirious and nondelirious patients show that the most common associated conditions are dementia or cognitive impairment, the use of psychotropic drugs, particularly those with anticholinergic properties, and urinary tract infections.

Table 6.1 highlights the causes of delirium that the physician should consider when evaluating patients. A more comprehensive listing is given in several reviews [22, 24]. Anticholinergic drugs, referring to medications that primarily interact with cholinergic receptors, are the biggest culprits among the medications. However, other medications such as some of the antidepressants, and the phenothiazine class of neuroleptics have anticholinergic properties. Noncholinergic medications that predispose to delirium include the benzodiazepines, both short acting (such as temazepan) and intermediate acting (such as lorazepam). Among the antihypertensives, the central alpha- and the beta-receptor blockers are associated with the greatest risk of delirium. Digitalis may cause delirium in the face of a normal serum level and in the absence of cardiotoxic effects.

The most important metabolic disturbances are fluid and electrolyte disturbances, which may be secondary to multiple causes. Hypercalcemia is a more common offender than hypocalcemia. Hypoglycemia resulting from insulin administration or

Table 6.1 Organic causes of delirium

Intoxication
Medications: anticholinergics, tricyclic antidepressants, lithium, sedative-hypnotics, neuroleptics, antihypertensive agents, anti-arrhythmic drugs, digitalis, anticonvulsants, antiparkinsonian agents, analgesics (opiates and non-narcotics), cimetidine, alcohol
Poisons: heavy metals, organic solvents, methyl alcohol, ethylene glycol
Withdrawal syndromes: alcohol, sedatives, and hypnotics
Metabolic
Electrolyte imbalance: elevated or decreased sodium, calcium, hypoglycemia, hyperglycemia
Acid–base imbalance: acidosis, alkalosis
Hypoxia
Failure of vital organs: liver, kidney, lung
Vitamin deficiency: thiamine (Wernicke's encephalopathy), folate, cyanocobalamin
Hyper- and hypothermia
Neurologic
Space-occupying lesions: tumor, subdural hematoma, aneurysm
Cerebrovascular diseases: thrombosis, embolism, hemorrhage, hypertensive encephalopathy, vasculitis
Epilepsy
Infectious
Intracranial: encephalitis and meningitis
Systemic: pneumonia, septicemia, influenza, urinary tract
Endocrine
Thyroid: thyrotoxicosis, myxedema
Parathyroid: hypo- and hyperparathyroidism
Cardiovascular
Congestive heart failure
Cardiac arrhythmia
Myocardial infarction

oral hypoglycemics should always be considered. Hyperglycemia may be caused by new-onset diabetes or to an exacerbation of diabetes in the form of the hyperglycemic hyperosmolar syndrome, which classically presents with delirium. Hypoxia-induced delirium usually occurs in the setting of an obvious respiratory or cardiac disorder. On the other hand, liver and renal failure may not be clinically obvious at the time of presentation. Thiamine is the most important vitamin deficiency. Folate and cyanocobalamin deficiencies can cause subacute presentations of delirium that develop over several weeks rather than over several days.

Strokes resulting from thrombosis, embolus, or hemorrhage may induce delirium. Both middle cerebral artery and posterior cerebral artery strokes may cause delirium without focal neurologic signs, but stoke is a rare cause of delirium in the absence of focal deficits [25]. Other space-occupying lesions and malignant hypertension also cause delirium.

Alzheimer's disease predisposes to delirium in the setting of another acute illness, but it does not cause delirium independently. However, patients with vascular dementia may exhibit sudden losses of cognitive abilities due to a recent lacunar infarct. Dementia of the Lewy Body type characteristically shows sudden fluctuations and hallucinations that can mimic delirium.

Infectious, endocrine, and cardiovascular disorders constitute the final groups of underlying causes. Localized infections of the urinary tract and lung in the absence of sepsis are most common. Sepsis from any cause may cause delirium. Pressure ulcers may be the source of infection in debilitated bedridden patients. Congestive heart failure, myocardial infarction, and cardiac arrhythmias can cause hypoperfusion that leads to delirium.

6.1.4 Risk Factors for Delirium

Investigators have shown an increased risk of developing delirium and increased severity of delirium with multiple risk factors, some of which are common across studies and others more controversial. Pre-existing cognitive impairment or dementia is the most important and certainly the most common risk factor for delirium as demonstrated in almost every study of delirium, irrespective of the clinical entity. Sometimes a history of dementia can be elicited, but in others, the physician will have to screen for cognitive impairment during the initial examination. Irrespective of the physical examination, obtaining history of cognitive function from a family member or associate is critical.

6.1.4.1 Medications

Pre-admission psychotropics and medications with anticholinergic properties have shown to be associated with delirium, but investigators have found contradictory relations between use of opioids and delirium. Some studies found no relation and others found narcotics and pain medications in general to be risk factors [4, 7]. Marcantonio et al. found a relation between delirium and meperidine use, as well as benzodiazepine use [23]. Note that withdrawal from alcohol and sedative hypnotic agents can cause delirium.

6.1.4.2 Multifactorial Risk Factor Assessment

Most patients exhibit multiple risk factors across multiple organ systems. Inouye and colleagues have identified several key risk factors for delirium in medical patients and others have identified risk factors specific for patients with fractures [10, 11]: Studies on patients with hip fracture or other surgery have found cognitive impairment, age, male gender, decreased functional status, depression, acute infections, exposure to opioid medications, and physical restraints to be significant [4, 5, 8, 10, 11, 15, 23, 26]. It is not surprising that the risk of delirium increases with the number of risk factors, allowing one to establish a low-risk group of 3–5%

with no risk factors, an intermediate risk group of 10% with one or two factors, and a high-risk group of greater than 50% with three or more risk factors. Note that the type of anesthesia and duration of the procedure have consistently been shown to be insignificant risk factors.

6.2 Evaluation of the Patient

Delirium is a clinical diagnosis. Neither abnormal laboratory tests, nor abnormal imaging studies establish the diagnosis of delirium, although they may be helpful in determining the causes of delirium. In evaluating patients with delirium, clinicians should systematically obtain a comprehensive database with a focus on the risk factors that increase vulnerability for delirium (referred to as predisposing factors), on factors that tend to precipitate delirium after admission to the hospital, and on the causes of delirium. The clinician must first distinguish delirium from other neuropsychiatric syndromes, of which the most important are dementia and depression.

Dementia refers to a chronic loss of cognitive function, but patients typically manifest a normal state of wakefulness. Although depression can cause cognitive deficits, disturbed mood is the dominant characteristic of this illness, and its history and onset are usually less rapid than delirium. In some instances, mania may simulate a hyperactive delirious state more closely than the other functional psychoses, but the presence of grandiosity and euphoria will help establish the correct diagnosis. The aforementioned functional syndromes may also have an organic basis, for example, a steroid-induced depression. In these instances, the syndromes are reclassified (such as organic affective disorder in the case of the steroid example), but the diagnostic features remain the same. Finally, acute Wernicke's aphasia can mimic delirium, but patients are alert, manifesting fluent (though rambling) speech.

Because of the frequent multiple co-morbidities and the atypical and nonspecific presenting symptoms in older adults, a comprehensive screening examination including a standard neurological examination is necessary. Although the Mini-Mental State Examination (MMSE) and other short mental status tests are helpful screening tools in the cognitively impaired elderly, they do not distinguish one syndrome from another. Since 40% of patients with hip fracture develop delirium, mental status screening is indicated in all elderly patients presenting with a fracture. All physicians should incorporate the following history and physical examination data in their clinical evaluation when assessing patients suspected of delirium.

6.2.1 History Taking

If a patient or family member describes a history of acute onset of abnormal behavior, abnormal speech, or deficits in memory or orientation, then several questions based on the criteria for delirium are pertinent. Rather than asking whether the patient has been confused, inquire about the specific cognitive deficits that result in confusion. What was the patient's premorbid mental status? Is there a remote and recent history of memory, orientation, or speech impairment? Have there been periods of lethargy or stupor? When did the process begin? Have the patient's symptoms fluctuated? Is there a history of falls, head trauma, focal neurologic symptoms, seizures, alcohol, or other drugs of abuse? What prescription and over-the-counter medications does the patient take?

6.2.2 *Physical Examination*

6.2.2.1 General Examination

A comprehensive screening examination is necessary to uncover concomitant illnesses such as a pneumonia, sepsis, dehydration, or congestive heart failure. Vision and hearing screening are necessary, particularly the former. The remainder of the physical evaluation must include a standard neurologic examination. Clinicians should screen for Parkinson's disease (which will influence mobility and may be associated with dementia) and focal weakness which would indicate underlying cerebrovascular disease. Evidence of psychomotor activity such as restlessness, tremulousness, or paucity of movement is noted.

6.2.3 *Mental Status Testing*

Attention. Since attention deficits have been shown to be the hallmark of delirium, clinicians must use tests that evaluate attention deficits [9, 21]. Attention deficits refer to the inability to focus, maintain, and shift attention. There are both positive and negative aspects of attention. Positive aspects include exploration, vigilance, and concentration. Negative aspects include distractibility, confusion, and neglect. Tests of awareness or state of arousal are based on direct observation while conducting the medical interview. Is the patient drowsy, stuporous, or comatose? Further evaluation is conducted by asking the patient to perform specific tasks: listing serial numbers forward and backward, spelling words backwards, and, for patients whose level of education is inappropriate for spelling and counting tests, reciting the days of the week backwards.

Cognition. Short-term memory and orientation, exemplary of cognitive deficits, can be tested by direct questioning of short-term items. Disorientation to time is tested by asking questions related to the day, date, month, and year. Disorientation to place is tested by asking about the city, state, country, and name of the hospital where the patient is being examined. In testing memory, registration is first tested by asking the patient to immediately repeat the names of three objects. Three minutes later ask the patient to repeat the same objects. Remote memory should be tested by asking about events with which the patient should be familiar: city of birth, age and birthdates of children, wedding anniversary, and other similar questions. A clock draw test, which combines elements of cognition, attention, and visual spatial skills, has been shown to be an effective screen for postoperative delirium in patients undergoing elective orthopedic surgery [2].

Perceptual disturbances in the form of frank psychotic symptoms – hallucinations, delusions, and paranoia can be observed during the physical examination or may be reported by family or nursing staff.

In summary, physicians should systematically evaluate the patient for the cardinal symptoms of delirium, which Inoye et al. described as elements of the Confusion Assessment Method (CAM) [13]: (1) acute onset and fluctuating course, (2) inattention, (3) disorganized thinking, and (4) altered level of consciousness. Using criteria (1) and (2) plus either (3) or (4), the CAM has a sensitivity and specificity over 90%. Since its development in a population of general medical patients, the CAM has been used in several studies of patients with hip fracture.

6.2.4 Preoperative Ancillary Tests

The purpose of preoperative testing is to uncover diseases and problems unrecognized by the history and physical examination or to confirm the diagnosis suspected by the history and examination. Several authors have recommended that physicians obtain multiple tests because of the broad range of illnesses that have been reported to be associated with delirium. However, rather than indiscriminately obtaining tests with marginal diagnostic value, such as an ANA, routine testing in all patients should include the tests marked as routine in Table 6.2. Additional tests should be selected according to the specific features of the clinical evaluation and the results of the routine testing.

Among the selective testing, the EEG, brain imaging, and the lumbar puncture deserve special comment. An EEG rarely yields helpful results except when associated with seizure activity.

An imaging study of the brain is almost always indicated in the setting of a fall. Therefore, most patients with a fracture should undergo brain imaging on admission. However, when delirium develops later in the hospital course, as is frequently the case, brain imaging is not always warranted, particularly if the cause of the delirium is known: e.g., dehydration, electrolyte disturbances, or a medication. Patients with a history of or signs of head trauma, those with focal neurologic symptoms or signs, and those without a reasonable explanation for delirium should undergo brain imaging.

A lumbar puncture should always be obtained when no organic cause of delirium is apparent. However, in the elderly patient with a known infection outside the central nervous system, such as pneumonia or urinary tract infection, the decision to perform a lumbar puncture becomes more complex. Clinical experience has

Table 6.2 Diagnostic studies used to investigate delirium

Routine procedures to be performed in all patients
Complete blood count
Blood chemistries: electrolytes (NA, K, Cl, CO_2), calcium, phosphate, glucose, blood urea nitrogen, liver enzymes, creatinine
Urinalysis
Chest X-ray
Oxygen saturation (with pCO_2 if acidosis is suspected)
Electrocardiogram
Special procedures to be performed in selected patients
Blood chemistries: magnesium, B_{12}, folate, thyroxine, thyroid-stimulating hormone
Blood levels of medications
Blood and urine toxic screens (drugs and poisons)
Blood cultures
Antinuclear antibody levels
Cerebrospinal fluid examination: cells, protein, glucose, culture, serology, pressures, electroencephalogram
Brain imaging: CT or MRI

shown that many elderly patients with localized infections develop delirium without spread of the infection to the central nervous system. Moreover, flexion of the cervical spine may not be helpful in diagnosing meningitis because of stiffness from osteoarthritis. In such cases, physicians will have to make an individualized decision on the utility of lumbar puncture.

6.3 Preventing and Managing Delirium

6.3.1 General

Randomized studies of delirium prevention in medical and fracture patients have shown that optimal success in preventing delirium is based on multicomponent, multidisciplinary team approaches using specialists with expertise in geriatric medicine [3, 8, 27–29]. This finding is not surprising since only the rare patient presents with one predisposing or precipitating factor. The preferred team approach incorporates some combination of a geriatric medicine specialist, physical medicine specialist or therapist, advanced nurse specialist, and a social worker, working as part of a structured program (Table 6.3). Core features of all studies have been treating acute medical problems, reducing harmful medications, mobilization, and administering analgesia on schedule instead of as needed. Outcomes of the multifactorial approach have included improved function, decreased nursing home admission, and in one study, decreased mortality. The severity of delirium is usually reduced in these studies but the incidence rate of delirium may not be affected.

Table 6.3 Summary of delirium prevention and management (based on a review of five intervention studies of fracture patients)

1. On day 1, consult with a geriatrics team comprising medical specialists in geriatrics (physician, nurse specialists, physical therapists, and social worker). This team conducts a comprehensive assessment, identifies risk factors for delirium, and provides a foundation for prevention and treatment
2. General care: Correct all metabolic abnormalities; treat acute medical problems; and provide anticoagulation
3. Eliminate all unnecessary medications, particularly benzodiapines, and anticholinergics
4. Modify the environment with the assistance of aides, family members, and orientation devices including visual and hearing aides
5. Treat pain beginning on day 1 with scheduled doses of acetaminophen or a nonsteroidal anti-inflammatory agent. Use narcotics as needed for breakthrough pain
6. Provide oxygen supplementation to maintain the oxygen saturation over 90%
7. Provide nutrition, with supplementation if necessary, either by mouth or with a feeding tube
8. Discontinue urinary catheterization by day 2
9. Mobilize patients beginning on postoperative day 1, using physical therapists and nurses
10. Treat psychotic symptoms and severe agitation with low-dose haloperidol, beginning with a scheduled low dose of 0.25–5 mg

Length of stay is not usually altered because of the variable factors and decision rules about discharge planning across distinct institutions.

Risk factors should be identified and corrected if possible. Acute medical problems such as ischemic heart disease, heart failure, arrhythmias, thromboemboli, respiratory complications, delirium, urinary tract infections, and fluid and electrolyte disturbances should be treated. Judicious use of analgesics is vital, but sometimes these agents will have to be discontinued because of delirium. Anticholinergic medications should be reduced or eliminated. Physical restraints, which can induce fear and anger and exacerbate motor restlessness, should be used only when necessary to facilitate evaluation and treatment. The use of physical restraints can be reduced by using an aide or family member to provide comfort and to redirect patients.

6.3.2 Nonpharmacologic management

Nonpharmacologic components of treatment are critical [26, 29]. McCusker et al. has identified environmental factors that can be modified: room changes, physical and medical restraints, and the absence of glasses [26]. Lighting should be modified to provide low light during the nighttime and bright light during the daytime hours. Room changes should be minimized, physical restraints eliminated if possible, and the patient should be given eye glasses and hearing aides. Continuity of personal contacts, such as a family member or sitter is important. Physical activity using physical therapists, nurses, and aides, or trained volunteers can be employed to prevent delirium or reduce its severity. Therefore mobilizing the patient as soon as possible not only is part of the rehabilitation, but part of the prevention and treatment of delirium. Mobility should be established by the first postoperative day and continued until discharge. Verbal reminders of the setting and time of day should be used frequently.

6.3.3 Pain Control

Pain is one of the major components of a wide range of neural, endocrine, metabolic, immunological, and inflammatory changes that constitute the stress response to surgery. Recent evidence has shown that surgical trauma induces processes of nervous system sensitization that contribute to and enhance postoperative pain and leads to chronic pain, providing a rational basis for pro-active, pre-operative analgesic strategies. Elderly patients are more sensitive to the effects of analgesia and sedatives, making the elderly more prone to the adverse consequences of high doses of analgesia required once pain is fully developed.

Once pain has developed, many techniques have been used with varying degrees of success. The optimal form of pain treatment is one that is applied pre-, intra-, and postoperatively to preempt the establishment of pain hypersensitivity both during and after surgery. Systemic opioid analgesia given on demand postoperatively is often poorly effective, and should no longer be used as the mainstay of treatment. Instead, perioperative analgesics should be administered on a routine schedule, usually for 3–5 days, starting on day 1 of the hospitalization [30]. Either acetaminophen or a nonsteroidal anti-inflammatory agent should be given on schedule, and supplemented by as needed medications, which can be narcotics [3, 27].

6.4 Pharmacologic Treatment of Delirium

Psychotropic medications are indicated to treat psychotic symptoms and to diminish agitation that interferes with care and evaluation. No psychotropic medication should be given unless necessary to accomplish the aforementioned goals. For example, the lethargic delirious patient with dehydration, hypernatremia, and a urinary tract infection that resulted in a fall and fracture requires fluid and electrolytes, not a psychotropic medication. Medications with anticholinergic effects should be avoided if possible. Benadryl should not be used because of its anticholinergic side effects and the sedating effects of the benzodiazepines, such as lorazepam, necessitates avoidance of this drug class. In most instances the drug of choice is a neuroleptic; the exception is in withdrawal states where sedative-hypnotics are the drugs of choice. One study on hip fracture patients used haldoperidol on admission, prior to the onset of delirium as part of a delirium prevention protocol, but this practice is not generally accepted [31]. In that study, the rate of delirium onset was not reduced but the rate of severity of delirium was reduced.

Among the neuroleptics, haloperidol has been used most often because of its low potential for sedation, low anticholinegic properties, and its useful antipsychotic properties in treating delusions, paranoia, and perceptual disturbances. Atypical antipsychotics have been used also, but there is great concern that the atypicals should be avoided in persons with diabetes or known atherosclerosis [32]. Clinicians should be mindful of the adverse effects of the neuroleptics: sedation, hypotension, extrapyramidal side effects, falls, and arrthymias. If neuroleptics are used, one must monitor for QT prolongation, and neuroleptic malignant syndrome (high fevers and muscle rigidity).

Haloperidol should be started as a low dose, 0.25–0.5 mg, used as standing dose for at least a couple of days, and supplemented by as needed treatment. Total reliance on as needed medications is inappropriate since delirium persists for at least a few days, if not much longer, and patients are incapable of asking for medications. In severe cases, 1.0–2 mg may be the starting dose with additional dosing as required. The total daily dose of haloperidol or other neuroleptic can be divided once, twice, or three times a day. Intramuscular haloperidol reaches peak absorption in 30–60 min, whereas the peak absorption after oral haloperidol may be 2–6 h.

References

1. Lawrence, V.A., et al., Medical complications and outcomes after hip fracture repair. Arch Intern Med, 2002. 162(18): p. 2053–7.
2. Fisher, B.W. and G. Flowerdew, A simple model for predicting postoperative delirium in older patients undergoing elective orthopedic surgery. J Am Geriatr Soc, 1995. 43(2): p. 175–8.
3. Marcantonio, E.R., et al., Reducing delirium after hip fracture: a randomized trial. J Am Geriatr Soc, 2001. 49(5): p. 516–22.
4. Dyer, C.B., C.M. Ashton, and T.A. Teasdale, Postoperative delirium. A review of 80 primary data-collection studies. Arch Intern Med, 1995. 155(5): p. 461–5.
5. Marcantonio, E.R., et al., Delirium is independently associated with poor functional recovery after hip fracture. J Am Geriatr Soc, 2000. 48(6): p. 618–24.
6. Marcantonio, E.R., et al., The relationship of postoperative delirium with psychoactive medications. JAMA, 1994. 272(19): p. 1518–22.
7. Williams-Russo, P., et al., Post-operative delirium: predictors and prognosis in elderly orthopedic patients. J Am Geriatr Soc, 1992. 40(8): p. 759–67.
8. Gustafson, Y., et al., Acute confusional states in elderly patients treated for femoral neck fracture. J Am Geriatr Soc, 1988. 36(6): p. 525–30.
9. Johnson, J.C., Identifying and recognizing delirium. Dementia Geriatr Cogn Disor, 1999. 10: p. 353–8.
10. Inouye, S.K. and P.A. Charpentier, Precipitating factors for delirium in hospitalized elderly persons. Predictive model and interrelationship with baseline vulnerability. JAMA, 1996. 275(11): p. 852–7.
11. Inouye, S.K., et al., A predictive model for delirium in hospitalized elderly medical patients based on admission characteristics. Ann Intern Med, 1993. 119(6): p. 474–81.
12. Carnes, M., et al., Physicians vary in approaches to the clinical management of delirium. J Am Geriatr Soc, 2003. 51(2): p. 234–9.
13. Inouye, S.K., et al., Clarifying confusion: the confusion assessment method. A new method for detection of delirium. Ann Intern Med, 1990. 113(12): p. 941–8.

14. McCartney, J.R. and L.M. Palmateer, Assessment of cognitive deficit in geriatric patients. A study of physician behavior. J Am Geriatr Soc, 1985. 33(7): p. 467–71.
15. de Jonghe, J.F., et al., Early symptoms in the prodromal phase of delirium: a prospective cohort study in elderly patients undergoing hip surgery. Am J Geriatr Psychiatry, 2007. 15(2): p. 112–21.
16. Marcantonio, E., et al., Delirium severity and psychomotor types: their relationship with outcomes after hip fracture repair. J Am Geriatr Soc, 2002. 50(5): p. 850–7.
17. Armstrong, S.C., K.L. Cozza, and K.S. Watanabe, The misdiagnosis of delirium. Psychosomatics, 1997. 38(5): p. 433–9.
18. American Psychiatric Association. Diagnostic and Statistical Manual of Mental Disorders. American Psychiatric Press, 2000(DSM-IV-TR 4th ed rev): p. 136–46.
19. O'keefe, S. and J. Lavan, The prognostic significance of delirium in older hospital patients. J Am Geriatr Soc, 1997. 45: p. 174–8.
20. Sandberg, O., et al., Clinical profile of delirium in older patients. J Am Geriatr Soc, 1999. 47(11): p. 1300–6.
21. Che'dru, F. and N. Geschwind, Disorders of high cortical functions in acute confusional states. Cortex, 1972. 8: p. 395–411.
22. Foreman, M.D., et al., Delirium in elderly patients: an overview of the state of the science. J Gerontol Nurs, 2001. 27(4): p. 12–20.
23. Marcantonio, E.R., et al., A clinical prediction rule for delirium after elective noncardiac surgery. JAMA, 1994. 271(2): p. 134–9.
24. Jacobson, S.A., Delirium in the elderly. Psychiatr Clin North Am, 1997. 20(1): p. 91–110.
25. Benbadis, S.R., C.A. Sila, and R.L. Cristea, Mental status changes and stroke. J Gen Intern Med, 1994. 9(9): p. 485–7.
26. McCusker, J., et al., Environmental risk factors for delirium in hospitalized older people. J Am Geriatr Soc, 2001. 49(10): p. 1327–34.
27. Milisen, K., et al., A nurse-led interdisciplinary intervention program for delirium in elderly hip-fracture patients. J Am Geriatr Soc, 2001. 49(5): p. 523–32.
28. Vidan, M., et al., Efficacy of a comprehensive geriatric intervention in older patients hospitalized for hip fracture: a randomized, controlled trial. J Am Geriatr Soc, 2005. 53(9): p. 1476–82.
29. Inouye, S.K., et al., A multicomponent intervention to prevent delirium in hospitalized older patients. N Engl J Med, 1999. 340(9): p. 669–76.
30. Feldt, K.S., M.B. Ryden, and S. Miles, Treatment of pain in cognitively impaired compared with cognitively intact older patients with hip-fracture. J Am Geriatr Soc, 1998. 46(9): p. 1079–85.
31. Kalisvaart, K.J., et al., Haloperidol prophylaxis for elderly hip-surgery patients at risk for delirium: a randomized placebo-controlled study. J Am Geriatr Soc, 2005. 53(10): p. 1658–66.
32. Schwartz, T.L. and P.S. Masand, Treatment of delirium with quetiapine. Prim Care Companion J Clin Psychiatry, 2000. 2(1): p. 10–12.

Chapter 7
Anesthesia and Postoperative Pain Control

Jonathan R. Gavrin

Abstract Fractures in the elderly are common. There is frequent need for surgical intervention. Anesthesiologists can safely use a variety of techniques to assist the orthopedic surgeon and help provide the kind of postoperative pain relief that is necessary for patients to recover successfully. General anesthesia, systemic analgesics, and regional techniques for operative anesthesia or postoperative pain relief all represent important tools in the total process, from injury to rehabilitation.

As a discipline, anesthesiology has been slow to embrace the idea of specialized geriatric care. The American Society of Anesthesiologists (ASA) and The Society for the Advancement of Geriatric Anesthesia (SAGA) have made progress in correcting that deficiency. There is a notable lack of evidence upon which to base anesthetic practices. Except for clear guidelines about neuraxial blockade when patients are anticoagulated, we are left to propose plans that draw on our knowledge of anesthesia broadly, interpreting it with what we know about physiologic changes that occur with aging. If we knew how anesthesia worked in the brain, and what its possible toxic effects on tissues were, it would be easier to posit explanations and justifications for what is best for geriatric patients.

What we do know is that older patients have decreased functional reserve in nearly all organ systems. They are more fragile than younger patients. However, age alone is not a significant risk factor for general anesthesia but the higher incidence of co-morbidities is, especially those that affect the most vital organs. Polypharmacy also is an issue. The nature of orthopedic injuries is such that the surgeon typically needs to intervene sooner rather than later. This can leave little time for extensive preoperative evaluation, so investigations should focus on functional status. In situations where further workup might alter anesthetic plans, and these are rare, the quickest and least invasive testing should be utilized. Routine tests have little value except when targeted at specific conditions or when needed for a baseline set of values; they rarely influence anesthetic management.

J.R. Gavrin (✉)
Department of Anesthesiology and Critical Care, Department of Medicine, Hospital of the University of Pennsylvania, Dulles 6, 3400 Spruce Street, Philadelphia, PA 19104, USA
e-mail: gavrinj@uphs.upenn.edu

R.J. Pignolo et al. (eds.), *Fractures in the Elderly*, Aging Medicine,
DOI 10.1007/978-1-60327-467-8_7, © Springer Science+Business Media, LLC 2011

All general anesthetics are cardiac depressants, contribute negatively to gas exchange in the lungs, and affect the brain in undefined ways. The liver and the kidney play a critical role in the clearance of intravenous anesthetic drugs and systemic analgesics that frequently have unpredictable distribution and protein binding because of changing body composition, often accompanied by poor nutritional status in elderly people. To avoid the need for general anesthesia some practitioners use regional techniques, although "casual empiricism" indicates that training programs have focused less and less on these methods in the past 15 years. Even with regional anesthesia, many patients will require sedation and get exposed to anesthetic drugs anyway. Some practitioners combine regional techniques with general anesthesia to avoid deep levels and to provide pain relief in the postoperative period. All practitioners should expect perioperative cardiovascular and neurologic instability to which older patients are predisposed. Interestingly, neither hypotension nor hypoxemia independently seems to cause adverse outcomes. No investigations have demonstrated that regional anesthesia is superior to general anesthesia for surgery, for postoperative analgesia, or for preventing postoperative cognitive dysfunction (POCD). Anesthesia providers should provide care with which they are familiar. Good postoperative analgesia plays a prominent role in reaching rehabilitative milestones; inadequate analgesia is a risk factor for the development of POCD. There are scant, but emerging, data to indicate that a "multimodal" approach to postoperative analgesia positively influences long-term recovery. However, this enthusiasm should be tempered by the fact that good systemic analgesia may do the same in most circumstances; many modalities and medications are available. The fundamental principles of good pain relief revolve around frequent and adequate assessment in an attempt to provide baseline analgesia plus the means by which to treat incident pain associated with activity.

The realities of the operating room, the time constraints surrounding surgical correction of orthopedic injuries, the skill sets of the involved practitioners, all dictate that decisions about perioperative care of geriatric patients should be made cooperatively, always taking into account patient preferences. The rule for the anesthesiologist in the operating room is to do what we do best – take things slowly, know our limits, and be vigilant. One hopes that recent efforts to promote geriatric anesthesia enjoy success.

Keywords Anesthesia • Pain relief • Geriatrics • Fractures • Older patients • Analgesia • Postoperative cognitive dysfunction • Preemptive analgesia

7.1 Introduction

Experts estimate that 25 years from now roughly 20% of the nation's population will be over 65 years of age and, of those, one in four will be over 85 years old [1]. Fractures in the elderly are common and many will need surgical intervention. It is imperative, then, that anesthesiologists be well prepared to provide perioperative care to older patients. Geriatricians will need to know the issues relevant to anesthesia so they may properly advise their patients. In one 10-year survey published in 1998, investigators found that the elderly surgical population grew by about 25% and the number of high risk elderly surgical patients increased by nearly 50% [2]. Longer life expectancy will make this trend more pronounced. It is only recently (within the last decade or two) that anesthesiologists have begun to specifically address the clinical issues pertaining to older adults. The Committee on Geriatric Anesthesiology, under the auspices of the American Society of Anesthesiologists (ASA), now publishes a syllabus on geriatric anesthesiology [3]. The Society for the Advancement of Geriatric Anesthesia (SAGA) is a complementary group of anesthesiologists with special interests in the same area [4].

To date, despite the large number of anesthetics and surgeries performed on older adults, there is no subspecialty in anesthesiology specific to geriatrics. There are accredited fellowships in cardiothoracic anesthesia, pain management, pediatric anesthesia, and critical care; and unaccredited, but formal, programs in regional anesthesia, obstetrical anesthesia, and neuroanesthesia – geriatric anesthesia has yet to come into its own as a subspecialty.

Compared to other areas of research there is a relative paucity of evidence-based literature on anesthesia for older adults. From the existing data, however, practitioners can draw some general conclusions based on changes that occur with aging. Extrapolating from what is known about the phenomenology of the perioperative period in the general population and in some studies targeting geriatric patients, this chapter will address the following topics related to anesthesia in the elderly:

1. Physiologic changes relevant to administration of anesthesia
2. Preoperative assessment
3. Intraoperative management
4. Postoperative analgesia
5. Postoperative cognitive dysfunction (POCD)

The discussion will describe multimodal approaches to the perioperative care of older patients with fractures, with special consideration given to postoperative pain relief.

The frequent need for early mobilization, the exaggerated problem of perioperative delirium in the elderly, and the variety of regional techniques available for orthopedic procedures make these particularly rich areas for outlining current practice and proposing future research. The author will address the crucial question of whether general or regional anesthesia is preferable in older populations, or whether combining techniques may offer advantages in providing intraoperative stability, managing postoperative pain, and facilitating rehabilitation. There is no "optimal" anesthetic for geriatric patients; every geriatric patient is unique. It is unclear how much the anesthetic itself contributes to POCD. Injury and surgery, with their resultant deleterious effects on mobility, function, and independence, may be the major contributors to POCD. The chapter will offer suggestions for the overall plan of perioperative care; with the growing recognition that anesthetic agents can be neurotoxic, this takes on added importance in older patients who, on average, have less neurologic reserve than younger patients.

7.2 Physiologic Changes that Influence Anesthesia in the Elderly

Although we know there is a universal decline in most organ function as we age, changes in a given older individual are unpredictable and variations among them encompass a wide range. When people are young, there is little variability in individual physiology but, as we age, the difference amongst individuals becomes unpredictable and can be profound [5]. In addition to organ function changes, or perhaps as a result, both pharmacokinetics (what the body does to a drug) and pharmacodynamics (what a drug does to the body) change with age. Co-morbidities, a general decrease in functional reserve, and issues surrounding polypharmacy, either iatrogenic or patient-initiated, influence anesthetic considerations.

7.2.1 Cardiac Changes with Age

Age-related changes in vascular compliance, hypertrophy of the ventricles, and impaired autonomic control all contribute to increased lability in blood pressure and increased risk of ischemic events in the elderly. Healthy young adults increase cardiac output, as a response to stress, primarily by increasing heart rate; older adults are much more dependent on Frank–Starling forces, increasing cardiac output primarily by increasing end-diastolic volumes and filling pressures, thus increasing myocardial work and oxygen requirement. The aging heart becomes less compliant and there is increased arterial resistance, making further demands on myocardium that has less reserve, e.g., due to arrhythmias or fluid overload [6–13]. These changes under stress occur despite the fact that, in the absence of intrinsic heart disease, resting cardiac output and contractility in older adults are unchanged [14].

7.2.2 Pulmonary Changes with Age

Aging causes changes in respiratory mechanics and homeostasis, including loss of chest wall compliance, increases in ventilation–perfusion (V/Q) mismatching, decreased ciliary function, and attenuated cough reflex [15–18]. Respiratory responses to hypercarbia and hypoxemia are attenuated in older adults; vital capacity and maximum minute ventilation also decrease [19]. In unstressed individuals these changes in lung function do not cause symptoms. General anesthesia alone, poorly controlled postoperative pain, inappropriate use of opioid analgesics, increased closing capacity, and the supine position may compromise respiratory parameters, further contributing to decreases in pulmonary functional reserve; these factors are most pronounced with thoracic and intra-abdominal procedures but also are significant in peripheral orthopedic procedures such as hip fracture fixation [20–23].

A special consideration with many orthopedic injuries, including some hip fractures, is that the patient lies in the lateral decubitus position (LDP) during surgery. This has important physiologic implications for anesthesia. In awake, spontaneously breathing patients, e.g., with neuraxial anesthesia, the dependent (lower) lung is perfused better than the nondependent (upper) lung and ventilation to the dependent lung is greater than that to the nondependent one. V/Q ratios remain fairly normal. Under general anesthesia, ventilation to the lower lung decreases while ventilation to the upper lung increases. Perfusion to the lower lung, however, remains higher than that to the upper lung due to gravity. The net result is an increase in V/Q mismatching due to a well-ventilated, poorly perfused nondependent lung and a poorly ventilated, well-perfused dependent lung [24]. Blunting of hypoxic pulmonary vasoconstriction by the vasodilating properties of general anesthetics can further exaggerate V/Q mismatching, contributing to increased pulmonary shunting. This can have serious implications for older patients who lack respiratory reserve.

7.2.3 Autonomic Nervous System Changes with Age

Both the parasympathetic and sympathetic responses are attenuated with aging. Plasma norepinephrine levels increase with age and correlate with increases in mean arterial blood pressure. The net effect is decreased responsiveness to acute stress and lability of cardiovascular parameters [25]. In the intraoperative period, changes in the autonomic nervous system associated with aging can degrade normal cardiovascular responses to vasodilating effects of anesthetics and may attenuate the response to vasoconstrictors or inotropes [26, 27]. Impaired thermoregulation places the older surgical patient at increased risk for hypothermia [28, 29]. Shivering, as a consequence, increases oxygen consumption and myocardial demand; lower body temperature affects the pharmacology of some anesthetic drugs, most notably neuromuscular blockers whose duration may be prolonged. Neuraxial blockade (epidural or intrathecal) causes vasodilation from the resultant sympathectomy; this exacerbates the problems faced by older patients who cool quickly, warm slowly, and are more susceptible to the hypotensive effects seen with such blocks [30–32].

7.2.4 Renal, Hepatic, and Pharmacologic Changes with Age

As renal mass decreases with aging so does renal function. Blood flow to the kidney and glomerular filtration rates decrease. Higher levels of atrial natriuretic peptide, coupled with lower levels of both aldosterone and renin activity, make the older patient less able to conserve sodium or excrete excess sodium and water [33, 34]. Serum creatinine levels are likely to remain in the "normal" range due to decreased muscle mass and less production of creatinine but creatinine clearance will have changed quite dramatically.

Changes in liver activity can be variable but hepatic function generally is preserved in the older patient. A decrease in hepatocyte mass parallels decreases in hepatic blood flow in such a way that homeostasis tends to persist. Oxidative mechanisms become less efficient so clearance of drugs such as diazepam is prolonged. Conjugative pathways, in particular glucuronidation, are preserved; lorazepam, hydromorphone, and morphine are glucuronidated [35, 36]. The glucuronide metabolites of lorazepam and hydromorphone are inactive but morphine-6-glucuronide (about 20% of the conjugated products) is 3–4 times as potent an analgesic, with a duration twice as long as the parent compound when given systemically and between 20 and 45 times as potent when given intracerebrally; morphine-3-glucuronide (about 80% of the conjugated products), the other major metabolite, appears to be inactive as an analgesic but may be responsible for some of the dysphoric side effects associated with morphine administration [37, 38]. The liver extensively metabolizes hydromorphone with ~95% of the dose conjugated to the inactive hydromorphone-3-glucuronide. With oral administration, mean exposure to hydromorphone increases fourfold with moderate hepatic impairment. Interestingly, after oral administration, mean exposure to hydromorphone is twofold in patients with moderate renal dysfunction (creatinine clearance 40–60 ml/min); with severe renal impairment mean exposure is threefold and terminal elimination times increase significantly [39–41]. Hepatic conjugative pathways have high capacity and a nearly dead liver will continue to glucuronidate the parent drug but will do so more slowly than an intact, healthy organ. Small changes in renal function will have profound effects on elimination of the active morphine-6-glucuronide and less, but clinically significant, effects on hydromorphone inactivation. Studies on lorazepam are inconclusive to date.

As the ratio of lean to fat body mass decreases and total body water increases with advanced age, there is less protein binding and more free serum drug available; this may account for some of the increased drug sensitivity seen in geriatric populations, particularly with relatively hydrophilic drugs such as neuromuscular blocking agents (NMBs). Lipid soluble drugs will be less available to the intravascular space. The sundry changes that affect drug distribution, metabolism, and clearance do so in unpredictable and idiosyncratic ways. In most circumstances, redistribution into lipid soluble tissues accounts for the rapid offset of hypnotic and analgesic drugs used in the operating room; adipose tissue also serves as a depot from which these drugs must egress before metabolism and ultimate clearance. It is difficult to anticipate the rates of hepatic and renal elimination, which account for most of the prolonged effects of intravenous anesthetic drugs but are less important in the short term. Because general anesthesia, by itself, decreases both hepatic and renal blood flow, limited organ reserve in older patients may lead to unanticipated complications with drug elimination, thus prolonging anesthetic effects.

With aging, then, comes a constellation of physiologic changes that can alter the pharmacokinetics and pharmacodynamics of medications in the perioperative period [42]. Rates and volumes of distribution change; redistribution between fat and lean mass is variable; elimination and clearance of drugs decrease in older adults. Predicting individual responses to the stresses of anesthesia and surgery is difficult, at best, but older age clearly appears to be an independent risk factor for increased pharmacodynamic effects of anesthetic drugs [43, 44]. The risk of opioid-induced respiratory depression is higher in older patients [45]. Interestingly, most older patients have similar intraoperative opioid requirements but typically require lower doses than younger patients in the postoperative period. This probably is due to decreased clearance and enhanced sensitivity [45–47]. Most practitioners expect exaggerated responses to anesthetic agents in the elderly and, appropriately, give less drug and allow for longer circulation and redistribution times; it is a great deal easier to give more drug if needed than to take it away. A common sense approach is always to "titrate to effect," allowing for longer times to peak drug effect and prolonged duration of action.

7.2.5 Neurologic Changes

Even though it can be difficult to predict the exact pharmacokinetics of anesthetic agents in the elderly, the central nervous system (CNS) changes coincident with aging are associated with increased pharmacodynamic effects that can make older adults more sensitive to anesthetic agents [42, 48–50]. Most significant perioperative morbidity is pulmonary or cardiac in origin. However, a variety of neurologic complications are encountered in the postoperative period in older patients. Many of these would be transient or relatively inconsequential in the younger patient with greater functional reserve. Almost everyone, for example, goes through a postoperative delirium after emergence from anesthesia; it usually is quite attenuated in young adults but can lead to prolonged morbidity in the elderly. Although autoregulation, blood flow, and metabolism remain relatively uncompromised with aging, degeneration and neuronal loss (centrally and peripherally) limit the functional reserve of geriatric patients [51, 52]. Any sort of cognitive dysfunction that interferes with orthopedic rehabilitation after fracture surgery can have devastating long-term results. Anesthesiologists should work with orthopedists to achieve a well-balanced postoperative analgesic regimen in order to maximize rehabilitation and minimize medication side effects. Importantly, practitioners should remember that inadequate analgesia is a major risk factor for disruption of normal circadian rhythms, with subsequent disorientation or frank delirium, leading to poor rehabilitation conditions.

The POCD is a well-described consequence of anesthesia and surgery and it is discussed in Sect. 7.5.6. Let it be said now, that there is emerging evidence that anesthetics are neurotoxic under certain conditions. It is, however, uncertain what contribution the anesthetic alone has in the development of POCD compared to the entirety of the stress response induced by the complex of injury, repair, and rehabilitation.

7.3 Preoperative Evaluation

Any orthopedist will confirm the fact that open fractures, or those that have compromised vascular or neurologic integrity, require prompt attention, within hours of injury; sometimes that involves a "washout" and either external fixation or traction; sometimes there needs to be open reduction and internal fixation. Surgical fixation of closed fractures often can wait, even for a few days. In the former cases, there is little luxury to do the "complete" preoperative workup, while in the latter the anesthesiologist can gather more information on pre-injury status and, perhaps, tailor an anesthetic for the patient. The goals of preoperative evaluation are to (a) define physiologic features that may affect perioperative management, (b) determine if, and what, medical interventions might optimize the patient's condition for anesthesia and surgery, (c) stratify risk and gather baseline data. In every case the anesthesiologist must, in concert with the orthopedist, perform a risk–benefit analysis based on the context of the injury. If, for example, an older person fractures an ankle while playing golf, it carries quite different implications than if a patient has a syncopal episode and sustains a fracture as a result. In the first instance, based upon good functional status, it is likely that the surgical case could proceed without any special diagnostic evaluations beyond baseline electrocardiogram (ECG), blood count, and electrolyte status. In the latter instance, it would be imperative to determine the cause of syncope as quickly as possible; were it due to such conditions as critical aortic stenosis, sick sinus syndrome, cardiac arrhythmia, or a thromboembolic event, for example, there would be serious implications for anesthetic management and postoperative care.

Age alone is not a disease and does not contribute as much to perioperative risk as co-morbidities do; historically, risk assessment has been disease oriented [53, 54]. The heterogeneity of geriatric populations, use of multiple medications, the existence of co-morbidities (up to 80% of geriatric surgical patients have co-morbidities) [55, 56] make it problematic to determine functional reserve and perioperative risk. Basal function in older adults may meet the demands of daily living, but functional reserve may be poor or inadequate to compensate for the stresses of anesthesia and surgery. Whether those perioperative risk factors can be altered in the direction of a favorable outcome is an open question, especially in the setting of the need for relatively immediate procedural intervention for orthopedic injuries. Whereas young people rarely experience catastrophic events in the perioperative period (unless they are multitrauma victims), older adults are at increased risk of significant myocardial, pulmonary, thromboembolic, and neurologic events. Less devastating, but equally important, complications from delirium, sepsis, falls, inability to ambulate, and malnutrition, to name a few, can have major implications in the recovery period and may lead to poor long-term results. At this point in time, the value of preoperative functional assessment is an area ripe for study; we simply do not know enough about older patients, especially "healthy" geriatric patients who are physiologically stressed by injury, anesthesia, and surgery.

So, how can anesthesiologists best prepare patients preoperatively? What sorts of preoperative evaluations will affect intraoperative management? It is well accepted that routine preoperative testing is not indicated in the majority of otherwise healthy patients; a small number of abnormalities will surface, and an even smaller number of anesthetic plans will change as a result [57–60]. Less is known specifically about the geriatric age group; one study on chest X-rays (CXRs) and one on ECGs revealed clinically significant abnormalities in 40–55% of patients 65 years or older but only a very small percentage (1–5%) delayed surgery [61–63]. Since surgical repair of fractures is constrained by time considerations, it seems highly improbable that batteries of routine preoperative evaluations will affect anesthetic management. Most practitioners, however, feel it is wise to get baseline CXRs, ECGs, a CBC, and electrolytes to better evaluate any changes in the intraoperative or postoperative period. Clinical history and physical exam are much more important and will help target those studies that may have added value in determining important co-morbidities such as diabetes and silent myocardial ischemia. A trans-thoracic cardiac echocardiogram is easy to perform, painless, and can help identify existing, or potential, issues that may affect cardiovascular stability during administration of anesthesia. More sophisticated testing, such as stress echocardiograms or radionuclide studies and cardiac catheterization, are impractical given the time constraints imposed by the need to intervene relatively quickly when someone suffers a fracture; there is little indication that such studies would change anesthetic management in any significant way.

7.4 Intraoperative Period

7.4.1 Introduction

Most research on anesthetics has concentrated on the events that occur during the finite time frame from induction through surgical anesthesia and into the immediate postoperative period but not beyond, with the notable exception of postoperative analgesia (see Sect. 7.5). We know a great deal about intraoperative cardio-pulmonary stability, time to emergence, postoperative nausea and vomiting, and time to discharge from the postanesthesia care unit (PACU). The use of prophylactic perioperative beta adrenergic blockade in patients at high risk for cardiac ischemia, for example, has become an accepted practice among anesthesiologists [64–66]. Investigators have looked at the effects of many drugs in elderly patients, including induction agents, volatile anesthetics, NMBs, opioid analgesics, benzodiazepines, and local anesthetics. There are unproven, but theoretical, advantages of using short-acting drugs in the elderly so much recent work has concentrated on this area. As Cook notes, "...perspective is needed." Even though induction may be more stable or awakening and discharge times may be shortened, these parameters might not have an effect on overall outcome; indeed, Cook cautions that "...changes on patient outcome [are] probably minimal" [67].

7.4.2 Regional vs. General Anesthesia

Does it make a difference whether a geriatric patient receives general or regional anesthesia? This is, perhaps, the most salient and vexing question related to anesthesia in older people. Decades ago, when drugs, monitoring, procedures to secure the airway, knowledge of the physiological consequences of anesthesia, and training in the specialty left much to be desired, mortality rates from general anesthesia were high; most practitioners (and patients) would have opted for a regional technique. Although some intra-thoracic and intra-abdominal surgeries can be done under regional anesthesia, all peripheral and some pelvic orthopedic procedures are possible with such techniques; axial skeletal fractures are the exception. It often is difficult to separate mortality due to surgical procedures or co-morbidities from those due exclusively to the anesthetic, but we know with certainty that general anesthesia is safer than ever. Initial studies from the 1950s suggested that mortality rates from general anesthesia were in the range of 1 in 10,000. Those rates now have fallen to about five or six deaths per million. Costs of malpractice have mirrored those numbers and now are in the same range as those for primary care doctors [68, 69]. Whereas there was major emphasis on teaching and utilizing regional techniques for surgical anesthesia in the middle of the twentieth century [70], most training programs now concentrate, instead, on regional techniques for postoperative analgesia after a general anesthetic for the surgery. Many residents finish training with little knowledge of, or facility in, peripheral techniques; instead, neuraxial analgesia provided by the epidural or intrathecal route are in common use. There are no data to support the hypothesis that regional anesthesia is safer than general anesthesia. Indeed, there even are mixed results and opinions about whether regional, specifically neuraxial anesthesia, reduces the incidence of POCD (see Sect. 7.5.6).

7.4.3 General Anesthesia in Older Adults with Fractures

No guidelines on this practice exist. However, general anesthesia in older patients never has been shown to be less safe than regional techniques except for suggestive data that neuraxial anesthesia is associated with slightly better oxygenation in the immediate postoperative period, less blood loss, and lower incidences of deep vein thrombosis (DVT) [71–77]; the last observation is based upon older studies and may not be applicable with the growing availability of more effective DVT prophylaxis regimens. The blood loss data may have some significance because increased blood transfusion is associated with higher rates of urinary tract infection after hip surgery [78]. Determined by the anesthesiologist's experience and comfort level, a wide variety of general anesthetic techniques are available and acceptable. Keeping in mind that anesthetic complications are more highly associated with co-morbidities than with age per se, individual practitioners should choose techniques that minimize perturbations in cardiovascular, pulmonary, and neurologic function. Preliminary data suggest a correlation between deeper levels of anesthesia and the development of POCD (see Sect. 7.5.6), so anesthesia providers should take this into account.

7.4.4 *Regional Anesthesia in Older Adults with Fractures*

Despite the fact that nearly every extremity fracture and many pelvic fractures are amenable to regional anesthesia and analgesia, anesthesiologists never should propose such techniques in the absence of a discussion with the orthopedic surgeon; postoperative anticoagulation strategies, positioning, duration of the procedure, and the surgeon's personal preference all are important. The variety of nerve blocks is shown in Table 7.1 [79–87].

Providers can do any of the blocks as single shots or with placement of a catheter, including continuous intrathecal blockade, a method that allows the anesthesiologist to bring the block on slowly to minimize changes in cardiovascular stability due to sympathectomy. Due to co-morbidities in the elderly and the growing use of various anticoagulants and thrombolytic therapies before and after surgery, regional anesthesia is not always possible in older populations. Table 7.2 summarizes consensus recommendations of the American Society for Regional Anesthesia (ASRA) on neural blockade in patients who are anticoagulated or on thrombolytic therapy [88, 89].

These are conservative recommendations and specifically apply only to neuraxial blockade because of the potentially devastating consequence of spinal hematoma. There are no consensus guidelines for the use of single-shot peripheral nerve blocks or indwelling catheters but it is probably prudent to apply the neuraxial guidelines. Many of the ASRA guidelines, although of general interest, have no applicability in acute orthopedic injuries because there will not have been time, or forewarning, to stop anticoagulants. In those cases, general anesthesia is preferred once bleeding parameters are sufficiently corrected for surgery to proceed safely.

Another important consideration is that many older people will require sedation as a supplement to regional anesthesia because they cannot tolerate being awake in one position for the duration of surgical fracture fixation or they simply do not want to hear the sound of hammers, drills, reamers, saws, and other orthopedic tools. Older people are more prone than younger ones to become disinhibited by benzodiazepines, such as midazolam; there is nothing better to ruin a good regional anesthetic than to have a disinhibited patient who may want to "help" the surgeon or simply cannot stay still. A better practice is to use low doses of the intravenous anesthetic propofol to achieve a proper balance between comfort and spontaneous respirations. Positioning also can complicate regional anesthesia, for example, shoulder surgery, because patients typically are in the "beach chair" position so emergency access to the airway is precarious; over-sedation to the point of loss of airway protection is a real risk. The prone position is a relative contraindication to regional anesthesia but depends upon length of procedure and the anatomy of the surgery; elbow fractures, for example, often are treated with the patient prone, arm hanging over the operating table, and can be complicated and long. Furthermore, positioning the patient might be too

Table 7.1 Neural blockade for orthopedic injuries

Type of block	Area anesthetized	Special complications
Interscalene brachial plexus	Shoulder and upper arm	Phrenic nerve paresis[a] [79–87]
Supraclavicular brachial plexus	Entire arm except proximal shoulder	Pneumothorax
Infraclavicular brachial plexus	Entire arm except proximal shoulder	Pneumothorax (rare)
Axillary brachial plexus	Forearm, hand (sometimes affects distal upper arm)	Intravascular injection
Bier block (intravenous regional anesthesia)	Hand and forearm (not recommended for lower extremity)	Local anesthetic toxicity from tourniquet failure
Elbow: ulnar, median, radial, lateral antebrachial cutaneous nerves	Sensory distribution of the specific nerve (each block is done separately)	None
Wrist: ulnar, median, radial	Sensory distribution of the specific nerve (each block is done separately)	None
Psoas compartment	Thigh to below knee	Intrathecal injection
Inguinal paravascular	Thigh to below knee	Intravascular injection
Femoral nerve	Thigh and medial aspect of lower leg	Intravascular injection
Sciatic nerve	Lower leg, except distal medial portion, plantar aspect of foot	None
Common peroneal nerve (at the knee)	Lateral aspect of lower leg, dorsum of foot	None
Tibial nerve (at the knee)	Plantar aspect of foot, lateral malleolus	None
Saphenous nerve (just distal to the knee)	Medial aspect of lower leg, medial malleolus	None
Ankle block	Foot	None
Neuraxial (intrathecal or epidural)	Entire area below the level of the block (epidural block occasionally misses the sacral roots)	Total spinal anesthetic intravascular injection Local anesthetic toxicity (with epidural only)

[a]Hemidiaphragmatic paresis occurs nearly 100% of the time and, although transient, is problematic in patients with limited pulmonary reserve

uncomfortable to perform a block – a painful hip fracture might prevent a patient from sitting up or lying in the LDP for a neuraxial block; one possible way to circumvent that is to perform a femoral nerve block first.

Many fractures will threaten neurovascular viability. There is potential advantage of sympathectomy and vasodilation for vascular compromise but anesthesiologists should exercise great caution if there is any hint of neural injury accompanying the fracture. For medico-legal reasons most anesthesiologists would be reluctant to use neural blockade in such instances. Masking of compartment syndromes by neural blockade, for example, with distal tibial fractures, is another concern (see Sect. 7.5.3).

Table 7.2 Summary of ASRA recommendations for regional anesthesia in anticoagulated patients [88, 89]

Type of anticoagulation	Recommendations
Thrombolytic/fibrinolytic therapy	1. Avoid neuraxial blockade 2. If thrombolytic therapy is initiated after placement of a catheter, limit infusions to minimize sensory and motor block 3. No specific recommendations for removal of catheter after thrombolytic is initiated. Fibrinogen level might help guide timing because it is one of the last clotting factors to recover
Unfractionated heparin	1. No contraindication with subcutaneous heparin alone 2. Risky in the presence of concurrent use of other anticoagulants 3. Subcutaneous heparin can cause thrombocytopenia after ~4 days – it is recommended to get a platelet count
Preoperative low molecular weight heparin (LMWH)	1. For prophylactic doses, placement should occur, at least, 10–12 h after the last dose 2. At high doses (1.5 mg/kg enoxaparin or equivalent every 12 h), placement should occur, at least, 24 h after the last dose 3. Antiplatelet or oral coagulant medications increase the risk of spinal hematoma 4. Traumatic (bloody) placement is not a cause to postpone surgery but LMWH therapy should be delayed 24 h
Postoperative LMWH	1. Safe to place preoperatively 2. With twice daily dosing The first dose of LMWH should be administered no earlier than 24 h after catheter placement Indwelling catheters should be removed prior to starting LMWH Continuous catheters may be removed the morning after surgery, with the first dose of LMWH given, at least, 2 h after catheter removal 3. With once daily dosing The first dose of LMWH should be given 6–8 h postoperatively The second postoperative dose of LMWH should be given no sooner than 24 h after the first dose Catheter removal should occur 10–12 h after the last dose of LMWH Subsequent dosing of LMWH should occur no earlier than 2 h after catheter removal
Oral anticoagulants	1. Chronic warfarin therapy should be stopped 4–5 days prior to neuraxial blockade (impractical with acute orthopedic injuries) 2. Concurrent use of medications that affect other components of the clotting cascade (including aspirin and other NSAIDs, ticlopidine, clopidogrel, unfractionated heparin, and LMWH) increases risk of spinal hematoma 3. For patients receiving a single dose of warfarin preoperatively, should check PT/INR 4. Catheter placement and removal should not occur if INR is >1.5 5. Neurologic surveillance should occur in all cases

(continued)

Table 7.2 (continued)

Type of anticoagulation	Recommendations
Antiplatelet regimens (including NSAIDs, aspirin, the thienopyridine derivatives ticlopidine, clopidogrel, and the GP Iib/IIIa antagonists abciximab, eptifibatide, and tirofiban)	1. No wholly acceptable test available, including bleeding time 2. Aspirin and other NSAIDs alone do not present increased risk 3. Wait 14 days after the last dose of ticlopidine 4. Wait 7 days after the last dose of clopidogrel 5. Concurrent use of other anticoagulants increases risk
Herbal therapies	No specific concerns have been identified in the absence of concurrent use of other anticoagulants
Direct thrombin inhibitors and fondaparinux	Unknown

It is worth including a few final notes about neural blockade. Neuraxial techniques are part of the basic skill set of any anesthesiologist. Exposure to peripheral neural blockade varies widely amongst training programs; it is unrealistic to expect every anesthesiologist to feel competent with these procedures. Older techniques of seeking paresthesias to locate particular nerves have given way to the use of nerve stimulators that increase accuracy and efficacy. Guided ultrasound techniques represent the most recent interventional aids and, though not available at all institutions, improve the chance, but do not guarantee, successful block [90–94]. In any case, the comfort level and experience of the anesthesiologist should not be discounted. In a trauma facility or one that performs many orthopedic procedures, it is reasonable to expect that most anesthesiologists will have the skills and confidence necessary to perform nerve blocks for nearly any procedure. In contrast, hospitals with little, or infrequent, exposure to orthopedic trauma may have anesthesiologists who lack the complete skill set.

7.5 Postoperative Care and Analgesia

7.5.1 General Principles of Analgesia

The most important principle of pain management after surgery, including fracture repair, is to provide baseline pain relief for when a patient is resting and breakthrough medications when patients engage in activities that cause increased pain over baseline. This has major implications for adequate postoperative mobilization in orthopedic patients. Poor pain relief has been shown to be a factor in the development of POCD (see Sect. 7.5.6) [95, 96] and likely correlates with lower activity levels. Systemic medications, regional neural blockade, and combinations of the two are ways to control postoperative pain due to orthopedic procedures. Many authors advocate the use of multimodal "balanced analgesia" in older patients [97–101]. There are many reasons for these recommendations, including sparing of systemic medications that may contribute to POCD, compromise organ function, or interfere with healing; emerging evidence for the efficacy of preemptive analgesia (see below); and better range of motion with regional techniques plus the use of systemic "breakthrough" analgesics if pain relief is inadequate during physical therapy. A priori, there is no way to determine which modalities will be most helpful to a particular patient. The author, therefore, recommends tailoring analgesic therapy to the patient and the condition, a decision that surgeons, therapists, and anesthesiologists should make together.

7.5.2 Systemic Analgesia

Acetaminophen, although not appropriate for acute postoperative pain, is an often forgotten drug and can be useful as an adjunct, especially as breakthrough medication in later stages of rehabilitation. The American Geriatrics Society suggests maximal doses of 4 g/day in patients with no renal or hepatic disease [102]. In frail patients, or in patients with hepatic disease, practitioners should adjust doses downward.

Nonsteroidal anti-inflammatory drugs (NSAIDs) have potent analgesic properties but their use in orthopedics is somewhat controversial. Animal data and some human data suggest that NSAIDs retard healing and contribute to nonunion of fractured bone [103–105]. Other studies have failed to show any significant differences in rates of healing or nonunion [106, 107]. Complicating interpretation of these data is the observation that NSAID use may be a reflection of persistent pain associated with nonunions rather than a cause [108]. A reasonable approach, advocated by many orthopedists, is to use NSAIDs for a limited time period, perhaps a few doses or for a few days, to help patients get over the acute pain associated with fracture repair [109, 110]. In geriatric populations, recommendations for the use of NSAIDs must be tempered by risks of co-morbidities, particularly gastrointestinal bleeding and compromised renal function.

Opioid analgesics remain the mainstay of systemic therapy for severe pain. In patients who are cognitively intact, patient-controlled analgesia (PCA) is the modality of choice for the first few days after fracture fixation. Investigators have shown that PCA, by giving patients the ability to titrate their own analgesia, preserves autonomy and self-control; provides better and more rapid analgesia; improves patient satisfaction; decreases sedation and anxiety; reduces nursing time; and decreases lengths of stay in hospital [111–117]. PCA has been shown to be safe [118], especially when used in conjunction with respiratory monitoring [119].

In those patients who cannot operate a PCA, intravenous opioids on a PRN basis can be problematic. If patients can verbalize pain reports, then titration of analgesics is logically easy but may be logistically difficult because nurses are not always readily available. Oral analgesics, because they have longer duration of action than parenteral ones, may be used for baseline pain relief with breakthrough medications being either oral or intravenous depending upon the stage of recovery and the severity of the pain. Nonverbal patients are difficult to assess for analgesic needs. A variety of observational tools is available to assess pain in nonverbal adults [120]. No single assessment tool has been shown to work in all contexts, so nurses and physicians must adapt and personalize assessment for each patient. Again, a combination regimen of a relatively long-acting oral opioid for baseline relief with breakthrough analgesia available for times when pain is poorly controlled would be reasonable in nonverbal patients. There is no formula for analgesics and "titration to effect" should be the rule.

Morphine, the gold standard opioid analgesic, can be delivered by almost any route imaginable. It has the advantage of coming in long- and short-acting oral formulations, making it possible to provide both sustained resting pain relief and incident pain relief with the same drug. Sustained release morphine preparations have effective half lives of 8–12 h; short-acting oral morphine has an effective half-life in the 3–4 h range. Practitioners should avoid morphine in patients who have significant renal compromise because of the active glucuronide metabolite (see Sect. 7.2.4).

Hydromorphone, oxycodone, hydrocodone, methadone, and levorphanol are synthetic opioids. Oxycodone comes in a sustained release preparation with an effective half-life of 8–12 h as well as the short-acting form that has an effective half life of 3–4 h; it, like morphine, often is used for both baseline pain relief and breakthrough analgesia. Hydromorphone does not come in a long-acting form and has an effective half-life of about 2–3 h making it difficult to use as a baseline analgesic but ideal for therapy sessions. Both methadone and levorphanol have analgesic effects that last 6–8 h; it is recommended that a pain specialist be consulted before using either of these potent and poorly understand opioid analgesics. Hydrocodone has similar potency to oxycodone and usually is prescribed as a combination drug with acetaminophen; it is a good medication for breakthrough pain but, because of potential acetaminophen toxicity, should not be used to provide baseline analgesia.

Meperidine, as an analgesic, has fallen out of favor, although it still is commonly used in low doses for shivering in the PACU. Its active metabolite, normeperidine, must be cleared by the kidneys and can accumulate quickly, in a matter of days, causing seizures with all their sequelae. Investigators have shown that meperidine, either systemically or by the epidural route, is associated with a higher incidence of POCD [121], another compelling reason to avoid this drug in geriatric populations.

Intravenous fentanyl should be reserved for specialized areas such as PACUs, intensive care units (ICUs), and operating rooms; its effects can be surprisingly profound and prolonged in older people despite its reputation as a short-acting opioid. It is a rare patient who will tolerate only intravenous fentanyl and no other opioid. Fentanyl transdermal patches have no role in acute postoperative pain management and can be dangerous because they are difficult to titrate and take hours to reach effective blood levels. They do have a useful role in pain syndromes that persist and are responsive to opioids.

How does one choose an opioid? In the absence of renal failure (in which case morphine is contraindicated), it is "dealers choice." There are anecdotal impressions that hydromorphone causes delirium less often than morphine and, therefore, should be the first line parenteral analgesic in older people. These impressions have never been substantiated. Opioid effects and side effects are idiosyncratic and unpredictable. The best way to know if a patient will respond positively to a particular opioid is to ask about past history of strong opioids; people know what works for them and what makes them feel sick or strange. In nonverbal patients, try to elicit an analgesic history from a family member or caretaker.

Pain after bony fracture and surgical intervention typically is intense for a period of days to weeks, depending upon the extent of the injury and the magnitude of the procedure. It then suddenly decreases and goes away, almost always coincident with positive rehabilitative milestones. If patients have pain beyond the expected time period after surgical intervention, they should consult with a pain specialist.

7.5.3 Regional Analgesia

Neural blockade to provide analgesia for orthopedic procedures is nearly identical to that for regional anesthesia (see Tables 7.1 and 7.2), with the notable exception that regional analgesia typically requires solutions of local anesthetic with lower concentrations, often infused in combination with opioids.

In the periphery, single-shot neural blockade is the standard but many specially trained anesthesiologists will place catheters to continuously infuse local anesthetic; these methods are available for both upper and lower extremity analgesia. In the neuraxis, the most versatile and effective method of continuous analgesia is by placement of an epidural catheter. This technique is valuable, and common, for lower extremity and pelvic fractures but it is unsuitable for upper extremity fractures. Sometimes epidural analgesia is combined with a spinal anesthetic, called "combined spinal epidural" or "CSE." The analogue of PCA for epidural analgesia is patient controlled epidural analgesia (PCEA), wherein patients receive continuous infusions of medication but also have the ability to provide themselves rescue medication via a patient-controlled pump. The evidence that regional techniques provide superior analgesia to systemic pain relievers is weak. Outcome data are lacking. The same patient limitations that apply to PCA also apply to the use of PCEA, viz. patients must be cognitively intact and understand the principles behind rescue dosing.

Normal practice is to use mixtures of low dose opioid and weak local anesthetic solutions in epidural catheters; drugs in the epidural space have a comparatively wide therapeutic index, can be administered safely by patient control, and often can be adjusted to provide analgesia without significantly altering motor function ("walking epidurals"). It is common practice to use either fentanyl or morphine as the opioid, although hydromorphone also is effective. There is good evidence that morphine has more pronounced local effects and fewer systemic effects than other opioids [122]. Intrathecal catheters are not in common use for postoperative pain relief due to inherent dangers associated with a narrow therapeutic index in the subarachnoid space; many practitioners recommend that patients with intrathecal catheters be monitored in an ICU setting because of the high risks of hypotension or respiratory depression. All neuraxial local anesthetics can cause hypotension due to sympathectomy; this easily is treated with ephedrine (5–10 mg intravenously) and fluids. Infusing local anesthetic through a peripheral catheter not only provides analgesia but also helps increase blood supply by promoting vasodilation; adding low dose opioids is an unproven, but theoretically sound, way to target peripheral opioid receptors, although the real effect may be from systemic absorption of the opioid.

An important area of concern to all orthopedists is compartment syndrome after trauma. That is no different in elderly adults than in other populations. There is hesitancy to use regional techniques in some conditions, e.g., for tibial nailing, fearing that local anesthetic blockade might mask the pain of a compartment syndrome [123]. Existing evidence is conflicting but case reports suggest it does occur [124–128]. Some case reports refute that conclusion [129] and one controlled study found that regional analgesia is not problematic in compartment syndromes [130]. It is essential to note that neuraxial opioids do not cause numbness or motor blockade [131]; if compartment syndrome is a major concern, then it is wise to use more dilute solutions of local anesthetic and higher concentrations of neuraxial opioids. In any case, practitioners should not rule out such techniques but should use good clinical judgment tempered by caution.

Regional analgesia has been the linchpin of preemptive techniques working, as it does, by binding to sodium channels and blocking transmission of nociceptive signals from the peripheral to the CNS.

7.5.4 Recommendations for Postoperative Analgesia

The most important factors determining postoperative analgesia are the skill sets of the practitioners, including the nurses who will provide postoperative care and patient preference. There is not enough evidence to recommend a specific practice [132]; the anesthesiologist should do what s/he feels comfortable doing and it should mesh with the surgeon's desires as well as the kind of available aftercare. Using a previous example, in a busy trauma center one would expect sophisticated regional techniques and a specialized team for pain management but in a community hospital there may be limits to resources. Just as there is no "optimal" anesthetic for older patients, there is no "cookbook" for postoperative analgesia. This author agrees with many others that multimodal, "balanced" analgesia tailored to individuals and their situations is the approach one would take in the best of all possible worlds [97–101]. If coagulation status is adequate, it is recommended to perform, at least, a one shot nerve block and, perhaps, place a catheter for continuous relief during the recovery period. Some patients will not tolerate such procedures without sedation and analgesia, sometime even deep sedation or general anesthesia. In those cases, practitioners should exercise great caution because only an awake patient can signal the danger of nerve infiltration, which is painful; risk to benefit analysis is warranted in every case. Although regional techniques have not been proven conclusively to be more effective, or prevent chronic pain, clinical experience certainly suggests that they are opioid sparing and contribute positively to rehabilitation [74]. If not possible for any of the reasons mentioned above, or the patient prefers not to have a regional intervention, then it is imperative to provide adequate systemic analgesia. To do that requires careful monitoring, continuous assessment, and appropriate dosing. Pain experience always is subjective and there is no laboratory test for it. In general, "believe what the patient says," or, in the case of nonverbal patients, make careful observations.

7.5.5 Preemptive Analgesia

Preemptive analgesia is an intervention at the time of surgery that attempts to attenuate, or eliminate, short-term, acute pain and the development of long-term, chronic neuropathic pain syndromes. Its importance is embodied in the belief that when pain is treated inadequately, "central sensitization" occurs, a process by which dorsal horn cells that mediate pain become hypersensitive; it is essential to remember that inhaled (volatile) anesthetics do not have analgesic properties but must be used in conjunction with pain relieving drugs and techniques [133, 134]. (The term "wind-up" also is used to describe this phenomenon and has attractive heuristic qualities.) Current understanding of pain mechanisms suggests that preemptive analgesia might succeed by interrupting nociceptive pathways at any point between skin and brain, maintaining analgesia at adequate levels intraoperatively and into the postoperative period to prevent central sensitization [135]. If preemptive analgesia works, anesthesiologists and surgeons can decrease pain and analgesic requirements postoperatively by intervening pre- or intraoperatively. It is reasonable to believe that such interventions would, if successful, lead to fewer postoperative side effects from analgesic medications. Although based on good theoretical science and a growing number of animal and human studies [136–145], it has been difficult to prove that preemptive analgesia is clinically significant [146] or that it alters outcomes [147–149].

There are many potential targets for preemptive analgesia from the incision site to the brain. Most research has focused on neural blockade but there is some evidence to suggest that systemic analgesics play an important role. An in-depth discussion of preemptive analgesia is beyond the scope of this chapter but its potential importance in recovery from orthopedic injuries is difficult to underestimate. Nearly every peripheral nerve is amenable to blockade, while pain from pelvic and lower extremity injuries can be controlled using neuraxial techniques. Regional techniques currently are thought to be the mainstays of preemptive analgesia, the most compelling data derived from studies on prevention of phantom limb pain with preoperative neuraxial blockade continued into the postoperative period [150–152].

Nociceptors in the skin, peripheral nerves, spinal cord, and brain are obvious targets to interrupt pain and all are used in practice. Skin infiltration with local anesthetic interrupts surface nociceptive activity. Several studies have indicated that skin infiltration prior to incision is effective but skin infiltration after wound closure yields no additional benefits except in the very short term [136, 141, 149]. Blockade of peripheral nerves interrupts signals further "downstream." Neuraxial blockade, either epidural or intrathecal, blocks transmission of nociceptive signals to the brain. NSAIDs work by reducing production of prostaglandins, one of the algogenic agents released by injured tissue (others are bradykinin, histamine, 5-hydroxytryptamine) that stimulate or sensitize nociceptors. Prostaglandins also play a role in the CNS transmission of pain [153–156]. Opioids, such as morphine or hydromorphone, work in the brain when given systemically and work at the dorsal horn when given intraspinally. Peripheral opioid receptors, including ones in the synovium, have taken on increasing interest [157–162]. Based on this literature and clinical impression, intra-articular morphine is in widespread use in orthopedic practices. Furthermore, *N*-methyl D-aspartate (NMDA) receptors mediate pain; ketamine, an anesthetic, potent analgesic, and NMDA receptor blocking agent, has been found to be safe in older populations [163, 164]. Its effectiveness in the population as a whole has been variable. Anecdotally, methadone, the only opioid that also has potent effects at the NMDA receptor, is used clinically for preemptive analgesia and has become an important modality in treating or preventing neuropathic pain syndromes, including phantom limb pain [165].

Based on the current state of knowledge, it is reasonable to recommend preemptive interventions as part of a multimodal approach to pain management [166]. Even though there is, as yet, no definitive proof of efficacy, the treatments do not cause harm; what data do exist, suggest that pre-incision interventions are most effective. This recommendation must be tempered by the knowledge that orthopedic pain cycles already have commenced by the time patients go to surgery. This is in direct contradistinction to study models of preemptive analgesia where there is little, or no, pain and stress prior to incision.

7.5.6 Postoperative Cognitive Dysfunction

Concerns about negative effects of anesthesia on cognitive function in older patients first appeared in the literature in 1955 [167]. Subsequently, POCD after cardiac surgery became a major topic of investigation [168]. Now, POCD is a well-recognized phenomenon affecting upwards of 30% of middle-aged and older adults in almost every postoperative context [66, 169–171]. Although less of a problem after minor procedures [172], POCD has far-reaching implications and potentially devastating consequences, from subtle memory loss to severe disability, loss of independence, and even death. Contributing factors include the stresses of injury, surgery, and rehabilitation; fever; medications; electrolyte abnormalities; organ failure; altered nutritional status; and, probably, hospitalization by itself with its coincident disruptions of normal activity and circadian rhythms [169, 173]. The only predictor of POCD definitively associated with anesthesia is age [174]. Intraoperative systemic hypotension and hypoxemia, somewhat counter-intuitively, do not correlate with POCD [175]. Emerging data, however, suggest that deep anesthesia and poor cerebral oxygenation are two major culprits [174, 176, 177]. More recent studies suggest that male gender and preoperative alcohol abuse also are strong risk factors [178, 179] but their specific relationship to anesthesia has yet to be elucidated. Of great relevance, no difference has been shown between general and regional anesthesia in a variety of clinical circumstances, not just those confined to orthopedic procedures [71, 74, 75, 180–183]. However, two important studies have shown high correlation between POCD and poorly controlled pain [95, 96].

References

1. Liu, L. and J. Leung. Perioperative complications in elderly patients. Syllabus on geriatric anesthesiology. 2001 August 2007 [cited 2007 August]; Available from: http://www.asahq.org/clinical/geriatrics/perio_comp.htm.
2. Klopfenstein, C.E., et al., The influence of an aging surgical population on the anesthesia workload: a ten-year survey. Anesthesia and Analgesia, 1998. 86(6): p. 1165–70.
3. Anesthesiology, C.o.G. Syllabus on geriatric anesthesiology. [web-based] 2001 [cited 2007 August]; Available from: http://www.asahq.org/clinical/geriatrics/syllabus.htm.
4. Anesthesia, S.f.t.A.o.G. Syllabus on geriatric anesthesia. 2007 [cited 2007 August]; Available from: http://10085.hostinglogin.com/saga1/.
5. Muravchick, S., The biology of aging and preoperative evaluation, in Geroanesthesia: principles for management of the elderly patient, L. Craven, Editor. 1997, Mosby-Year Book, Inc: St. Louis. p. 1–34.
6. Cleroux, J., et al., Decreased cardiopulmonary reflexes with aging in normotensive humans. American Journal of Physiology, 1989. 257: p. H961–8.
7. Collins, K., et al., Functional changes in autonomic nervous responses with ageing. Age Ageing, 1980. 9: p. 17–24.
8. Franklin, S., et al., Hemodynamic patterns of age-related changes in blood pressure. The Framingham Heart Study. Circulation, 1997. 96: p. 308–15.
9. Landahl, S., et al., Age-related changes in blood pressure. Hypertension, 1986. 8: p. 1044–9.
10. Aronow, W.S., et al., Resting left ventricular ejection fraction in elderly patients without evidence of heart disease. American Journal of Cardiology, 1989. 63(5): p. 368–9.
11. Kawaguchi, M., et al., Combined ventricular systolic and arterial stiffening in patients with heart failure and preserved ejection fraction: implications for systolic and diastolic reserve limitations. Circulation, 2003. 107(5): p. 714–20.
12. Rodeheffer, R.J., et al., Postural changes in cardiac volumes in men in relation to adult age. Experimental Gerontology, 1986. 21(4–5): p. 367–78.
13. Rodeheffer, R.J., et al., Exercise cardiac output is maintained with advancing age in healthy human subjects: cardiac dilatation and increased stroke volume compensate for a diminished heart rate. Circulation, 1984. 69(2): p. 203–13.
14. Folkow, B. and A. Svanborg, Physiology of cardiovascular aging. Physiological Review, 1993. 73: p. 725–64.
15. Kitamura, H., T. Sawa, and E. Ikezono, Postoperative hypoxemia: the contribution of age to the maldistribution of ventilation. Anesthesiology, 1972. 36: p. 244–52.

16. Kronenberg, R. and C. Drage, Attenuation of the ventilatory and heart rate responses to hypoxia and hypercapnia with aging in normal men. Journal of Clinical Investigation, 1973. 52: p. 1812–8.
17. Lynne-Davies, P., Influence of age on the respiratory system. Geriatrics, 1977. 32: p. 57–60.
18. Zaugg, M. and E. Lucchinetti, Respiratory function in the elderly. Anesthesiology Clinics of North America, 2000. 18: p. 47–56, vi.
19. Peterson, D.D., et al., Effects of aging on ventilatory and occlusion pressure responses to hypoxia and hypercapnia. American Review of Respiratory Disease, 1981. 124(4): p. 387–91.
20. Arunasalam, K., et al., Ventilatory response to morphine in young and old subjects. Anaesthesia, 1983. 38: p. 529–33.
21. Clayer, M. and J. Bruckner, Occult hypoxia after femoral neck fracture and elective hip surgery. Clinical Orthopaedics and Related Research, 2000. (4): p. 265–71.
22. Sari, A., et al., The magnitude of hypoxemia in elderly patients with fractures of the femoral neck. Anesthesia and Analgesia, 1986. 65: p. 692–4.
23. Allen, S., Respiratory considerations in the elderly surgical patient. Clinics in Anesthesiology, 1986. 4: p. 899–930.
24. Benumof, J. and D. Alfery, Anesthesia for thoracic surgery, in Anesthesia, R. Miller, Editor. 2000, Elsevier Churchill Livingstone: Philadelphia. p. 1686–8.
25. Pfeifer, M.A., et al., Differential changes of autonomic nervous system function with age in man. American Journal of Medicine, 1983. 75(2): p. 249–58.
26. Phillips, P., G. Hodsman, and C. Johnston, Neuroendocrine mechanisms and cardiovascular homeostasis in the elderly. Cardiovascular Drugs Therapy, 1991. 4(Suppl 6): p. 1209–13.
27. Rowe, J. and B. Troen, Sympathetic nervous system and aging in man. Endocrine Reviews, 1980. 1(167–179).
28. Ozaki, M., et al., The threshold for thermoregulatory vasoconstriction during nitrous oxide/sevoflurane anesthesia is reduced in the elderly. Anesthesia and Analgesia, 1997. 84(5): p. 1029–33.
29. Kurz, A., et al., The threshold for thermoregulatory vasoconstriction during nitrous oxide/isoflurane anesthesia is lower in elderly than in young patients. Anesthesiology, 1993. 79(3): p. 465–9.
30. Carpenter, R.L., et al., Incidence and risk factors for side effects of spinal anesthesia. Anesthesiology, 1992. 76(6): p. 906–16.
31. Frank, S.M., et al., Epidural versus general anesthesia, ambient operating room temperature, and patient age as predictors of inadvertent hypothermia. Anesthesiology, 1992. 77(2): p. 252–7.
32. Frank, S.M., et al., Core hypothermia and skin-surface temperature gradients. Epidural versus general anesthesia and the effects of age. Anesthesiology, 1994. 80(3): p. 502–8.
33. Lamb, E.J., S.E. O'Riordan, and M.P. Delaney, Kidney function in older people: pathology, assessment and management. Clinica Chimica Acta, 2003. 334(1–2): p. 25–40.
34. Lindeman, R.D., Renal physiology and pathophysiology of aging. Contributions to Nephrology, 1993. 105: p. 1–12.
35. Jansen, P.L.M., Liver disease in the elderly. Best Practice and Research in Clinical Gastroenterology, 2002. 16(1): p. 149–58.
36. Wakabayashi, H., et al., Evaluation of the effect of age on functioning hepatocyte mass and liver blood flow using liver scintigraphy in preoperative estimations for surgical patients: comparison with CT volumetry. Journal of Surgical Research, 2002. 106(2): p. 246–53.
37. Krzanowska, E.K., et al., Potency ratios of morphine and morphine-6beta-glucuronide analgesia elicited from the periaqueductal gray, locus coeruleus or rostral ventromedial medulla of rats. Brain Research, 1998. 799(2): p. 329–33.
38. Shimomura, K., et al., Analgesic effect of morphine glucuronides. Tohoku Journal of Experimental Medicine, 1971. 105(1): p. 45–52.
39. Dean, M., Opioids in renal failure and dialysis patients. Journal of Pain and Symptom Management, 2004. 28(5): p. 497–504.

40. Kurella, M., W.M. Bennett, and G.M. Chertow, Analgesia in patients with ESRD: a review of available evidence. American Journal of Kidney Diseases, 2003. 42(2): p. 217–28.
41. Lotsch, J., Opioid metabolites. Journal of Pain and Symptom Management, 2005. 29(5 Suppl): p. S10–24.
42. Lamy, P. and T. Wiser, Geriatric anesthesia, in Pharmacotherapeutic considerations in the elderly surgical patient, M. Katlic, Editor. 1990, Urban & Schwarzenberg, Inc: Baltimore. p. 209–39.
43. Bressler, R. and J.J. Bahl, Principles of drug therapy for the elderly patient. Mayo Clinic Proceedings, 2003. 78(12): p. 1564–77.
44. Turnheim, K., When drug therapy gets old: pharmacokinetics and pharmacodynamics in the elderly. Experimental Gerontology, 2003. 38(8): p. 843–53.
45. Cepeda, M.S., et al., Side effects of opioids during short-term administration: effect of age, gender, and race. Clinical Pharmacology and Therapeutics, 2003. 74(2): p. 102–12.
46. Aubrun, F., et al., Postoperative morphine consumption in the elderly patient. Anesthesiology, 2003. 99(1): p. 160–5.
47. Woodhouse, A. and L.E. Mather, The influence of age upon opioid analgesic use in the patient-controlled analgesia (PCA) environment. Anaesthesia, 1997. 52(10): p. 949–55.
48. Dundee, J., et al., Sensitivity to propofol in the elderly. Anaesthesia, 1986. 41: p. 482–5.
49. Jacobs, J., et al., Aging increases pharmacodynamic sensitivity to the hypnotic effects of midazolam. Anesthesia and Analgesia, 1995. 80: p. 143–8.
50. Homer, T., et al., The effect of increasing age on thiopental disposition and anesthetic requirement. Anesthesiology, 1983. 62: p. 714–24.
51. Morris, J. and D. McManus, The neurology of aging: normal versus pathologic change. Geriatrics, 1991. 46: p. 47–48.
52. Creasey, H. and S.I. Rapoport, The aging human brain. Annals of Neurology, 1985. 17: p. 2–10.
53. Arvidsson, S., et al., Predicting postoperative adverse events. Clinical efficiency of four general classification systems. The project perioperative risk. Acta Anaesthesiologica Scandinavica, 1996. 40: p. 783–91.
54. Tiret, L., et al., Complications associated with anaesthesia – a prospective survey in France. Canadian Anaesthesia Society Journal, 1986. 33: p. 336–44.
55. Thomas, D. and C. Ritchie, Preoperative assessment of older adults. Journal of American Geriatric Society, 1995. 43: p. 811–21.
56. Vaz, F. and D. Seymour, A prospective study of elderly general surgical patients: I. Pre-operative medical problems. Age Ageing, 1989. 18: p. 309–15.
57. Kaplan, E., et al., The usefulness of preoperative laboratory screening. JAMA, 1985. 253: p. 3576–81.
58. Narr, B., et al., Outcomes of patients with no laboratory assessment before anesthesia and a surgical procedure. Mayo Clinic Proceedings, 1997. 72: p. 505–9.
59. Perez, A., et al., Value of routine preoperative tests: a multicentre study in four general hospitals. British Journal of Anaesthesia, 1985. 74: p. 250–6.
60. Turnbull, J. and C. Buck, The value of preoperative screening investigations in otherwise healthy individuals. Archives of Internal Medicine, 1987. 147: p. 1101–5.
61. Sewell, J.M., L.L. Spooner, A.K. Dixon, and D. Rubenstein, Screening investigations in the elderly. Age Ageing, 1981. 10: p. 165–8.
62. Seymour, D., R. Pringle, and W. MacLennan, The role of the routine pre-operative electrocardiogram in the elderly surgical patient. Age Ageing, 1983. 12: p. 97–104.
63. Seymour, D., R. Pringle, and J. Shaw, The role of the routine pre-operative chest X-ray in the elderly general surgical patient. Postgraduate Medical Journal, 1982. 58: p. 741–5.
64. Berg, C., et al., Perioperative beta-blocker therapy and heart rate control during noncardiac surgery. American Journal of Surgery, 2007. 194(2): p. 189–91.
65. Feringa, H.H.H., J.J. Bax, and D. Poldermans, Perioperative medical management of ischemic heart disease in patients undergoing noncardiac surgery. Current Opinion in Anaesthesiology, 2007. 20(3): p. 254–60.

66. Levine, W.C., V. Mehta, and G. Landesberg, Anesthesia for the elderly: selected topics. Current Opinion in Anaesthesiology, 2006. 19(3): p. 320–4.
67. Cook, D. Geriatric anesthesia. American Geriatrics Society RASP Project 2003 [cited 2007 August]; Available from: http://www.frycomm.com/ags/rasp/chapter.asp?ch=2.
68. Fleisher, L., Risk of anesthesia, in Miller's anesthesia, R. Miller, Editor. 2005, Elsevier Churchill Livingstone: Philadelphia. p. 893–925.
69. Rosenberg, H. Mortality associated with anesthesia. circa 2001 [cited 2007 August]; Available from: http://expertpages.com/news/mortality_anesthesia.htm.
70. Moore, D., Regional block: a handbook for use in the clinical practice of medicine and surgery. 1953, Charles C. Thomas: Springfield, IL.
71. Covert, C.R. and G.S. Fox, Anaesthesia for hip surgery in the elderly. Canadian Journal of Anaesthesia, 1989. 36(3 Pt 1): p. 311–9.
72. Mitchell, D., et al., Prevention of thromboembolic disease following total knee arthroplasty. Epidural versus general anesthesia. Clinical Orthopaedics and Related Research, 1991. (269): p. 109–12.
73. Wickstrom, I., I. Holmberg, and T. Stefansson, Survival of female geriatric patients after hip fracture surgery. a comparison of 5 anesthetic methods. Acta Anaesthesiologica Scandinavica, 1982. 26(6): p. 607–14.
74. Williams-Russo, P., et al., Randomized trial of epidural versus general anesthesia: outcomes after primary total knee replacement. Clinical Orthopaedics and Related Research, 1996 (331): p. 199–208.
75. Williams-Russo, P., et al., Cognitive effects after epidural vs general anesthesia in older adults. A randomized trial. JAMA, 1995. 274(1): p. 44–50.
76. Wu, C.L., et al., Effect of postoperative epidural analgesia on morbidity and mortality after total hip replacement surgery in medicare patients. Regional Anesthesia and Pain Medicine, 2003. 28(4): p. 271–8.
77. Wu, C.L., et al., Effect of postoperative epidural analgesia on morbidity and mortality following surgery in medicare patients. Regional Anesthesia and Pain Medicine, 2004. 29(6): p. 525–33; discussion 515–9.
78. Koval, K.J., et al., Does blood transfusion increase the risk of infection after hip fracture? Journal of Orthopaedic Trauma, 1997. 11(4): p. 260–5; discussion 265–6.
79. Emery, G., et al., Incidence of phrenic nerve block and hypercapnia in patients undergoing carotid endarterectomy under cervical plexus block. Anaesthesia and Intensive Care, 1998. 26(4): p. 377–81.
80. Knoblanche, G.E., The incidence and aetiology of phrenic nerve blockade associated with supraclavicular brachial plexus block. Anaesthesia and Intensive Care, 1979. 7(4): p. 346–9.
81. Urmey, W.F., K.H. Talts, and N.E. Sharrock, One hundred percent incidence of hemidiaphragmatic paresis associated with interscalene brachial plexus anesthesia as diagnosed by ultrasonography. Anesthesia and Analgesia, 1991. 72(4): p. 498–503.
82. Bigeleisen, P.E., Anatomical variations of the phrenic nerve and its clinical implication for supraclavicular block. British Journal of Anaesthesia, 2003. 91(6): p. 916–7.
83. Dullenkopf, A., et al., Diaphragmatic excursion and respiratory function after the modified Raj technique of the infraclavicular plexus block. Regional Anesthesia and Pain Medicine, 2004. 29(2): p. 110–4.
84. Bashein, G., H.T. Robertson, and W.F. Kennedy Jr., Persistent phrenic nerve paresis following interscalene brachial plexus block. Anesthesiology, 1985. 63(1): p. 102–4.
85. Bennani, S.E., et al., An attempt to prevent spread of local anaesthetic to the phrenic nerve by compression above the injection site during the interscalene brachial plexus block. European Journal of Anaesthesiology, 1998. 15(4): p. 453–6.
86. Pere, P., The effect of continuous interscalene brachial plexus block with 0.125% bupivacaine plus fentanyl on diaphragmatic motility and ventilatory function. Regional Anesthesia, 1993. 18(2): p. 93–7.
87. Pere, P., et al., Effect of continuous interscalene brachial plexus block on diaphragm motion and on ventilatory function. Acta Anaesthesiologica Scandinavica, 1992. 36(1): p. 53–7.

88. Medicine, A.S.o.R.A.a.P. Regional anesthesia in the anticoagulated patient: defining the risk. Second Consensus Conference on Neuraxial Anesthesia and Anticoagulation 2002 [cited 2007 August]; Consensus statement]. Available from: http://www.asra.com/consensus-statements/2.html.
89. Horlocker, T.T., et al., Regional anesthesia in the anticoagulated patient: defining the risks (the second ASRA Consensus Conference on Neuraxial Anesthesia and Anticoagulation). Regional Anesthesia and Pain Medicine, 2003. 28(3): p. 172–97.
90. Gray, A.T., Ultrasound-guided regional anesthesia: current state of the art. Anesthesiology, 2006. 104(2): p. 368–73.
91. Horlocker, T.T. and D.J. Wedel, Ultrasound-guided regional anesthesia: in search of the holy grail.[comment]. Anesthesia and Analgesia, 2007. 104(5): p. 1009–11.
92. Marhofer, P. and V.W.S. Chan, Ultrasound-guided regional anesthesia: current concepts and future trends. Anesthesia and Analgesia, 2007. 104(5): p. 1265–9.
93. Marhofer, P., M. Greher, and S. Kapral, Ultrasound guidance in regional anaesthesia. British Journal of Anaesthesia, 2005. 94(1): p. 7–17.
94. Peterson, M.K., F.A. Millar, and D.G. Sheppard, Ultrasound-guided nerve blocks.[comment]. British Journal of Anaesthesia, 2002. 88(5): p. 621–4.
95. Lynch, E.P., et al., The impact of postoperative pain on the development of postoperative delirium. Anesthesia and Analgesia, 1998. 86(4): p. 781–5.
96. Wang, Y., et al., The effects of postoperative pain and its management on postoperative cognitive dysfunction. American Journal of Geriatric Psychiatry, 2007. 15(1): p. 50–59.
97. Busch, C.A., et al., Efficacy of periarticular multimodal drug injection in total knee arthroplasty. A randomized trial. Journal of Bone and Joint Surgery – American Volume, 2006. 88(5): p. 959–63.
98. Kehlet, H. and J.B. Dahl, The value of "multimodal" or "balanced analgesia" in postoperative pain treatment. Anesthesia and Analgesia, 1993. 77(5): p. 1048–56.
99. Kelly, D.J., M. Ahmad, and S.J. Brull, Preemptive analgesia I: physiological pathways and pharmacological modalities. Canadian Journal of Anaesthesia, 2001. 48(10): p. 1000–10.
100. Kelly, D.J., M. Ahmad, and S.J. Brull, Preemptive analgesia II: recent advances and current trends. Canadian Journal of Anaesthesia, 2001. 48(11): p. 1091–101.
101. Skinner, H.B., Multimodal acute pain management. American Journal of Orthopedics, 2004. 33(5 Suppl): p. 5–9.
102. Adults, A.G.S.A.P.o.P.P.i.O., The management of persistent pain in older adults. JAGS, 2002. 50(6 Suppl): p. S205–24.
103. Burd, T.A., M.S. Hughes, and J.O. Anglen, Heterotopic ossification prophylaxis with indomethacin increases the risk of long-bone nonunion. Journal of Bone and Joint Surgery – British Volume, 2003. 85(5): p. 700–5.
104. Endo, K., et al., Cyclooxygenase-2 inhibitor delays fracture healing in rats. Acta Orthopaedica, 2005. 76(4): p. 470–4.
105. Giannoudis, P.V., et al., Nonunion of the femoral diaphysis. The influence of reaming and non-steroidal anti-inflammatory drugs. Journal of Bone and Joint Surgery – British Volume, 2000. 82(5): p. 655–8.
106. Clarke, S. and F. Lecky, Best evidence topic report. Do non-steroidal anti-inflammatory drugs cause a delay in fracture healing? Emergency Medicine Journal, 2005. 22(9): p. 652–3.
107. Mullis, B.H., et al., Effect of COX-2 inhibitors and non-steroidal anti-inflammatory drugs on a mouse fracture model. Injury, 2006. 37(9): p. 827–37.
108. Bhattacharyya, T., et al., Nonsteroidal antiinflammatory drugs and nonunion of humeral shaft fractures. Arthritis and Rheumatism, 2005. 53(3): p. 364–7.
109. Langford, R.M. and V. Mehta, Selective cyclooxygenase inhibition: its role in pain and anaesthesia. Biomedicine and Pharmacotherapy, 2006. 60(7): p. 323–8.
110. Wheeler, P. and M.E. Batt, Do non-steroidal anti-inflammatory drugs adversely affect stress fracture healing? A short review. British Journal of Sports Medicine, 2005. 39(2): p. 65–9.
111. Dolin, S.J., J.N. Cashman, and J.M. Bland, Effectiveness of acute postoperative pain management: I. Evidence from published data. British Journal of Anaesthesia, 2002. 89(3): p. 409–23.

112. Everett, B. and Y. Salamonson, Differences in postoperative opioid consumption in patients prescribed patient-controlled analgesia versus intramuscular injection. Pain Management Nursing, 2005. 6(4): p. 137–44.
113. Kluger, M.T. and H. Owen, Patients' expectations of patient-controlled analgesia. Anaesthesia, 1990. 45(12): p. 1072–4.
114. Lehmann, K.A., Recent developments in patient-controlled analgesia. Journal of Pain and Symptom Management, 2005. 29(5 Suppl): p. S72–89.
115. Ripamonti, C. and E. Bruera, Current status of patient-controlled analgesia in cancer patients. Oncology, 1997. 11(3): p. 373–80, 383–4; discussion 384–6.
116. Rowbotham, D.J., The development and safe use of patient-controlled analgesia [comment]. British Journal of Anaesthesia, 1992. 68(4): p. 331–2.
117. Shapiro, B.S., D.E. Cohen, and C.J. Howe, Patient-controlled analgesia for sickle-cell-related pain. Journal of Pain and Symptom Management, 1993. 8(1): p. 22–8.
118. Sidebotham, D., M.R. Dijkhuizen, and S.A. Schug, The safety and utilization of patient-controlled analgesia. Journal of Pain and Symptom Management, 1997. 14(4): p. 202–9.
119. Maddox, R.R., C.K. Williams, and M. Fields, Respiratory monitoring in patient-controlled analgesia. American Journal of Health-System Pharmacy, 2004. 61(24): p. 2628.
120. Organization, W.H. Tools and techniques to assess pain and other symptoms in elderly patients. Cancer Pain Release 2007 [cited 2007 August]; Available from: http://www.whocancerpain.wisc.edu/eng/17_1-2/Tools.html.
121. Marcantonio, E.R., et al., The relationship of postoperative delirium with psychoactive medications. JAMA, 1994. 272(19): p. 1518–22.
122. Bernards, C.M., et al., Epidural, cerebrospinal fluid, and plasma pharmacokinetics of epidural opioids (part 2): effect of epinephrine. Anesthesiology, 2003. 99(2): p. 466–75.
123. Barre, J., P. Lefort, and M. Payen, [Locoregional anesthesia for injuries of the lower limbs]. Cahiers d Anesthesiologie, 1996. 44(3): p. 197–201.
124. Dunwoody, J.M., C.C. Reichert, and K.L. Brown, Compartment syndrome associated with bupivacaine and fentanyl epidural analgesia in pediatric orthopaedics. Journal of Pediatric Orthopedics, 1997. 17(3): p. 285–8.
125. Morrow, B.C., I.N. Mawhinney, and J.R. Elliott, Tibial compartment syndrome complicating closed femoral nailing: diagnosis delayed by an epidural analgesic technique – case report. Journal of Trauma-Injury Infection and Critical Care, 1994. 37(5): p. 867–8.
126. Pacheco, R.J., et al., Gluteal compartment syndrome after total knee arthroplasty with epidural postoperative analgesia. Journal of Bone and Joint Surgery – British Volume, 2001. 83(5): p. 739–40.
127. Price, C., J. Ribeiro, and T. Kinnebrew, Compartment syndromes associated with postoperative epidural analgesia. A case report. Journal of Bone and Joint Surgery – American Volume, 1996. 78(4): p. 597–9.
128. Sorrentino, F., et al., [Missed compartment syndrome after anterior cruciate ligament-plasty following continuous peridural anesthesia]. Unfallchirurg, 1998. 101(6): p. 491–4.
129. Beerle, B.J. and R.J. Rose, Lower extremity compartment syndrome from prolonged lithotomy position not masked by epidural bupivacaine and fentanyl. Regional Anesthesia, 1993. 18(3): p. 189–90.
130. Montgomery, C.J. and L.B. Ready, Epidural opioid analgesia does not obscure diagnosis of compartment syndrome resulting from prolonged lithotomy position. Anesthesiology, 1991. 75(3): p. 541–3.
131. Mubarak, S.J. and N.C. Wilton, Compartment syndromes and epidural analgesia. Journal of Pediatric Orthopedics, 1997. 17(3): p. 282–4.
132. Grape, S. and M.R. Tramer, Do we need preemptive analgesia for the treatment of postoperative pain? Best Practice and Research. Clinical Anaesthesiology, 2007. 21(1): p. 51–63.
133. Gottschalk, A. and D.S. Smith, New concepts in acute pain therapy: preemptive analgesia. American Family Physician, 2001. 63(10): p. 1979–84.
134. Katz, J., et al., Preemptive analgesia. Clinical evidence of neuroplasticity contributing to postoperative pain. Anesthesiology, 1992. 77(3): p. 439–46.

135. Frerichs, J.A. and L.R. Janis, Preemptive analgesia in foot and ankle surgery. Clinics in Podiatric Medicine and Surgery, 2003. 20(2): p. 237–56.
136. Bugedo, G.J., et al., Preoperative percutaneous ilioinguinal and iliohypogastric nerve block with 0.5% bupivacaine for post-herniorrhaphy pain management in adults. Regional Anesthesia, 1990. 15(3): p. 130–3.
137. Cooper, J., et al., Sciatic nerve blockade improves early postoperative analgesia after open repair of calcaneus fractures. Journal of Orthopaedic Trauma, 2004. 18(4): p. 197–201.
138. Farris, D.A. and M.A. Fiedler, Preemptive analgesia applied to postoperative pain management. AANA Journal, 2001. 69(3): p. 223–8.
139. Kararmaz, A., et al., Intraoperative intravenous ketamine in combination with epidural analgesia: postoperative analgesia after renal surgery. Anesthesia and Analgesia, 2003. 97(4): p. 1092–6.
140. Katz, J., et al., Postoperative morphine use and hyperalgesia are reduced by preoperative but not intraoperative epidural analgesia: implications for preemptive analgesia and the prevention of central sensitization. Anesthesiology, 2003. 98(6): p. 1449–60.
141. Ke, R.W., et al., A randomized, double-blinded trial of preemptive analgesia in laparoscopy. Obstetrics and Gynecology, 1998. 92(6): p. 972–5.
142. Lee, I.O. and I.H. Lee, Systemic, but not intrathecal, ketamine produces preemptive analgesia in the rat formalin model. Acta Anaesthesiologica Sinica, 2001. 39(3): p. 123–7.
143. Richmond, C.E., L.M. Bromley, and C.J. Woolf, Preoperative morphine pre-empts postoperative pain. Lancet, 1993. 342(8863): p. 73–5.
144. Tverskoy, M., et al., Postoperative pain after inguinal herniorrhaphy with different types of anesthesia. Anesthesia and Analgesia, 1990. 70(1): p. 29–35.
145. Yukawa, Y., et al., A prospective randomized study of preemptive analgesia for postoperative pain in the patients undergoing posterior lumbar interbody fusion: continuous subcutaneous morphine, continuous epidural morphine, and diclofenac sodium. Spine, 2005. 30(21): p. 2357–61.
146. McQuay, H.J., Pre-emptive analgesia: a systematic review of clinical studies. Annals of Medicine, 1995. 27(2): p. 249–56.
147. Grube, J.O., M.P. Milad, and J. Damme-Sorenen, Preemptive analgesia does not reduce pain or improve postoperative functioning. Journal of the Society of Laparoendoscopic Surgeons, 2004. 8(1): p. 15–8.
148. Moiniche, S., et al., The effect of balanced analgesia on early convalescence after major orthopaedic surgery. Acta Anaesthesiologica Scandinavica, 1994. 38(4): p. 328–35.
149. Ong, C.K.S., et al., The efficacy of preemptive analgesia for acute postoperative pain management: a meta-analysis. Anesthesia and Analgesia, 2005. 100(3): p. 757–73.
150. Katz, J., Phantom limb pain [erratum appears in Lancet 1998 Feb 21;351(9102):604]. Lancet, 1997. 350(9088): p. 1338–9.
151. Katz, J., Prevention of phantom limb pain by regional anaesthesia. Lancet, 1997. 349(9051): p. 519–20.
152. Bach, S., M.F. Noreng, and N.U. Tjellden, Phantom limb pain in amputees during the first 12 months following limb amputation, after preoperative lumbar epidural blockade. Pain, 1988. 33(3): p. 297–301.
153. Devoghel, J., Small intrathecal doses of lysine acetylsalicylate relieve intractable pain in man. Journal of International Medical Research, 1983. 11: p. 90–91.
154. Ramwell, P., J. Shaw, and R. Jessup, Spontaneous and evoked release of prostaglandins from frog spinal cord. American Journal of Physiology, 1966. 211: p. 998–1104.
155. Willer, J., T. De Brouke, and B. Bussel, et al., Central analgesic effect of ketoprofen in humans: Electrophysiologic evidence for a supraspinal mechanism in a double-blind cross over study. Pain, 1989. 38: p. 1–7.
156. Yaksh, T., Central and peripheral mechanisms for the antialgesic action of acetylsalicylic acid, in Acetylsalicylic acid; new uses for an old drug, H. Barnett, J. Hirsh, and J. Mustard, Editors. 1982, Raven Press: New York. p. 137–51.

157. Lawrence, A.J., et al., Evidence for analgesia mediated by peripheral opioid receptors in inflamed synovial tissue. European Journal of Clinical Pharmacology, 1992. 43(4): p. 351–5.
158. Parsons, C.G., et al., Peripheral opioid receptors mediating antinociception in inflammation. Activation by endogenous opioids and role of the pituitary-adrenal axis. Pain, 1990. 41(1): p. 81–93.
159. Smith, T.W. and P. Buchan, Peripheral opioid receptors located on the rat saphenous nerve. Neuropeptides, 1984. 5(1–3): p. 217–20.
160. Stein, C., et al., Peripheral opioid receptors mediating antinociception in inflammation. Evidence for involvement of mu, delta and kappa receptors. Journal of Pharmacology and Experimental Therapeutics, 1989. 248(3): p. 1269–75.
161. Stein, C., M. Schafer, and A.H. Hassan, Peripheral opioid receptors. Annals of Medicine, 1995. 27(2): p. 219–21.
162. Tverskoy, M., et al., The peripheral effect of fentanyl on postoperative pain. Anesthesia and Analgesia, 1998. 87(5): p. 1121–4.
163. Stefansson, T., I. Wickstrom, and H. Haljamae, Hemodynamic and metabolic effects of ketamine anesthesia in the geriatric patient. Acta Anaesthesiologica Scandinavica, 1982. 26(4): p. 371–7.
164. Neumark, J. and I. Halbgebauer, [Ketamine-halothane combination anesthesia in geriatric and accident surgery]. Wiener Medizinische Wochenschrift, 1973. 123(31): p. 495–8.
165. Bergmans, L., et al., Methadone for phantom limb pain. Clinical Journal of Pain, 2002. 18(3): p. 203–5.
166. Gottschalk, A. and E.A. Ochroch, Preemptive analgesia: what do we do now? Anesthesiology, 2003. 98(1): p. 280–1; author reply 281.
167. Bedford, P., Adverse cerebral effects of anaesthesia on old people. Lancet, 1955. 269: p. 259–63.
168. Newman, M., et al., Longitudinal assessment of neurocognitive function after coronary-artery bypass surgery. New England Journal of Medicine, 2001. 344: p. 395–402.
169. Johnson, T., et al., Postoperative cognitive dysfunction in middle-aged patients. Anesthesiology, 2002. 96(6): p. 1351–7.
170. Maze, M. and M. Todd, Special issue on postoperative cognitive dysfunction: selected reports from the journal-sponsored symposium. Anesthesiology, 2007. 106(3): p. 418–20.
171. Moller, J.T., et al., Long-term postoperative cognitive dysfunction in the elderly ISPOCD1 study. ISPOCD investigators. International Study of Post-Operative Cognitive Dysfunction. Lancet, 1998. 351(9106): p. 857–61.
172. Canet, J., et al., Cognitive dysfunction after minor surgery in the elderly. Acta Anaesthesiologica Scandinavica, 2003. 47(10): p. 1204–10.
173. Bowman, A.M., Sleep satisfaction, perceived pain and acute confusion in elderly clients undergoing orthopaedic procedures. Journal of Advanced Nursing, 1997. 26(3): p. 550–64.
174. Monk, T., et al., Predictors of postoperative cognitive dysfunction following major surgery. Anesthesiology, 2001. 95: p. A50.
175. Biedler, A., et al., Postoperative cognition disorders in elderly patients. The results of the "International Study of Postoperative Cognitive Dysfunction" ISPOCD 1. Anaesthesist, 1999. 48: p. 12884–95.
176. Monk, T., et al., Cerebral oxygen desaturations are associated with postoperative cognitive dysfunction in elderly patients. Anesthesiology, 2002. 96: p. A40.
177. Lennmarken, C., et al., Confirmation that low intraoperative BIS[a] levels predict increased risk of postoperative mortality. Anesthesiology, 2003. 99(Suppl): p. A303.
178. Williams-Russo, P., et al., Post-operative delirium: predictors and prognosis in elderly orthopedic patients. Journal of the American Geriatrics Society, 1992. 40(8): p. 759–67.
179. Hudetz, J., et al., Postoperative cognitive dysfunction in older patients with a history of alcohol abuse. Anesthesiology, 2007. 106(3): p. 423–30.

180. Bryson, G. and A. Wyand, Evidence-based clinical update: general anesthesia and the risk of delirium and postoperative cognitive dysfunction. Canadian Journal of Anaesthesia, 2006. 53(7): p. 669–677.
181. Rasmussen, L., et al., Does anaesthesia cause postoperative cognitive dysfunction? A randomised study of regional versus general anaesthesia in 438 elderly patients. Acta Anaesthesiologica Scandinavica, 2003. 47(3): p. 260–6.
182. Rasmussen, L., Postoperative cognitive dysfunction: incidence and prevention. Best Practice and Research Clinical Anaesthesiology, 2006. 20(2): p. 315–30.
183. Wu, C.L., et al., Postoperative cognitive function as an outcome of regional anesthesia and analgesia. Regional Anesthesia and Pain Medicine, 2004. 29(3): p. 257–68.

Chapter 8
Postoperative Complications

Jung-Hoon Kim

Abstract Not long ago, old patients were frequently denied surgical intervention exclusively based on their age. However, as perioperative management improved significantly over the past decades, many elderly patients with multiple comorbidities have undergone surgical procedures, requiring specialized perioperative care. Contrary to the conventional thought that major complications or death occur intraoperatively, most adverse events arise postoperatively, particularly within the first 24 h, and morbidity and mortality rates are twice as high compared to the intraoperative period. In this chapter, we will discuss several common postoperative complications that present in the elderly.

Keywords Postoperative complication • Hypertension • Heart failure • Arrhythmias • Anemia • Bleeding • Hematoma • Falls • Electrolyte imbalance • Nutrition • Infection • Pressure ulcers • Deep vein thrombosis • Pulmonary embolism • Delirium

8.1 Cardiac Complications

Cardiopulmonary complications are the most frequent type of postoperative complications, followed by thromboembolic, infectious, and hematologic complications [1]. Hypertension, heart failure, and arrhythmias are common cardiovascular complications in older persons after surgery. Evaluation of postoperative

J.-H. Kim (✉)
University of Pennsylvania, Department of Medicine, Division of Geriatric Medicine, 3615 Chestnut Street, Ralston-Penn Center, Philadelphia, PA USA
e-mail: jung-hoon.kim@uphs.upenn.edu

R.J. Pignolo et al. (eds.), *Fractures in the Elderly*, Aging Medicine,
DOI 10.1007/978-1-60327-467-8_8, © Springer Science+Business Media, LLC 2011

hypertension should include non-cardiovascular etiologies such as assessment of pain, urinary retention, anxiety, delirium, electrolyte imbalance as well as a review of medications, assessment of volume status, and evaluation of fluid administration. Antihypertensive drugs can be continued throughout the perioperative period. In particular, perioperative beta-blocker therapy can decrease mortality rates; thus beta-blocker therapy may be continued or initiated preoperatively in patients with coronary artery disease or risk factors for coronary artery disease if there are no contraindications such as beta-blocker sensitive asthma or bradycardia [2, 3]].

When non-cardiovascular causes are ruled out for the etiology of postoperative hypertension, alpha- or beta-adrenergic receptor blockers, calcium channel blockers, or angiotensin-converting enzyme inhibitors can be administered orally or intravenously [3]. The potential adverse effects of certain antihypertensive agents should be considered and monitored carefully. For example, hydralazine, a potent vasodilator, should be avoided in patients with hypertrophic cardiomyopathy because rapid vasodilation and reflex tachycardia induced by it can compromise diastolic filling. In addition, the negative chronotropic effect of beta-blockers can mask the physiologic compensatory response of tachycardia due to intravascular volume depletion.

Older patients with congestive heart failure (CHF), coronary artery disease, or longstanding hypertension are also predisposed to postoperative volume overload, as their cardiac reserve is narrow and can be easily compromised. Studies have shown that CHF is associated with increased morbidity and mortality after noncardiac surgery in patients aged 65 years and older [4, 5]. CHF can develop as a result of any conditions that give rise to excessive intravascular volume overload. Acute cardiac ischemia, tachy- or brady-arrhythmia, and iatrogenic volume overload from intravenous fluid therapy are common causes of postoperative CHF. When patients present with acute symptoms or signs of CHF such as shortness of breath, edema, weight gain, tachypnea, abnormal respiratory sounds, hypoxia, new S3 gallop, or elevated JVP, meticulous evaluation and treatment should be conducted immediately.

The approach to CHF treatment is reducing vascular volume and cardiac afterload. Diuretics and vasodilators are commonly used for systolic heart failure. Occasionally, positive inotropic agents are needed. Although it is often difficult to accurately evaluate volume status in older patients based on physical examination, laboratory, and imaging studies, more invasive monitoring by Swan–Ganz catheter has no proven mortality benefit in high-risk patients [6–8].

In older adults, the mortality of perioperative myocardiac infarction (MI) has been reported to be as high as 40% and the incidence of postoperative MI is associated with a high prevalence of underlying coronary artery disease [9]. Thus, early recognition and proper treatment is critical in the treatment of perioperative MI. The most common cause of postoperative MI is thought to be thrombosis due to coagulation cascade activation by surgery [10]. Older patients do not always present with "typical" features of myocardial ischemia such as chest pain. It can manifest with subtle mental status changes, gastrointestinal symptoms, shortness of breath, or even without any symptoms. Especially, in cognitively impaired patients who are unable to communicate effectively, electrocardiograms should be included in the assessment of postoperative complications.

Cardiac arrhythmias are correlated with MI and heart failure. Postoperative arrhythmias can be an indicator of new cardiac ischemia or heart failure and arrhythmia itself can lead to these complications [11, 12]. Therefore, when new arrhythmia develops postoperatively, the diagnostic work-up is directed toward investigation of possible underlying causes. Often, non-cardiac problems such as electrolyte imbalance (hypokalemia, hypomagnesemia) or infections can give rise to arrhythmia. Common arrhythmias in the postoperative settings are supraventricular tachycardia, atrial fibrillation, and ventricular tachyarrhythmia [12–15]. Polanczyk et al. identified risk factors for perioperative supraventricular tachycardia to be valvular disease, age greater than 70, prior history of supraventricular tachycardia, asthma, heart failure, and premature atrial complexes on preoperative electrocardiogram. Adenosine, beta-blockers, and calcium channel blockers can be used to control ventricular rate as well as promote conversion to sinus rhythm. When atrial fibrillation is diagnosed, anticoagulation should be considered to reduce the risk of stroke, especially if it persists more than 24 h. Electrical or chemical cardioversion, and rate control with beta-blockers or calcium channel blockers are the mainstays of treatment for atrial fibrillation, with each method having different indications, advantages and disadvantages [16, 17].

8.2 Anemia, Bleeding, and Hematoma

Anemia is very common in the elderly. About 9.5% of people aged 65 and older were reported to have anemia, with the incidence and prevalence increasing with age, according to the National Health and Nutrition Examination Survey (NHANES) III study [18]. More specifically, estimates of the prevalence in geriatric patients undergoing orthopedic surgery range from 5 to 45% depending on the definitions of anemia each study applied [19, 20]. Currently the World Health Organization criteria, defining normal hemoglobin values as ≥12 g/dl for women and ≥13.0 g/dl for men, is widely accepted and adopted in most studies.

As most elderly patients have multiple contributing etiologies for anemia, it is difficulty to identify the most likely etiology, especially if it is present in a preoperative evaluation. In the NHANES III study, causes of anemia were deficiencies of iron, folate, and B12, renal insufficiency, anemia of chronic inflammation, and unexplained anemia. However, the most common causes of newly developed anemia following surgery are acute or chronic blood loss, followed by nutritional deficiency and anemia of chronic disease [21]. Regardless of the underlying reasons, a limited physiologic reserve and diminished response to blood loss render the elderly population vulnerable to postoperative hematologic complications including anemia. Wu et al. [22] found that preoperative anemia is associated with a higher 30-day mortality rate.

Blood transfusion is commonly used to rapidly restore hemoglobin levels when patients present with symptoms of anemia or are hemodynamically compromised. However, due to a lack of reliable evidence, there are no clear guidelines, as yet, for blood transfusion therapy. National Clearinghouse Guidelines provide thresholds for postoperative hemoglobin transfusion; transfusion is usually unnecessary at hemoglobin levels >10 g/dl, but required at hemoglobin levels <7 g/dl. Patients with cardiovascular disease, or those expected to have covert cardiovascular disease (e.g., elderly patients or those with peripheral vascular disease), are likely to benefit from transfusion when their hemoglobin level falls below 9 g/dl [23]. Although deficiency of iron, folate, or vitamin B12 can be easily corrected through oral or parenteral therapy, some geriatric patients do not tolerate oral iron well due to gastrointestinal symptoms, requiring intravenous iron. Several small studies on the roles of perioperative intravenous iron and/or erythropoietin therapy showed safety and moderate effectiveness in reduction of allogenic transfusion but large randomized studies are still required [24–26]. In addition, intraoperative blood conservation techniques using cell recovery devices and acute normovolemic hemodilution procedures are other options to utilize the patient's own blood and reduce the need of allogenic blood transfusion [27–30].

Several case reports have described bleeding from surgical wounds and neuropathy induced by hematomas leading to significant postoperative morbidity [31–33]. Therefore, it is important to detect early signs and symptoms of postoperative bleeding and hematoma (e.g., unusual pain, ecchymosis, marked swelling, decreasing hemoglobin, any neural deficit). Surgical decompression or conservative management, as well as restoration of appropriate hemoglobin levels, should be instituted when appropriate for the treatment of postoperative bleeding and hematoma.

It is not always simple to manage anticoagulation therapy during the perioperative period. In addition, preventing deep vein thrombosis with prophylactic anticoagulation may not be safe in certain situations. Perioperative management of anticoagulation for deep vein thrombosis prophylaxis is discussed in detail in Chap. 5.

8.3 Falls

About 30% of persons 65 years and older experience at least one fall every year, 1.8 million elderly people visit emergency departments for treatment, and more than 13,000 people die as a result of falls [34]. Injuries from falls can vary from bruises and minor contusions to severe soft tissue wounds and fractures [35]. Hip fractures are almost always associated with falls either in the community or inpatient setting [36, 37]. People admitted to hospitals or residing in nursing homes have three times higher incidence of falls than community dwellers. The rate of falls in elderly inpatients ranges from 2.2 to 27% and incidence of falls peak at the second postoperative week when patients begin to resume ambulatory function [38].

Many studies have identified the risk factors for falls. These can be categorized into intrinsic and extrinsic factors. Intrinsic risk factors supported by many studies are age greater than 75, a history of falls, cognitive impairment, functional disability, gait and balance disorders, comorbidities, and visual impairment [39]. Extrinsic factors include environmental factors and polypharmacy or high-risk medications. Stevens et al. identified several environmental hazards (uneven surfaces, cluttered environment, rugs, poor illumination, use of restraints, Foley's catheter placement, IV poles) associated with falls [40, 41]. Of note, use of bed side rails does not decrease or prevent falls and fall-related injuries [42]. Also polypharmacy or "high-risk" medications such as opioids, antihistamines, selective serotonin reuptake inhibitors, tricyclic antidepressants, sedatives, and anticoagulants are considered a strong predictor of falling [43]. The risk of falling increases when multiple risk factors are combined. Tinetti et al. [44] reported that the percentage of falling in persons with four or more risk factors increased from 27 to 78% compared with those with none or just one risk factor.

When a patient sustains a fall, a comprehensive physical examination and a review of predisposing risk factors should be performed. Vital signs including orthostatic blood pressure should be measured since syncopal episodes resulting from comorbidities or deconditioning from operations are closely related to falls. Special attention should be taken in neurologic evaluation, of which evaluation of gait and balance is an essential part. Mental and psychological status exams should not be excluded since delirium plays a significant role in the risk of falling in acute settings.

At least 24–48 h of close monitoring is warranted to detect delayed complications of falls, especially in the hospital setting. Along with treatment of injuries, strategies for the prevention of future falls should be sought after falls. Several randomized controlled trials [45–48] have demonstrated that multidisciplinary and multifactorial programs show a modest reduction of the incidence of falls. These multifaceted approaches contain general and individualized safety precautions. Avoidance of physical restraints and unnecessary IV or Foley's catheter placement, encouragement of early ambulation, availability of a call light, the use of low-rise beds and floor mats, proper illumination, and scheduled toileting are examples of general safety measurements [49, 50].

A review of medications to reduce those that pose a high risk and encouragement of physical activities to enhance balance and gait are also crucial components of individualized fall prevention strategies. The individualized assessment and development of fall prevention strategies are important and beneficial, especially for patients with cognitive impairment, osteoporosis, brain injury, or other predisposing diseases that make them vulnerable to falls and fractures [51]. Education for patients and care givers, and discharge instructions for fall prevention should also be ensured in the transition from hospital to primary care.

A more detailed description of the approach to falls can be found in Chap. 3 dedicated to falls.

8.4 Electrolyte Imbalances, Fluctuating Volume Status, and Nutritional Considerations

The kidneys play an important role in the homeostasis of fluid and electrolytes, as well as in drug metabolism. The aging kidneys contribute to decreased glomerular filtration rate, reduced urine concentration ability, and impaired thirst mechanism. Normal physiologic changes of the kidneys with aging, in addition to acute, "non-physiologic stress" from surgery, predispose older patients to develop fluid and electrolyte imbalances. In this section, several common electrolyte imbalances and the importance of postoperative nutrition in older patients will be discussed.

8.4.1 Hyponatremia

As older people have limited cardiopulmonary reserve they are very vulnerable to subtle volume changes postoperatively. A common electrolyte imbalance in patients is hyponatremia [52]. Etiologies can be multifactorial, including medications (diuretics, NSAIDS) and underlying heart (CHF), renal (salt wasting nephropathy), adrenal (adrenal insufficiency), or thyroid (hypothyroidism) diseases. Clinically, hyponatremia is associated with three different states of extracellular fluid (ECF) volume: decreased ECF volume (e.g., gastrointestinal losses, adrenal and renal salt-wasting conditions), increased ECF volume (e.g., heart failure), or normal ECF volume (e.g., syndrome of inappropriate antidiuretic hormone or SIADH) [53]. The most common cause of hyponatremia is SIADH, but regardless of the underlying cause, it is related to an excessive release of antidiuretic hormone, which can be stimulated in the postoperative period by pain, narcotics, nausea, and anesthesia. This hormone mediates retention of free water by increasing reabsorption of water in the kidneys and reducing the concentration of sodium in the body. Moreover, a diminished ability to eliminate excess fluid in older persons exacerbates water retention. Sunderam et al. [54] reported that the mortality rate doubled in elderly patients 65 years of age or older with hyponatremia. The most common manifestation of hyponatremia is alteration in neurologic function, such as mild cognitive impairment, seizure, and coma due to brain edema. Improvement of neurologic symptoms usually follows days after hyponatremia is corrected.

SIADH can be caused by numerous conditions, such as infection, pulmonary and central nervous system disorders, and medications [55]. Well-recognized medications widely taken by the elderly that may cause SIADH include diuretics (thiazide, furosemide), antidepressants (SSRIs, trazodone, venlafaxine, duloxetine), antipsychotics (haloperidol, quetiapine), antihypertensives (ACE-I, ARB, carvediol), drugs for urinary incontinence (tolterodine, oxybutynin), proton pump inhibitors, and donepezil. Physicians should be aware of these potential offending drugs and administer them cautiously during the immediate postoperative period. The diagnosis of SIADH is made after excluding other hyponatremic conditions;

low plasma osmolality (<275 mosmol/kg) and inappropriate urine concentration (urine osmolality > 100 mosmol/kg) are of pathognomic value [56].

Although treatment for older patients is not different from younger ones, slow correction and frequent monitoring are the key to avoid iatrogenic cardiovascular and/or neurologic complications.

8.4.2 Hypernatremia

Hypernatremia can occur as a result of loss of free water or gain of sodium. Older adults have a decreased ability to concentrate urine and an impaired thirst mechanism, which predisposes to the development of hypernatremia especially in acute settings. Those patients with cognitive impairment or who are not ambulatory are at the highest risk for hypernatremia as well as those with infections, fever, and neurologic disorders. Mortality in these patients has been reported to be as high as 70% [57]. In a retrospective analysis of 15,187 geriatric inpatients, Snyder et al. described the incidence of hypernatremia to be 1%; the most common cause was surgery (21%), followed by febrile illness (20%) [58]. Common medications associated with the development of hypernatremia are diuretics, lithium, demeclocycline, phenytoin, ofloxacin, and amphotericin B. These drugs should be used cautiously in older patients.

A study of the symptoms of hypernatremia in 150 geriatric patients found that tachycardia, low blood pressure secondary to volume depletion and cognitive dysfunction due to neuronal cell shrinkage were the most common presenting signs [59]. The declining cognitive function associated with hypernatremia may be difficult to notice in elderly patients who have a preexisting cognitive impairment. Therefore, frequent monitoring of electrolytes and close observation of mental status is very important to prevent these events and initiate early treatment. The free water deficit should be replaced slowly, usually over 72 h.

8.4.3 Potassium Imbalance

Many elderly patients have a high risk of potassium imbalance as nephrotoxic insults in the settings of chronic kidney disease are common in the postoperative period. Often drugs such as NSAIDS, angiotensin converting enzyme inhibitors, potassium supplements, and beta-blockers can lead to hyperkalemia [53]. Many older patients on diuretics take potassium supplementation. Thus, close monitoring of potassium is important especially when those patients are not receiving diuretics postoperatively to manage intravascular volume.

Since hypokalemia affects the cardiovascular, neurologic, muscular, and renal systems, early identification and treatment are keys to minimize morbidity and mortality. There are many potential etiologies of hypokalemia in elderly patients during the postoperative period (such as vomiting, diarrhea, and nasogastric suction) all of which can induce metabolic alkalosis, shifting potassium into cells. Renal loss from the use of diuretics, underlying kidney disease, and endocrine problems are also common causes. Correction of underlying condition(s) and appropriate potassium repletion are the major approaches in the treatment of hypokalemia.

8.4.4 Imbalances in Calcium and Other Electrolytes

There are multiple causes for hypercalcemia and hypocalcemia in the elderly and these are not commonly associated with postoperative complications. However, since many older patients who have sustained fractures are likely to have underlying osteoporosis, physicians should ensure that patients take adequate amounts of calcium and vitamin D to reduce the risk of future fractures. Currently as of 2009, a total of 1,200 mg of daily calcium from dietary and supplemental sources is recommended by the National Osteoporosis Foundation.

Renal insufficiency, poor or excessive dietary intake, and certain medications can contribute to alterations in other electrolytes. For example, a high-calcium diet may inhibit zinc absorption which is an essential dietary element for proper wound healing [53, 60], and hypocalcemia cannot be corrected without correction of hypomagnesemia [53]. Hence, monitoring of calcium and magnesium is imperative in ill geriatric patients.

8.4.5 Nutrition

Older patients are predisposed to under- or malnourishment in the postoperative period. Up to 20% of patients with hip fractures [61, 62] were reported to have malnutrition. In particular, protein depletion adversely affects the outcome of surgery and is associated with poor wound healing and decreased 1 year survival [63, 64]. Patients with low serum albumin (<3.5 g/dl) and low total lymphocyte count (<1,500 cells/μl) have longer hospital stays (2.9 times), higher 1 year mortality (3.9 times), and are less likely to return to their pre-fracture level of functional (4.6 times) [65]. By contrast, patients with hip fractures who had received aggressive postoperative nutritional protein supplementation had shorter hospitalizations, appropriate weight gains, and declines in postoperative complications [66–69].

Most patients should be advised to resume oral intake as early as within 12 h postoperatively. Intake of supplementary formula was found to have a beneficial effect on surgery outcome [70]. If adequate oral intake is not achieved, temporary nasogastric tube feeding should be considered as an alternative or supplementary method [71, 72], although tolerability may be low. It may be prudent to consult with a dietician to meet patient-specific nutritional requirements.

8.5 Infections: Surgical Site Infection, Urinary Tract Infection, and Pneumonia

Elderly patients may have decreased immune function resulting from both age-related declines in immunity and comorbidities. Therefore, typical signs and symptoms of infection (for example fever) may be absent in frail older adults with serious infections, and it is not uncommon that they present with confusion, falls, or non-specific decline in functional status. If these occur in demented patients, it becomes very difficult for physicians to differentiate infection from underlying mental illness; thus, physical and psychological changes in the elderly should be carefully monitored postoperatively.

8.5.1 Surgical Site Infection

Surgical site infection is a serious postoperative complication. A recent study by Kaye et al. [73] demonstrated that elderly patients with postoperative surgical site infection had three times higher mortality and their hospital stays were 2 weeks longer on average. *Staphylococcus aureus* was the most common pathogen in surgical site infection, followed by coagulase negative *Staphylococcus*, *Enterococcus* spp., *Streptococcus*, *E. coli* and *Pseudomonas*. Of note, 58.2% of the staphylococci were methicillin resistant. Interestingly, one of the significant predictors of surgical site infection in the elderly after orthopedic procedures is the location from which patients arrive, including nursing homes, assisted living facilities, or other hospitals. This may be explained by the diminished general health status compared to those who live at home [74]. However, contrary to general belief, factors related to frailty such as decreased daily living activities, comorbidities, and duration of hospitalization prior to surgery were not reported to be independent risk factors for a surgical infection after orthopedic surgery [74].

A decreased incidence of surgical wound infections in patients with hip fracture was observed with the use of antibiotics prior to surgery [75]. Gillespie et al. reviewed 22 trials of prophylactic antibiotic use for femoral neck and other long bone fractures and demonstrated that deep wound infection was decreased by 64% and urinary tract infection by 44% [76]. Hence, appropriate use of antibiotics may reduce the incidence of common postoperative infections. The optimal timing for administration of antibiotics is within the 2 h prior to surgery and until 24 h after surgery [77, 78].

8.5.2 Pulmonary Complications: Pneumonia

In the elderly, a diminished ability to protect the airway from aspiration, and their decreased vital capacity, makes them prone to developing postoperative pulmonary infections. Atelectasis is a common predisposing factor to the development of pneumonia. Arozullah et al. proposed a clinical prediction model for postoperative pneumonia in noncardiac surgical patients based on a database study of 160,000 veterans [79]. Patients were divided into five risk classes based on risk index scores generated from predisposing factors such as type of operation, age, functional status, weight loss, chronic obstructive pulmonary disease, general anesthesia, impaired sensorium, cerebral vascular accident, blood urea nitrogen level, recent transfusion, emergency surgery, long-term steroid use, smoking, and alcohol use. Pneumonia rates were 0.2% among those with 0–15 risk points, 1.2% for those with 16–25 risk points, 4.0% for those with 26–40 risk points, 9.4% for those with 41–55 risk points, and 15.3% for those with more than 55 risk points. This index may be useful in identification of high-risk patients and in providing early preventative measures, including percussion, voluntary cough, incentive spirometry, and encouragement of early ambulation [80].

8.5.3 Urinary Tract Infection

Postoperative urinary tract infections are common problems amongst the elderly [81]. The incidence of urinary tract infection after hip fracture surgery was reported to be between 23 and 25% [82–84]. After the second day of catheterization, the risk of UTI increases by 5–10% [85, 86].

The most common organisms associated with short-term catheter use during an operative procedure are usually from skin colonization, and include *Escherichia coli*, enterococci, *Pseudomonas*, *Klebsiella*, *Enterobacter*, *Staphylococcus epidermidis*, *Staphylococcus aureus*, and *Serratia*. The gold standard diagnostic test in patients with an indwelling catheter is urine culture after documentation of significant pyuria by urinalysis (usually >50 WBC/hpw). The growth of 10^5 or more organisms per milliliter of urine can diagnose UTI with a 90% specificity and a 37% sensitivity [87]. Treatment of UTI is straightforward but separate consideration should be paid to asymptomatic bacteriuria, which does not need to be treated except in patients who are undergoing implantation of a prosthesis, are immunocompromised, or harbor strains that have a high incidence of bacteremia (e.g., *S. marcescens*) [88]. Treatment with appropriate antibiotics for 10–14 days, depending upon the severity of symptoms and rapidity of response, is generally recommended for UTIs associated with indwelling catheters [89]. Choice of antibiotics should be based upon the culture results. If treatment is needed before culture results are available, the urine Gram stain, previous culture results, or hospital-specific antimicrobial sensitivity patterns should be considered when initiating empiric antibiotics.

Removing indwelling urinary catheters within 24 h of surgery has been shown to reduce the incidence of urinary retention [90]. One randomized controlled trial also demonstrated that intermittent urinary catheterization rather than indwelling catheterization accelerated recovery of the normal voiding pattern by 4 days [91].

Physicians also need to pay attention to common medications that can contribute to urinary retention such as sedatives and anticholinergics.

8.6 Pressure Ulcers

A pressure ulcer is defined by The National Pressure Ulcer Advisory Panel (NPUAP) as localized injury to the skin and/or underlying tissue, usually over a bony prominence, as a result of pressure, or pressure in combination with shear and/or friction [92]. The incidence of pressure ulcer in patients with hip fractures is reported to range from 10 to 40% [93, 94]. Common sites of occurrence are the ischium (28%), sacrum (17–27%), trochanter (12–19%), and heel (9–18%) [92, 95–98]. In geriatric patients, the occiput and the thoracic kyphotic areas can also be involved, as those hospitalized are often likely to lie in a supine position for a long period of time. Pressure ulcers are detected by their appearance and location overlying a bony prominence, but need to be distinguished from ulcers associated with by diabetic neuropathy, vascular insufficiency, and cellulitis.

The NPUAP published an update to pressure ulcer staging in 2007. These are: Stage 1, Intact skin with non-blanchable redness of a localized area usually over a bony prominence. Stage 2, Partial thickness loss of dermis presenting as a shallow open ulcer with a red pink wound bed, without slough. Stage 3, Full thickness tissue loss. Subcutaneous fat may be visible, but bone, tendon, or muscle is not exposed. Undermining and tunneling may also be seen. Stage 4, Full thickness skin loss with exposed bone, tendon or muscle. These ulcers often include undermining and tunneling. (Table 8.1) Unstageable: Full thickness tissue loss in which the base of the ulcer is covered by slough (yellow, tan, gray, green, or brown) and/or eschar (tan, brown, or black) in the wound bed.

Pathogenesis of pressure ulcers is multifactorial, usually as a result of a combination of external factors (pressure, shearing forces, friction, moisture) and host factors [99]. The host factors include immobility, incontinence, nutritional compromise, skin perfusion, and neurologic diseases [100–104]. Haleem et al. [105] identified risk factors for pressure ulcers in patients with hip fractures as increased age, diabetes mellitus, a lower mental status test score, a lower mobility score, lower admission hemoglobin, and an intra-operative drop in blood pressure.

Table 8.1 Progression of Pressure Ulcers

Stages	Features
Stage 1	Intact skin with non-blanchable redness
Stage 2	Partial thickness loss of dermis
Stage 3	Full thickness skin loss without exposure of bone, tendon or muscle
Stage 4	Full thickness skin loss with exposed bone, tendon or muscle

An increased risk of nosocomial infections and prolonged hospitalization is associated with development of pressure ulcers during inpatient stays [93, 106]. Infection is the most common major complication of pressure ulcers. It can present as superficial infection or seriously as cellulitis, osteomyelitis, and sepsis. Commonly isolated organisms are Proteus mirabilis, group D streptococci, Escherichia coli, Staphylococcus species, Pseudomonas species, and Corynebacterium organisms [107]. Although infection of pressure ulcers is usually indicated by local signs such as warmth, erythema, tenderness, discharge, and the presence of a foul odor [108], delayed wound healing can be the only sign of infection. In the elderly, systemic signs (leukocytosis, fever) are not always present [109].

Distinguishing between bacterial colonization and invasion is challenging as almost all pressure ulcers have bacterial colonization and it precedes the development of infection. Wound swab culture is a simple procedure that is often used to guide antibiotic selection for patients who are not candidates for invasive diagnostic procedures such as bone or tissue biopsy. However, guidelines on the treatment of pressure ulcers by the Agency for Healthcare Research and Quality recommend against using swab cultures to define the microbiology of a pressure ulcer as it merely reflects bacterial colonization [110]. The gold standard method of wound culture is still culturing deep tissue specimens sampled from a surgically cleaned and debrided ulcer, along with blood cultures if necessary. The general concepts of wound care are keeping the wound moist and intact skin dry, as well as removing dead tissue. Currently, hydrocolloid dressings have been supported by many experts because of their excellent effect on rapid wound healing, fewer dressing requirements, and cost-effectiveness [111].

Necrotic tissue prevents wound healing and provides an environment for bacteria to grow; so it should be debrided. There are several debridement methods including enzymatic, autolytic, mechanical, surgical, and biosurgical (e.g., using larvae-sterile maggots of the green bottle fly, *Lucilia sericata*) [112]. The choice of method should be based on a consideration of the patient's ability to tolerate the procedure, as some of these (e.g., mechanical, surgical) may cause pain [111, 113].

The strategy of pressure ulcer prevention consists of skin care measures, relief of skin pressure using pressure-relieving devices or frequent position changes, and good nutrition (increased protein intake 1.25–1.50 g/kg) [111]. Placing pillows under the legs, applying transparent film dressings on the heels, and changing the patient's position regularly and frequently are good examples of pressure ulcer prevention for the heel [111, 113, 114]. Active utilization of pressure-relieving devices such as foam, gel, low air loss, or air-fluidized mattresses also helps to prevent ulcers and accelerate wound healing in high-risk patients. Education of patients, caregivers, and care providing staff are critical parts of pressure ulcer prevention.

8.7 Pain Management

Insufficient postoperative pain management can lead to delayed ambulation and a prolonged hospital stay. Conversely, adequate pain control can have a positive impact on the rapid resumption of functional status [115]. Choosing the right analgesics is sometimes challenging to physicians because older patients are vulnerable to side effects of analgesics and drug interactions, and in cognitively impaired patients it is very difficult to assess the response to medications. Therapy with "round the clock" non-narcotics such as acetaminophen along with short-acting opioids for breakthrough pain has been shown to be effective for pain control in geriatric hip fracture patients [116]. Prevention of analgesic-induced side effects is as important as good pain control. When opioids are used, good bowel regimens should be included to avoid constipation.

See Chap. 7 for a comprehensive overview of peri-operative pain management.

8.8 Deep Vein Thrombosis, Pulmonary Embolism, and Fat Embolism

8.8.1 Deep Vein Thrombosis

Deep Vein Thromboses (DVTs) are common in patients with fractures. The incidence rate in patients after hip fracture surgery was reported to be 27% [117, 118] and the rate of fatal pulmonary embolism was 1.4–2.5% for the first 3 months after hip fracture surgery [117].

The Seventh American College of Chest Physicians Consensus Conference on Antithrombotic and Thrombolytic Therapy recommends the use of unfractionated heparin, low molecular weight heparin, fondaparinux, or warfarin (INR target range 2–3), starting before orthopedic surgery and continuing until the recovery of full ambulation [119, 120]. Among these agents, fondaparinux has the best efficacy among DVT prevention modalities [121]. Platelet count should be regularly monitored to detect heparin-induced thrombocytopenia in patients on heparin products (unfractionated or LMWH). Aspirin alone is not recommended for DVT prophylaxis.

See Chap. 5 for a detailed review of DVT prophylaxis.

8.8.2 Pulmonary Embolism

One of the most serious complications following orthopedic surgery is pulmonary embolism (PE). Immobilization from orthopedic procedures, underlying diseases such as heart failure, malignancy, myeloproliferative disease, and age itself pose a high risk for developing thrombosis and subsequent PE in the elderly. PE develops most commonly as a result of migration of thrombi from the deep venous system of the lower extremity [122]. The incidence of PE increases with age with an annual incidence of 1.8 per 1,000 among persons of age 65–69 as compared with 3.1 in those age 85–89 [123]. Especially after orthopedic surgery, the incidence of PE is reported to be as high as 30% for total hip replacement surgery, 7% for total knee replacement surgery, and 24% for hip fracture surgery [124].

Elderly patients with PE can present with a wide variety of symptoms and signs from mild shortness of breath to sudden cardiopulmonary arrest. Since the symptoms and signs of PE are nonspecific and difficult to differentiate from patients' underlying cardiopulmonary diseases, it is often mis- or under-diagnosed. Morpurgo et al. reported in 200 autopsy cases that 78% of massive or submassive PE had not been detected by physicians [125]. The most common symptoms and signs include dyspnea at rest or on exertion, cough, pleuritic pain, orthopnea, calf or thigh swelling or pain, tachypnea, tachycardia, and abnormal lung sounds such as crackles and decreased breath sounds [126]. Therefore, when assessing a patient presenting with unexplained tachypnea, tachycardia, or change in mental status in postoperative periods, PE should be included in the differential diagnosis.

The diagnosis of PE can be challenging due to the lack of specificity and sensitivity of these presentations. Therefore, a scoring system that provides a pretest probability has been developed to guide clinicians to consider further diagnostic tests to prove the diagnosis of PE [127]. However, since a clinician's subjective judgment strongly influences the scores, the objectivity and validity of this scoring system are still being debated. Therefore, diagnostic tests should be performed when clinical suspicion is present. These can be categorized into laboratory tests and imaging studies. Currently, imaging studies such as a ventilation–perfusion lung scan (V/Q scan) and single- or multi-detector computed tomographic angiography (CT angiography) play a more important role than other laboratory tests in the diagnosis of PE.

The V/Q scan uses a pattern of a mismatch of perfusion with ventilation and the results are displayed as normal, high, intermediate, and low probabilities. Until recently, this was long considered one of the definitive diagnostic tests for PE. The Prospective Investigation of Pulmonary Embolism Diagnosis (PIOPED) study demonstrated that the predictive value of the V/Q scan varies depending on clinical suspicion. For example, when a high-probability V/Q scan is combined with a high clinical pretest probability, the likelihood of PE was 96%, but only 56–88% had confirmed PE when a high probability V/Q scan is associated with a low clinical pretest probability. In one study, there are up to 70% of patients who remain undiagnosed even after the V/Q scan is performed [128]. Therefore, additional tests are required in many situations and the study itself is not often feasible in certain patients who are not able to follow the instructions of scan protocols. These limitations make CT angiography a more preferable choice for a diagnosis of PE. A study reported that single detector CT angiography had a sensitivity of 70% and a specificity of 88% with 84% negative predictive value, and 76% a positive predictive value [129]. Although it has limited sensitivity in detecting subsegmental emboli, it has additional advantage in detecting other pulmonary diseases. Also, a negative CT angiography was able to function as a decision-making point for the safe withdrawal of anticoagulation therapy [130].

Pulmonary angiography is a definitive diagnostic test for PE but because it has several disadvantages including its invasiveness and high intravenous contrast exposure, it should be reserved until other test results turn up undiagnostic and the angiography results will change treatment plans. Ultrasonography and color-flow Doppler may be helpful for patients with nondiagnostic V/Q scan and CT angiography. Patients with positive test results of ultrasonography can receive anti-coagulation therapy regardless of V/Q scan or CT angiography results.

The most common EKG findings are sinus tachycardia and right-sided strain pattern, but classic patterns like S1Q3T3 (S wave in Lead I, Q wave in Lead III, T wave inversion in Lead III) are seen in less than 20% of cases [131]. The chest X-ray can be normal but the classic "hampton hump" sign caused by pleural infarction can also be seen. The D-dimer test has been intensively investigated as a role for a non-invasive, radiation-free test for DVT and PE. However, the specificity of this test has been questioned and been shown to depend upon the type of assay [132, 133]. Furthermore, the specificity was found to be lower in geriatric patients. Therefore, this test should be used in conjunction with other imaging studies [134–136]. Arterial blood gas studies are also nonspecific. Arterial hypoxemia and an increased alveolar–arterial (A–a) gradient are common findings but these cannot be used in diagnosis of PE since an elevated A–a gradient is not uncommon in a geriatric population [136].

Treatment for PE consists of supportive care, anticoagulation, and close monitoring of bleeding complications from anticoagulation therapy. Adequate intravascular volume, which can be compromised due to a decreased cardiac output and supplementary oxygen should be ensured. In addition, immediate anticoagulation therapy with either unfractionated or low-molecular-weight heparin should not be delayed until the completion of the diagnostic work-up when there is moderate-to-high clinical suspicion of PE, because the mortality rate is highest within the first few hours of clot development.

Oral anticoagulation with warfarin should also be started with heparin therapy and heparin can be discontinued when warfarin reaches therapeutic range, usually with an INR of 2–3. Duration of warfarin therapy depends on possible underlying etiologies. If PE occurs with reversible risk factors such as surgery and immobilization, warfarin therapy should be maintained for 3–6 months. However, patients with recurrent thromboembolism or irreversible risk factors such as Factor V Leiden mutation, protein C and S deficiency, or antiphospholipid antibodies should receive warfarin for a longer period of time. Patients with a first episode of idiopathic thromboembolism should be treated with warfarin for at least 6 months [137, 138].

Thrombolytic therapy should be considered for hemodynamically unstable patients. Although there is no proven mortality benefit from thrombolytic therapy, many studies have demonstrated hemodynamic and radiographic improvement in critically ill patients.

When a patient with PE is not a candidate for anticoagulation therapy due to absolute contraindications such as recent surgery, active bleeding, or hemorrhagic stroke, or when there is a foreseeable fatal clot burden from recurrent thromboembolism, an inferior vena cava filter (IVC filter or Greenfield filter) insertion should be considered [137–140].

8.8.3 Fat Embolism

Fat embolism (FE) is a potentially fatal condition causing high mortality and morbidity in trauma patients. It can develop as a result of entrance of fat droplets into the circulatory system. The majority of cases are associated with major trauma such as long bone and pelvic fractures. The incidence of fat embolism has been reported from 0.9 to 23% in patients with fractures [141, 142]. A higher incidence was associated with multiple fractures and closed fractures [143, 144].

Clinical manifestations of FE consist of a classic triad: respiratory abnormalities, skin rash, and neurologic changes [144, 145]. These symptoms and signs usually present 24–72 h after the trauma. Frequently, respiratory abnormalities such as tachypnea, hypoxia, and dyspnea precede other skin and neurologic problems. FE often leads to respiratory failure requiring mechanical ventilation. When these fat emboli go to the central nervous system and the skin after escaping the pulmonary circulation, neurologic changes, including confusion, disorientation, personality change, vision change, paresis, and seizures can develop, followed by the occurrence of skin rash such as characteristic petechial rash in the conjunctiva, skin folds, and oral mucous membrane [146].

Diagnosis is usually made based on typical clinical features. However, this is often challenging because there is no definitive test to rely on. Thus, several diagnostic criteria, for example, Lindeque's criteria, Gurd's criteria, and a fat embolism index have been proposed. But, the sensitivity and specificity of these criteria still remain unclear [147, 148].

Laboratory tests may be helpful. An unexplained drop of hematocrit, thrombocytopenia due to intravascular coagulopathy, and hypocalcemia due to calcium binding to fatty acids can be present.

There are several radiographic changes suggestive of FE but not very specific to this condition. The chest X-ray findings vary from normal to diffuse or patchy air space consolidation. The signs of alveolar edema, hemorrhage, and inflammatory changes can be seen on chest CT scan [145, 149]. It may also be useful to confirm the presence of fat globules in urine or sputum in diagnosis of FE [148].

No specific treatment has been developed for FE, which conversely emphasizes the importance of prevention. Early immobilization and operative fixation of fractures and application of surgical techniques that minimizes an increase of intraosseous pressure are reported to reduce the incidence of FE [150]. Prophylaxis with corticosteroids decreased the incidence and severity of FE in several studies [147, 151] but the routine use of prophylactic corticosteroid is still controversial. Once the diagnosis of FE is highly considered, supportive care is a mainstay of treatment plans. Adequate oxygenation and hydration, and proper prophylaxis of DVT and GI bleeding, should be ensured [152]. Overall mortality is reported to be approximately 7% [153].

8.9 Postoperative Cognitive Dysfunction: Delirium

Delirium may be the most common postoperative complication in geriatric patients. The incidence was reported to be as high as 62% among hip fracture patients [154]. It is often underdiagnosed and undertreated [155]. There is growing evidence that delirium is associated with increasing mortality, prolonged length of hospital stay, high likelihood of post-discharge nursing home placement, poor functional recovery, and even increased risk of death 2 years after hospital discharge [156–158]. The most common risk factors are advanced age, dementia, sensory impairment, a history of alcohol abuse, electrolyte imbalance, use of psychotropic medications, and changes in sleep–wake cycle [159, 160].

Clinicians can diagnose delirium by utilizing the Confusion Assessment Method (CAM) which incorporates the four key features of delirium. These components are: (1) acute change in mental status and fluctuating course; (2) inattention; (3) disorganized thinking; and (4) altered level of consciousness. The diagnosis of delirium requires the presence of components 1 and 2, and either 3 or 4 [161, 162]. Once delirium is suspected, a comprehensive history and thorough physical examination with a focused neuropsychiatric exam, review of medications, assessment of pain, and targeted diagnostic laboratory tests are essential.

The major principles in the prevention and treatment of delirium consist of identification and correction of reversible risk factors. Removing physical restraints as well as unnecessary Foley catheter and intravenous lines, resuming ambulation, minimizing environmental changes, and verbal and visual reorientation are important. When pharmacologic treatment is considered, high-potent antipsychotics are preferred due to their favorable side effect profiles [159, 160, 163]. Chapter 6 provides a detailed overview of post-operative delirium.

References

1. McLaughlin M et al. Preoperative status and risk of complications in patients with hip fractures. J Gen Intern Med 2006;21:219–225.
2. Siddiqui AK, Ahmed S, Delbeau H, Conner D, Maffana J. Lack of physician concordance with guidelines on the perioperative use of beta-blockers. Arch Intern Med 2004;164(6):664–667.

3. Eagle KA, Berger PB, Calkins H, et al. ACC/AHA guideline update for perioperative cardiovascular evaluation for noncardiac surgery-executive summary. Circulation 2002; 105(10):1257–1267.
4. Hernandez AF, Whellan DJ, Stroud S, Sun JL, O'Connor CM, Jollis JG. Outcomes in heart failure patients after major noncardiac surgery. J Am Coll Cardiol 2004;44(7):1446–1453.
5. Dunlop WE, Rosenblood L, Lawrason L, Birdsall L, Rusnak CH. Effects of age and severity of illness on outcome and length of stay in geriatric surgical patients. Am J Surg 1993;165(5):577–580.
6. Shah MR, Hasselblad V, et al. Impact of the pulmonary artery catheter in critically ill patients: meta-analysis of randomized clinical trials. JAMA 2005;294:1664–1670.
7. Binanay C, Califf RM, Hasselblad V, et al. ESCAPE investigators and ESCAPE study coordinators. Evaluation study of congestive heart failure and pulmonary artery catheterization effectiveness: the ESCAPE trial. JAMA 2005;294:1625–1633.
8. Shah MR, O'Connor CM, Sopko G, et al. Evaluation study of congestive heart failure and pulmonary artery catheterization effectiveness (ESCAPE): design and rationale. Am Heart J 2001;141:528–535.
9. Mangano DT. Perioperative cardiac morbidity. Anesthesiology 1990;72:153–184.
10. Souders J, Rooke A. Perioperative care for geriatric patients. Ann Longterm Care 2005;13: 17–29.
11. Goldman L. Cardiac risks and complications of noncardiac surgery. Ann Intern Med 1983;98:513–514.
12. Pedersen T, Eliasen K, Henriksen E. A prospective study of risk factors and cardiopulmonary complications associated with anaesthesia and surgery: risk indicators of cardiopulmonary morbidity. Acta Anaesthesiol Scand 1990;34:144–155.
13. Polanczyk CA, Goldman L, Marcantonio ER, Orav EJ, Lee TH. Supraventricular arrhythmia in patients having noncardiac surgery: clinical correlates and effect on length of stay. Ann Intern Med 1998;129:279–285.
14. Pedersen T, Eliasen K, Henriksen E. A prospective study of risk factors and cardiopulmonary complications associated with anaesthesia and surgery: risk indicators of cardiopulmonary morbidity. Acta Anaesthesiol Scand 1990;34:144–155.
15. McLaughlin M et al. Preoperative status and risk of complications in patients with hip fractures. J Gen Intern Med 2006;21:219–225.
16. Khoo CW, Lip GY. Acute management of atrial fibrillation. Chest 2009;135(3):849–859.
17. Naccarelli GV, Wolbrette DL, Khan M, Bhatta L, Hynes J, Samii S, Luck J. Old and new antiarrhythmic drugs for converting and maintaining sinus rhythm in atrial fibrillation: comparative efficacy and results of trials. Am J Cardiol 2003;91(6A):15D–26D.
18. Guralnik JM, Eisenstaedt RS, Ferrucci L, Klein HG, Woodman RC. Prevalence of anemia in persons 65 years and older in the United States: evidence for a high rate of unexplained anemia. Blood 2004;104(8):2263–2268.
19. Haljamae H, Stefansson T, Wickstrom I. Preanesthetic evaluation of the female geriatric patient with hip fracture. Acta Anaesthesiol Scand 1982;26:393–402.
20. Gruson KI, Aharonoff GB, Egol KA, et al. The relationship between admission hemoglobin level and outcome after hip fracture. J Orthop Trauma 2002;16:39–44.
21. Kulier A, Gombotz H. Perioperative anemia. Anaesthesist 2001;50(2):73–86.
22. Wu WC et al. Preoperative hematocrit levels and postoperative outcomes in older patients undergoing noncardiac surgery. JAMA 2007;297(22):2481–2488.
23. National Guideline Clearinghouse. (1) Perioperative blood transfusion for elective surgery. A national clinical guideline. (2) Perioperative blood transfusion for elective surgery. Update to printed guideline. Available at: http://www.guideline.gov. Last accessed on November 11, 2010.
24. Munoz M et al. Role of parenteral iron in transfusion requirements after total hip replacement. A pilot study. Transfus Med 2006;16(2):137–142.
25. Garcia-Erce JA et al. Perioperative stimulation of erythropoiesis with intravenous iron and erythropoietin reduces transfusion requirements in patients with hip fracture. A prospective observational study. Vox Sang 2005;88(4):235–243.

26. Cuenca J et al. Perioperative intravenous iron, with or without erythropoietin, plus restrictive transfusion protocol reduce the need for allogeneic blood after knee replacement surgery. Transfusion 2006;46(7):1112–1119.
27. Goodnough LT, Monk TG, Sicard G, et al. Intraoperative salvage in patients undergoing elective abdominal aortic aneurysm repair: an analysis of cost and benefit. J Vasc Surg 1996;24(2):213–218.
28. Monk TG, Goodnough LT, Brecher ME, et al. A prospective randomized comparison of three blood conservation strategies for radical prostatectomy. Anesthesiology 1999;91(1):24–33.
29. Bryson GL, Laupacis A, Wells GA. Does acute normovolemic hemodilution reduce perioperative allogeneic transfusion? A meta-analysis. The international study of perioperative transfusion. Anesth Analg 1998;86(1):9–15.
30. Monk TG, Goodnough LT. Acute normovolemic hemodilution. Clin Orthop Relat Res 1998;357:74–81.
31. Oldenberg M, Muller RT. The frequency, prognosis and significance of nerve injuries in total hip arthroplasty. Int Orthop 1997;21(1):1–3.
32. Farrell CM, Springer BD et al. Motor nerve palsy following primary total hip arthroplasty. J Bone Joint Surg Am 2005;87(12):2619–2625.
33. Fleming RE, Michelsen CB, Stinchfield FE. Sciatic paralysis. A complication of bleeding following hip surgery. J Bone Joint Surg Am 1979;61:37–39.
34. Centers for Disease Control and Prevention. Fatalities and injuries from fall among older adults – United States, 1993-2003 and 2001-2005. MMWR Morb Mortal Wkly Rep 2006;55:1221–1224.
35. Kannus P, Sievanen H, Palvanen M et al. Prevention of falls and consequent injuries in elderly people. Lancet 2005;**366**:1885–1893.
36. Nyberg L, Gustafson Y, Berggren D, Brannstrom B, Bucht G. Falls leading to femoral neck fractures in lucid older people. Incidence of falls in three different types of geriatric care. A Swedish prospective study. J Am Geriatr Soc 1996;44:156–160.
37. Nyberg L, Gustafson Y, Janson A, Sandman PO, Eriksson S. Incidence of falls in three different types. Scand J Soc Med 1997;25(1):8–13.
38. Pils K, Neumann F, Meisner W, Schano W, Vavrovsky G, Van der Cammen TJ. Predictors of falls in elderly people during rehabilitation after hip fracture – who is at risk of a second one? Z Gerontol Geriatr 2003;36(1):16–22.
39. Tinetti ME. Preventing falls in elderly persons. N Engl J Med 2003;348:42–49.
40. Grey-Micelli D, Capezuti E, Zwicker D, Mezey M, Fulmer T, eds. Preventing falls in acute care: evidence-based geriatric nursing protocols for best practice, 3rd ed. New York, NY: Springer Publishing Company, 2008, pp 161–198.
41. Stevens M, Holman CD, Bennett N. Prevential falls in older people: impact of an intervention to reduce environmental hazards in home. J Am Geriatr Soc 2001;49:1442–1448.
42. Capezuti E, Maislin G, Strumpf N, Evans LK. Side rail use and bed-related fall outcome among nursing home residents. J Am Geriatr Soc 2002;50:90–96.
43. Leigzig RM, Cumming RG, Tinetti ME. Drugs and falls in older people: a systematic review and meta-analysis: I. Psychotropic drugs. J Am Geriatr Soc 1999;47:30–35.
44. Tinetti ME, Speechley M, Ginter SF. Risk factors for falls among elderly persons living in the community. *N Engl J Med* 1988;**319**:1701–1707.
45. Haines TP, Bennell KL, Osborne RH, Hill KD. Effectiveness of targeted falls prevention programmes in a subacute setting. A randomised controlled trial. BMJ 2004;328: 676–679.
46. Healey F, Monro A Cockram A, et al. Using targeted risk factor reduction to prevent falls in older hospital inpatients. A randomised controlled trial. Age Ageing 2004;33:390–395.
47. Reuben DB, Borok GM, Wolde-Tsadik G, et al. A randomized trial of comprehensive geriatric assessment in the care of hospitalized patients. NEJM 1995;332(20):1345–1350.
48. Berggren M, Stenvall M, Olofsson B, Gustafson Y. Evaluation of a fall-prevention program in older people after femoral neck fracture: a one-year follow-up. Osteoporosis Int 2008;19(6):801–809.

49. Tinetti ME. Multifactorial fall-prevention strategies: time to retreat or advance. J Am Geriatr Soc 2008;56:1563–1570.
50. Chang JT, Ganz DA. Quality indicators for fall and mobility problems in vulnerable elders. J Am Geriatr Soc 2007;55(Suppl 2):S327–S334.
51. Naqvi F, Lee S, Fields S. An evidence-based review of the NICHE guideline for preventing falls in older adults in an acute setting. Geriatrics 2009;64:10–26.
52. Gordon M. Restoring functional independence in the older hip fracture patient. Geriatrics 1989;44(12):48–53; see also pp 56, 59.
53. Luckey AE, Parsa CH. Fluid and electrolytes in the elderly. Arch Surg 2003;138(10):1055–1060.
54. Sunderam SG, Mankikar GD. Hyponatraemia in the elderly. Age Ageing 1983;12:77–80.
55. Hirshberg B, Ben-Yehuda A. The syndrome of inappropriate antidiuretic hormone secretion in the elderly. Am J Med 1997;103:270–273.
56. Laczi F. Etiology, diagnostics and therapy of hyponatremias. Orv Hetil 2008;149(29):1347–1354.
57. Miller PD, Krebs RA, Neal BJ, McIntyre DO. Hypodipsia in geriatric patients. Am J Med 1982;73:354–356.
58. Snyder NA, Feigal DW, Arieff AI. Hypernatremia in elderly patients: a heterogeneous, morbid, and iatrogenic entity. Ann Intern Med 1987;107:309–319.
59. Chassagne P, Druesne L, Capet C, et al. Clinical presentation of hypernatremia in elderly patients: a case control study. J Am Geriatr Soc 2006;54(8):1225–1230.
60. Portale AA, Lonergan ET, Tanney DM, Halloran BP. Aging alters calcium regulation of serum concentration of parathyroid hormone in healthy men. Am J Physiol 1997;272: E139–E146.
61. Garcia Lazaro M, Montero Perez-Barquero M, Carpintero Benitez P. The role of malnutrition and other medical factors in the evolution of patients with hip fracture. An Med Intern 2004;21(11):557–563.
62. Lichtblau S. Treatment of hip fractures in the elderly – the decision process. Mt Sinai J Med 2002;69(4):250–260.
63. Huddleston JM, Whitford KJ. Medical care of elderly patients with hip fractures. Mayo Clin Proc 2001;76(3):295–298.
64. Lavernia CJ, Sierra RJ, Baerga L. Nutritional parameters and short term outcome in arthroplasty. J Am Coll Nutr 1999;18(3):274–278.
65. Koval KJ, Maurer SG, Su ET, et al. The effects of nutritional status on outcome after hip fracture. J Orthop Trauma 1999;13(3):164–169.
66. Bastow MD, Rawlings J, Allison SP. Benefits of supplementary tube feeding after fractured neck of femur: a randomised controlled trial. BMJ 1983;287:1589–1592.
67. Hartgrink HH, Wille J, Konig P, Hermans J, Breslau PJ. Pressure sores and tube feeding in patients with a fracture of the hip: a randomized clinical trial. Clin Nutr 1998;17:287–292.
68. Sullivan DH, Nelson CL, Bopp MM, Puskarich-May CL, Walls RC. Nightly enteral nutrition support of elderly hip fracture patients: a phase I trial. J Am Coll Nutr 1998;17:155–161.
69. Tidermark J., Ponzer S., Carlsson P., et al. Effects of protein-rich supplementation and nandrolone in lean elderly women with femoral neck fractures. Clin Nutr 2004;23(4): 587–596.
70. Avenell A, Handoll HH. Nutritional supplementation for hip fracture aftercare in older people. Cochrane Database Syst Rev 2006;(4):CD001880.
71. Bastow MD, Rawlings J, Allison SP. Benefits of supplementary tube feeding after fractured neck of femur: a randomised controlled trial. BMJ 1983;287:1589–1592.
72. Hartgrink HH, Wille J, Konig P, Hermans J, Breslau PJ. Pressure sores and tube feeding in patients with a fracture of the hip: a randomized clinical trial Clin Nutr 1998;17:287–292.
73. Kaye KS, Anderson DJ, Sloane R, Chen LF, Choi Y, Link K, Sexton DJ, et al. The effect of surgical site infection on older operative patients. J Am Geriatr Soc 2009;57:46–54.
74. Kaye KS, Sloane R, Sexton DJ et al. Risk factors for surgical site infections in older people. J Am Geriatr Soc 2006;54:391–396.
75. Zuckerman JD. Hip fracture. N Engl J Med 1996;334(23):1519–1525.
76. Gillespie WJ, Walenkamp G. Antibiotic prophylaxis for surgery for proximal femoral and other closed long bone fractures. Cochrane Database Syst Rev 2001;1(1):CD000244.

77. Classen DC, Evans RS, Pestotnik SL, Horn SD, Menlove RL, Burke JP. The timing of prophylactic administration of antibiotics and the risk of surgical-wound infection. N Engl J Med 1992;326:281–286.
78. March L, Chamberlain A, Cameron I, Cumming R, Kurrle S, Finnegan T, et al. Prevention, treatment, and rehabilitation of fractured neck of femur. Report from the Northern Sydney Area Fractured Neck of Femur Health Outcomes Project. 1996. Available at: http://www.mja.com.au/public/issues/iprs2/march/fnof.pdf, accessed February 15, 2006.
79. Tambyah PA, Maki DG. The relationship between pyuria and infection in patients with indwelling urinary catheters: a prospective study of 761 patients. Arch Intern Med 2000;160(5):673–677.
80. Arozullah AM, Khuri SF, Henderson WG, et al. Development and validation of a multifactorial risk index for predicting postoperative pneumonia after major noncardiac surgery. Ann Intern Med 2001;135(10):847–857.
81. Skelly JM, Guyatt GH, Kalbfleisch R, Singer J, Winter L. Management of urinary retention after surgical repair of hip fracture. Can Med Assoc J 1992;146:1185–1189.
82. Sigel A, Schrott KM. Disturbances of micturition after general surgical operations. Langenbecks Arch Chir 1977;345:563–564.
83. Johansson I, Athlin E, Frykholm L, Bolinder H, Larsson G. Intermittent versus indwelling catheters for older patients with hip fractures. J Clin Nurs 2002;11:651–656.
84. Southwell-Keely JP, Russo RR, March L, Cumming R, Cameron I, Brnabic AJ. Antibiotic prophylaxis in hip fracture surgery: a metaanalysis. Clin Orthop 2004;(419):179–184.
85. Smith NK, Albazzaz MK. A prospective study of urinary retention and risk of death after proximal femoral fracture. Age Ageing 1996;25:150–154.
86. Schaeffer AJ. Catheter-associated bacteriuria. Urol Clin North Am 1986;13(4):735–747.
87. Sedor J, Mulholland SG. Hospital-acquired urinary tract infections associated with the indwelling catheter. Urol Clin North Am 1999;26(4):821–828.
88. Nicolle LE. Asymptomatic bacteriuria: when to screen and when to treat, Infect Dis Clin North Am 2003(17):367–394.
89. Stamm WE. Guidelines for prevention of catheter-associated urinary tract infections. Ann Intern Med 1975;82(3):386–390.
90. Skelly JM, Guyatt GH, Kalbfleisch R, Singer J, Winter L. Management of urinary retention after surgical repair of hip fracture. Can Med Assoc J 1992;146:1185–1189.
91. Morrison RS, Chassin MR, Siu AL. The medical consultant's role in caring for patients with hip fracture. Ann Intern Med 1998;128:1010–1020.
92. The National Pressure Ulcer Advisory Panel Updated Staging System. Available at http://www.npuap.org/pr2.htm. Last accessed on November 11, 2010.
93. Allman RM, Goode PS, Burst N, Bartolucci AA, Thomas DR. Pressure ulcers, hospital complications, and disease severity: impact on hospital costs and length of stay. Adv Wound Care 1999;12:22–30.
94. Baumgarten M, Margolis D, Berlin JA, et al. Risk factors for pressure ulcers among elderly hip fracture patients. Wound Repair Regen 2003;11:96–103.
95. Abrussezze RS. Early assessment and prevention of pressure ulcers. In: Lee BY, ed. Chronic ulcers of the skin. New York, NY: McGraw-Hill, 1985, pp 1–9.
96. Allman RM. Pressure ulcers among the elderly. N Engl J Med 1989;320(13):850–853.
97. Fuhrer MJ, Garber SL, Rintala DH, et al. Pressure ulcers in community-resident persons with spinal cord injury: prevalence and risk factors. Arch Phys Med Rehabil 1993; 74(11):1172–1177.
98. Garber SL, Campion LJ, Krouskop TA. Trochanteric pressure in spinal cord injury. Arch Phys Med Rehabil 1982;63(11):549–552.
99. Reuler JB, Cooney TG. The pressure sore: pathophysiology and principles of management. Ann Intern Med 1981;94(5):661–666.
100. Barbenel JC, Ferguson-Pell MW, Kennedy R. Mobility of elderly patients in bed. Measurement and association with patient condition. J Am Geriatr Soc 1986;34(9):633–636.
101. Lowthian PT. Underpadsin the prevention of decubiti. In: Kenedi RM, Cowden JM, Scales JT, eds. Bedsore biomechanics. Baltimore, MD: University Park Press, 1976, p 141.

102. Berlowitz DR, Wilking SV. Risk factors for pressure sores. A comparison of cross-sectional and cohort-derived data. J Am Geriatr Soc 1989;37(11):1043–1050.
103. Bliss M, Simini B. When are the seeds of postoperative pressure sores sown? Often during surgery. BMJ 1999;319:863.
104. Inouye SK, Studenski S, Tinetti ME, Kuchel GA. Geriatric syndromes: clinical, research, and policy implications of a core geriatric concept. J Am Geriatr Soc 2007;55(5): 780–791.
105. Haleem S, Heinert G, Paker MJ. Pressure sores and hip fractures. Injury 2008;39(2):219–223.
106. Nuffield Institute of Health, University of Leeds, NHS Centre for Review and Dissemination. How effective are pressure relieving interventions for the prevention and treatment of pressure sores? Effective Health Care Bull 1995;2:1–15.
107. Peromet M, Labbe M, Yourassowsky E, et al. Anaerobic bacteria isolated from decubitus ulcers. Infection 1973;1(4):205–207.
108. Livesley NJ, Chow AW. Infected pressure ulcers in elderly individuals. Clin Infect Dis 2002;35(11):1390–1396.
109. Brown NK, Thompson DJ. Nontreatment of fever in extended-care facilities. N Engl J Med 1979;300(22):1246–1250.
110. Agency for Health Care Policy and Research (AHCPR). Treatment of pressure ulcers. Rockville (MD). US Department of Health and Human Services, Public Health Service, Clinical Practice Guideline Number 15. AHCPR Publication No. 95–0652. 1994.
111. Pompei P, Murphy JB, eds. Geriatric review syllabus: a core curriculum in geriatric medicine, 6th ed. New York, NY: American Geriatric Society, 2006.
112. Mumcuoglu KY. Clinical applications for maggots in wound care. Am J Clin Dermatol 2001(4):219–227.
113. Bergstrom N, Bennett MA, Carlson CE, et al. Treatment of pressure ulcers. Clinical practice guideline no. 15. Rockville, MD: US Department of Health and Human Services, Public Health Service, Agency for Health Care Policy and Research, 1994, pp 47–49.
114. Lyder CH, Preston J, Grady JN, et al. Quality of care for hospitalized Medicare patients at risk for pressure ulcers. Arch Intern Med 2001;161(12):1549–1554.
115. Souders J, Rooke A. Perioperative care for geriatric patients. Ann Longterm Care 2005;13(6):17–29.
116. Marcantonio ER, Flacker JM, Wright RJ, et al. Reducing delirium after hip fracture: a randomized trial. J Am Geriatr Soc 2001;49(5):516–522.
117. Todd CJ, Freeman CJ, Camilleri-Ferrante C, et al. Differences in mortality after fracture of hip: the east Anglian audit. BMJ 1995;310:904–908.
118. Anderson FA Jr, Wheeler HB, Goldberg RJ, et al. A population-based perspective of the hospital incidence and case-fatality rates of deep vein thrombosis and pulmonary embolism. The Worcester DVT study. Arch Intern Med 1991;151:933–938.
119. Barsoum WK, Helfand R, Krebs V, et al. Managing perioperative risk in the hipfracture patient. Cleve Clin J Med 2006;73(Suppl 1):S46–S50.
120. Geerts WH, Pineo GF, Heit JA, et al. Prevention of venous thromboembolism: the seventh ACCP conference on antithrombotic and thrombolytic therapy. Chest 2004;126(3 Suppl):338S–400S.
121. Shorr AF, Kwong LM, Sarnes M, et al. Venous thromboembolism after orthopedic surgery: implications of the choice for prophylaxis. Thromb Res 2007;121(1):17–24.
122. Moser K., Pulmonary thromboembolism. In: Wilson J, Harrison TR, et al, eds. Harrison's principles of internal medicine, 12th ed, vol 1. New York, NY: McGraw-Hill, 1991, pp 1090.
123. Kniffin WD, Baron J, Barrett J, et al. The epidemiology of diagnosed pulmonary embolism and deep venous thrombosis in the elderly. Arch Intern Med 154:861–866.
124. Geerts WH, Heit JA, Clagett GP, et al. Prevention of venous thromboembolism. Chest 2001;119:132S–1325S.
125. Morpurgo M, Schmid C, Mandelli V. Factors influencing the clinical diagnosis of pulmonary embolism: analysis of 229 postmortem cases. Int J Cardiol 1998;65(Suppl I):S79–S82.

126. Stein PD, Beemath A, Matta F, et al. Clinical characteristics of patients with acute pulmonary embolism: data from PIOPED II. Am J Med 2007;120:871–879.
127. Wells PS, Ginsberg JS, Anderson DR et al. Use of a clinical model for safe management of patients with suspected pulmonary embolism. Ann Intern Med 1998;129:997–1005.
128. The PIOPED Investigators. Value of the ventilation/perfusion scan in acute pulmonary embolism: results of the prospective investigation of pulmonary embolism diagnosis (PIOPED). JAMA 1990;263(20):2753–2759.
129. Stein PD, Hull RD, Pineo GF. The role of newer diagnostic techniques in the diagnosis of pulmonary embolism. Curr Opin Pulm Med 1999;5:212–215.
130. Lindeque B, Schoeman H, Dommisse G, Boeyens MC, Vlok AL. Fat embolism and the fat embolism syndrome. J Bone Joint Surg 1987;69B:128–131.
131. Rodger M, Markropoulos D et al. Diagnostic value of the electrocardiogram in suspected pulmonary embolism. Am J Cardiol 2000;86(7):807–809.
132. Moores LK, Jackson WL, Shorr AF, Jackson JL. Meta-analysis: outcomes in patients with suspected pulmonary embolism managed with computed tomographic pulmonary angiography. Ann Intern Med 2007;141:866–874.
133. Egermayer P, Town GI, Turner JG, et al. Usefulness of D-dimer, blood gas, and respiratory rate measurements for excluding pulmonary embolism. Thorax 1998;53:830–834.
134. Tapson VF, Carroll BA, Davidson BL, et al. American Thoracic Society. Clinical practice guideline: the diagnostic approach to acute venous thromboembolism. Am J Respir Crit Care Med 1999;160:1043–1066.
135. The Task Force on Pulmonary Embolism, European Society of Cardiology. Guidelines on the diagnosis and management of acute pulmonary embolism. Eur Heart J 2000;21:1301–1336.
136. Ginsberg JS, Wells PS, Kearon C, et al. Sensitivity and specificity of a rapid whole-blood assay for D-dimer in the diagnosis of pulmonary embolism. Ann Intern Med 1998;129(12):1006–1011.
137. Schulman S, Granqvist S, Holmstrom M, et al. The duration of oral anticoagulant therapy after a second episode of venous thromboembolism. The duration of anticoagulation trial study group. N Engl J Med 1997;336(6):393–398.
138. Ramzi DW, Leeper KV. DVT and pulmonary embolism: part II. Treatment and prevention. Am Fam Physician 2004;69(12):2841.
139. Levine M, Hirsh J, Weitz J, et al. A randomized trial of a single bolus dosage regimen of recombinant tissue plasminogen activator in patients with acute pulmonary embolism. Chest 1990;98(6):1473–1479.
140. Hirsh J, Dalen JE, Anderson DR, et al. Oral anticoagulants: mechanism of action, clinical effectiveness, and optimal therapeutic range. Chest 1998;114(5 Suppl):445S–469S.
141. Mageral F, Tscherne H. Zur Diagnose, Therapie und proplylaxe der fettembolie. Langenbecks Arch Klin Chir 1966;314:29.
142. Ganong RB. Fat emboli syndrome in isolated fractures of the tibia and femur. Clin Ortho 1993;291:208–214.
143. Collins JA, Hudson TL, Hamacher WR et al. Systemic fat embolism in four combat causalities. Ann Surg 1968;167:493–499.
144. Johnson MJ, Lucas GL. Fat embolism syndrome. Orthopedics 1996;19:41.
145. Fulde GW, Harrison P. Fat embolism – a review. Arch Emerg Med 1991;8:233–239.
146. Kaplan RP, Grant JN, Kaufman AJ. Dermatologic features of the fat embolism syndrome. Cutis 1986;38:52–55.
147. Lindeque B, Schoeman H, Dommisse G, Boeyens MC, Vlok AL. Fat embolism and the fat embolism syndrome. J Bone Joint Surg 1987;69B:128–131.
148. Gurd AR. Fat embolism: an aid to diagnosis. J Bone Joint Surg Br 1970;52b:732–737.
149. Van den Brande FGJ, Hellemans S, De Schepper A, et al. Post-traumatic severe fat embolism syndrome with uncommon CT findings. Anaesth Intensive Care 2006;34:102–106.
150. Riska EB, Van Bonsdorff H, Hakkien S, Japonia O, Kilivoyo O, Papillainen T. Prevention of fat embolism by early fixation of fractures in patients with multiple injuries. Injury 1976;8: 110–116.

151. Schonfeld SA, Ploysongsang Y, DiLisio R, et al. Fat embolism prophylaxis with corticosteroids. Ann Intern Med 1983;99:438–443.
152. Mellor A, Soni N. Fat embolism. Anaesthesia 2001;56:145–154.
153. Bulger EM, Smith DG, Maier RV, Jurkovich GJ. Fat embolism syndrome. A 10-year review. Arch Surg 1997;132(4):435–439.
154. Bitsch M, Foss N, Kristensen B, et al. Pathogenesis of and management strategies for postoperative delirium after hip fracture: a review. Acta Orthop Scand 2004;75(4):378–389.
155. Morrison RS, Chassin MR, Siu AL. The medical consultant's role in caring for patients with hip fracture. Ann Intern Med 1998;128(12 Pt 1):1010–1102.
156. Bellelli G, Frisoni GB, Pagani M, et al. Does cognitive performance affect physical therapy regimen after hip fracture surgery? Aging Clin Exp Res 2007;19(2):119–124.
157. Feil D, Marmon T, Unutzer J. Cognitive impairment, chronic medical illness, and risk of mortality in an elderly cohort. Am J Geriatr Psychiatry 003;11(5):551–560.
158. Kiely DK, Bergmann MA, Murphy KM, et al. Delirium among newly admitted post-acute facility patients: prevalence, symptoms, and severity. J Gerontol A Biol Sci Med Sci 2003;58(5): M441–M445.
159. Bitsch M, Foss N, Kristensen B, et al. Pathogenesis of and management strategies for postoperative delirium after hip fracture: a review. Acta Orthop Scand 2004;75(4):378–389.
160. Marcantonio ER, Flacker JM, Wright RJ, et al. Reducing delirium after hip fracture: a randomized trial. J Am Geriatr Soc 2001;49(5):516–522.
161. Ely EW, Inouye SK, Bernard GR, et al. Delirium in mechanically ventilated patients: validity and reliability of the confusion assessment method for the intensive care unit. JAMA 2001;286(21):2703–2710.
162. Inouye SK, Van Dyck CH, Alessi CA, et al. Clarifying confusion: the Confusion Assessment Method: a new method for detection of delirium. Ann Intern Med 1990;113(12):941–948.
163. Trzepacz P, Breitbart W, Franklin J, et al. Practice guideline for the treatment of patients with delirium. American Psychiatric Association; Available at: http://www.psychiatryonline.com/pracGuide/pracGuideTopic_2.aspx

Part III
Common Fractures in the Elderly

Chapter 9
Hand and Wrist Fractures in the Elderly

Laura C. Wiegand, Atul F. Kamath, Nick D. Pappas, and David J. Bozentka

Abstract Hand and wrist fractures are a relatively common injury in the elderly population, often resulting from a low-energy fall or a fragility fracture. Initial closed reduction and stabilization in a splint are most often performed in the emergency room or location of initial presentation. Non-surgical management of hand and wrist fractures is typically reserved for non-displaced or minimally displaced fractures. Operative treatment is almost always recommended for open fractures, fractures with associated soft tissue defects, and those fractures associated with neurovascular injury. Surgery is also often recommended for unstable fractures, intra-articular fractures, or fractures in which closed reduction and casting fails to achieve and/or maintain adequate alignment. It is important to consider the patient's age, functional status, medical comorbidities, and concomitant injuries in the decision of whether or not to proceed with surgery. Techniques of operative stabilization include external fixation, closed reduction and percutaneous pinning, open reduction, and internal fixation. One of the challenges of treating hand and wrist fractures is the need for immobilization to facilitate fracture healing, which results in muscle atrophy and joint stiffness. Rehabilitation after a hand or wrist fracture is especially important in order to decrease the risk of complications and maximize functional recovery from the injury. Prevention of future falls and the evaluation and treatment of osteoporosis are additional important aspects of the management of hand and wrist fractures in the elderly.

Keywords Fracture • Distal radius • Hand • Internal fixation • Fragility • Osteoporosis • Splinting • Rehabilitation

---

D.J. Bozentka (✉)
Department of Orthopaedic Surgery, Hospital of the University of Pennsylvania,
34th and Spruce Streets, 2nd Floor, Silverstein Building, Philadelphia, PA 19104, USA
and
Department of Orthopaedic Surgery, Penn Presbyterian Medical Center,
Cupp 1, 39th and Market Streets, Philadelphia, PA 19104, USA
e-mail: david.bozentka@uphs.upenn.edu

R.J. Pignolo et al. (eds.), *Fractures in the Elderly*, Aging Medicine,
DOI 10.1007/978-1-60327-467-8_9,

9.1 Basic Anatomy

9.1.1 Carpus

The carpus is composed of eight small bones that are organized in two rows of four carpal bones. Each of these bones has unique features that aid in its identification radiographically. The proximal row includes the scaphoid (navicular), lunate, triquetrum, and pisiform from radial to ulnar. The scaphoid is boat-shaped and has a notable tubercle distally. The lunate is shaped like a half moon and the triquetrum is pyramidal. Lastly, the pisiform is a small circular bone found on the volar surface of the triquetrum.

The distal carpal row is composed of the trapezium, trapezoid, capitate, and hamate from radial to ulnar. The trapezium is four sided and has a rectangular shape. The trapezoid is wedge shaped and the smallest of the distal row. The capitate is more rounded and the largest of the carpal bones. The hamate is also wedge shaped and has a hook-like process volarly.

The carpal bones are stabilized by intrinsic (interosseous) and extrinsic (extraosseous) ligaments. The intrinsic ligaments arise from and insert on the carpal bones. In the proximal row, the two most important interosseous ligaments are the scapholunate and the lunotriquetral. They not only hold their respective bones together but also allow for small amounts of rotational motion. The extrinsic ligaments arise outside the carpus and insert on the carpal bones. The most significant of the extrinsic ligaments of the proximal row is the volar ligaments and include the radioscaphoid-capitate, long radiolunate, and short radiolunate. These ligaments anchor the proximal row to the distal radius and ulna. While these ligaments stabilize the radiocarpal joint radially, the ulnocarpal ligaments (including the ulnolunate, ulnotriquetral, and ulnocapitate) provide support ulnarly. The key dorsal ligaments are the dorsal transverse intercarpal, which runs from the scaphoid to the triquetrum, and the dorsal radiocarpal ligament, which connects the radius to the triquetrum.

The radiocarpal joint is composed of the distal radius, ulna, and proximal carpal row. The distal radius has a separate facet for articulation with both the scaphoid and lunate. The angle of inclination of the distal radius is roughly 22° while its height radially is approximately 11 mm relative to its most ulnar surface (see Fig. 9.1). The articular surface of the distal radius is tilted volarly at an angle of approximately 11° [1].

The distal radioulnar joint (DRUJ) is another important articulation that allows rotation of the wrist. The distal ulna is surrounded by a structure called the triangular fibrocartilage complex (TFCC). The TFCC stabilizes the DRUJ and absorb forces directed from the carpus to the ulnar head. It is composed of volar and dorsal radioulnar ligaments, ulnotriquetral and ulnolunate ligaments, the ulnar collateral ligament, a meniscus homolog, and the articular disk [2].

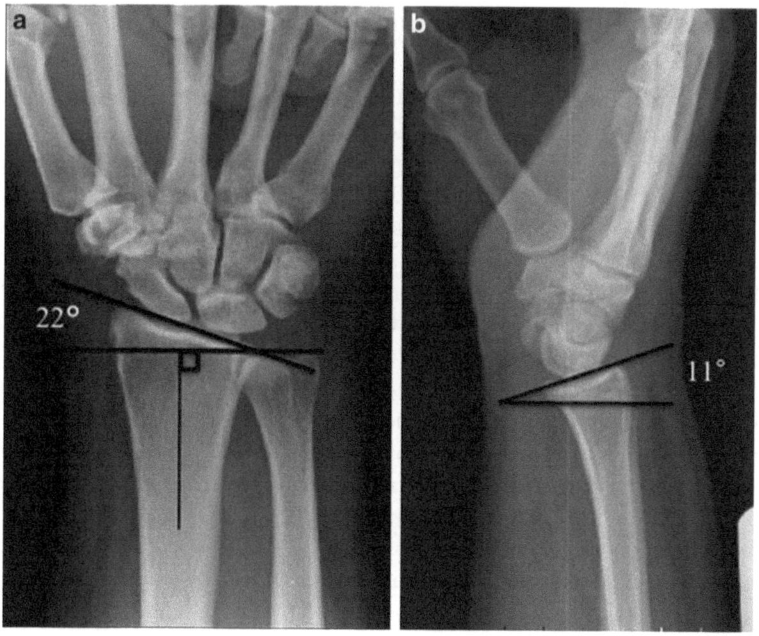

Fig. 9.1 (**a**) The angle of inclination of the distal radius is approximately 22°. (**b**) The volar tilt of the articular surface of the distal radius is approximately 11° (these images are courtesy of UPenn Orthopaedic Hand Service)

9.2 Phalangeal and Metacarpal Structures

Each digit is composed of three phalanges (proximal, middle, and distal) with the exception of the thumb, which has only a proximal and distal phalanx. The proximal phalanges articulate directly with the digit's respective metacarpal head. The phalanges decrease in size as one moves from proximal to distal. Their heads are bicondylar in shape, unlike those of the aforementioned metacarpals. Collateral ligaments stabilize the interphalangeal joints laterally and medially.

The metacarpus is composed of five elongated bones each with a head, neck, body, and base area. All of the metacarpal heads are cam shaped, such that the diameter from palmar to dorsal is larger than from the head to neck junction. The metacarpal–phalangeal joints (MCP) are stabilized medially and laterally by collateral ligaments, which originate dorsally on the metacarpal head and attach volarly on the proximal phalanx. The cam shape of the metacarpal heads renders the collateral ligaments tighter in flexion and looser in extension. In addition, the volar surface of the MCP joint contains fibrous thickenings of the joint capsule, collectively known as volar plates, which stabilize the joint and prevent hyperextension.

9.3 Basic Physical Examination

Proper diagnosis of any hand or wrist fracture begins with a detailed history that includes answers to certain key questions which begins by exploring the chief complaint. Typically a patient will complain of pain in a specific area of the hand. A good plan is to have the patient localize the pain by pointing with one finger to the area of maximal discomfort. The examiner should determine the mechanism of injury. A high-energy injury will tend to lead to more comminution and a more unstable fracture compared to a low-energy injury such as a fall from standing height. One should also inquire about the patient's age, hand dominance, activity level, type of work, and relevant past medical history such as previous hand or wrist trauma, diabetes, or rheumatoid arthritis.

The physical examination is performed in a systematic fashion by starting with inspection, followed by palpation and an assessment of the range of motion of all joints of the hand and wrist. It is particularly important to evaluate the joint above and the joint below the area of injury. Due to the small size of the structures in the hand, palpation with the back end of a pen or pencil may help further localize the area of maximal tenderness. Motor and sensory function of the upper extremity should be recorded. A vascular examination of the radial and brachial pulses is included.

Radiographically, one should obtain plain films showing a minimum three views including posteroanterior (PA), lateral, and oblique. It is important to order X-rays of the hand for injuries to the metacarpals and views of the finger for symptoms more distally to best evaluate the digits. Occasionally, a special view may be requested depending on the patient's symptomatology and the suspected diagnosis. For example, if the clinician suspects a hook of the hamate fracture, a carpal tunnel view is obtained. The X-ray beam is directed along the palm of the hand with the volar wrist placed on the cassette and held in maximal extension.

Additional, sophisticated imaging might be necessary for certain types of suspected injuries. For example, a patient with unexplained anatomic snuff box tenderness 2 weeks after a fall onto an outstretched hand might merit an MRI to rule out a scaphoid fracture. CT scan can be useful for the diagnosis of hook of the hamate fractures or evaluating the injury pattern of intra-articular distal radius fractures.

9.4 Common Fractures and Their Management

9.4.1 Distal Radius Fractures

Distal radius fractures are one of the most commonly encountered fractures in the elderly population. The typical mechanism is a fall onto an outstretched hand. In general, distal radius fractures are commonly referred to by certain eponyms, which include Colles (dorsal displacement), Smith (volar displacement), Barton's (radial rim fracture with either volar or dorsal displacement of the carpus), or Chauffeur's (radial styloid) fractures. Distal radius fractures are also classified based on whether they are intra- or extra-articular.

Treatment options for distal radius fractures are dependent on several variables, such as the patient's age, activity level, and future interests. However, the degree of displacement is often tantamount to these. Recall from the anatomy section that the angle of inclination of the distal radius is roughly 22° while its radial height is approximately 11 mm and volar tilt is approximately 11°. These numbers are used to gauge whether a reduction, open or closed, is necessary. Despite lack of a consensus, most would consider acceptable alignment for an active patient to be neutral volar tilt, a congruent DRUJ, <2 mm of intra-articular step off at radiocarpal joint, radial shortening < 5 mm, and radial inclination > 15° [3].

Closed reduction maneuvers may vary depending on the characteristics of the fracture. Recreating the mechanism that caused the deformity, traction, then reversing the mechanism is a rule of thumb. For example, since a Colles fracture occurs via a wrist hyperextension mechanism, the reduction is performed by wrist hyperextension, longitudinal traction, and then wrist flexion. The latter maneuver is performed to lever the dorsally displaced fragment back into position. Alternately, for a Smith fracture, the wrist is flexed initially then extended for the reduction maneuver. After successful reduction, the patient can be immobilized in a sugar tong plaster splint.

A few serious complications can occur after a distal radius fracture, both in the short and long term. After the initial trauma, an acute carpal tunnel syndrome can develop, especially if repeated closed reductions are attempted. In acute carpal tunnel syndrome, the patient typically develops progressive numbness in the median nerve distribution several hours after the injury. If this numbness gets progressively worse, immediate carpal tunnel release is necessary. Acute carpal tunnel syndrome should be distinguished from median nerve contusion. Unlike acute carpal tunnel syndrome, median nerve contusion causes numbness in the median nerve distribution which is stable. Rupture of the extensor pollicis longus tendon is a long-term complication that can occur, particularly with non-displaced distal radius fractures.

When closed reduction attempts fail to achieve appropriate alignment, surgery is often recommended. Closed reduction and percutaneous pinning is more appropriate for extra-articular and non-comminuted fractures. New developments in locking distal radius plating have made either volar or dorsal plating a better option for older patients (see Fig. 9.2). For comminuted distal radius fractures in which there is significant bony or soft tissue loss, external fixation is also an option.

9.4.2 *Carpus*

The scaphoid is the most frequently fractured bone in the carpus. It is typically injured by a fall onto an outstretched hand. Fractures of the scaphoid are often

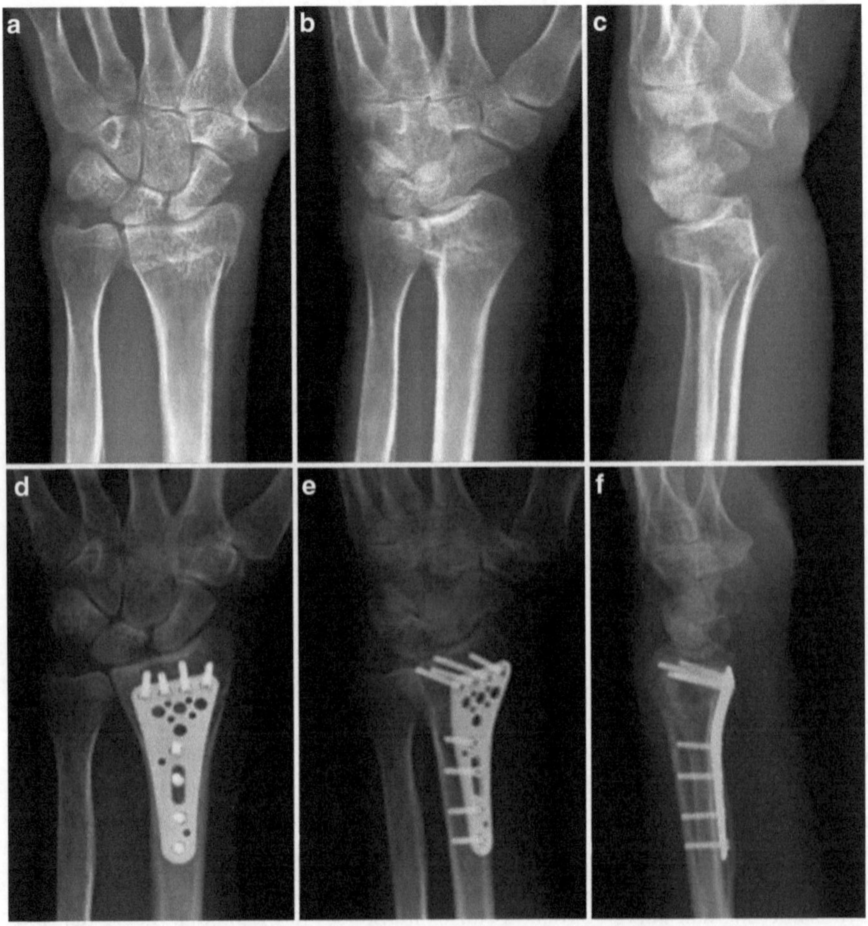

Fig. 9.2 Distal radius fracture. Preoperative X-rays of a distal radius fracture. (**a**) AP X-ray, (**b**) oblique X-ray, (**c**) lateral X-ray. Post-operative X-rays after distal radius open reduction and internal fixation with a volar plate. (**d**) AP X-ray, (**e**) oblique X-ray, (**f**) lateral X-ray (these images are courtesy of UPenn Orthopaedic Hand Service)

described based on anatomic location as tubercle, proximal pole, waist, or distal pole. All scaphoid fractures can be problematic but fractures of the proximal pole have the worst outcomes. Since the scaphoid has a retrograde blood supply from the radial artery that enters dorsally and distally, a proximal pole fracture is particularly susceptible to nonunion and avascular necrosis.

Scaphoid fractures are often elusive because they may not show up on initial radiographs. If a patient complains of radially sided wrist pain and has anatomic snuffbox tenderness after wrist trauma, they should be placed in a thumb spica splint and follow up for repeat radiographs in 2–3 weeks. At that time bone resorption may be evident if there was indeed a fracture. Ultimately, one may need either an MRI or CT scan of the wrist with 1 mm cuts through the plane of the scaphoid to diagnose an occult scaphoid fracture. Bone scan is another medium that can be used although the study is less specific.

The lunate is less commonly fractured than the scaphoid but like the scaphoid it has a tenuous blood supply. Osteonecrosis of the lunate (Kienbock's Disease) is a well-described condition thought to result from either an acute trauma causing disruption of the blood supply or repetitive stress from negative ulnar variance, which places increased stresses on the lunate. Patients typically present with central wrist pain and may have negative plain radiographs. An MRI should be obtained if the diagnosis is suspected.

Triquetral fractures typically present as a dorsal avulsion that is best seen on a plain lateral radiograph. These injuries can typically be treated with a removable splint while a fracture of the body is treated with 4–6 weeks of cast immobilization [3].

Trapezial fractures are relatively uncommon. There are two types: trapezial body and trapezial ridge fractures. Body fractures are intra-articular and therefore often require open reduction and internal fixation (ORIF). Trapezial ridge fractures can occur by either direct trauma or via pull of the flexor retinaculum and involve either the tip or the base of the trapezium. Tip fractures can be treated with cast immobilization for 3–6 weeks while base fractures may require excision since they frequently result in painful non-union.

Capitate fractures are rather rare but often have poor outcomes. Non-displaced fractures can be treated with cast immobilization. Proximal pole fractures are more worrisome, even if non-displaced, and can result in avascular necrosis due to a tenuous blood supply which is retrograde.

Hamate fractures can involve either the body or hook, the latter being exceedingly more common. Non-displaced body fractures can be treated with cast immobilization, while displaced or unstable fractures may require ORIF. Fractures of the hook of hamate occur following direct trauma to the hypothenar eminence. They are commonly seen in golfers or in other athletic activities that require racquets or sticks such as tennis, hockey, or baseball. Patients present with pain over the ulnar side of the wrist, diminished grip strength, and may even complain of numbness in the ulnar nerve distribution. The hook of the hamate is best visualized on plain film by a carpal tunnel view or CT scan. While non-displaced hook of the hamate fractures can be treated with 4–6 weeks of cast immobilization, displaced fractures or painful non-unions of the hook should be excised.

Pisiform fractures are also rather uncommon. These can usually be treated in a short arm cast. A painful non-union may require excision.

9.4.3 Phalangeal Fractures

Distal phalanx fractures come in three types: tuft, shaft, and intra-articular fractures. Fractures of the tuft are generally the result of a crush injury. Their surrounding soft tissue envelope usually renders them stable. Most distal phalanx fractures can be treated non-operatively with an aluminum finger splint. However, soft tissue injury can often be a concern with these injuries, especially damage to the underlying nail bed. If there is a high likelihood of a nail bed injury with a displaced fracture of the distal phalanx and a large subungual hematoma, the nail plate should be removed in order to repair the nail matrix [3].

Fractures of the proximal and middle phalanx can be categorized into the following: base, shaft, neck, and condylar. Non-displaced or even minimally displaced fractures can be treated non-operatively with buddy tape, aluminum, or plaster splinting. If a patient is placed in a plaster splint, one must immobilize the wrist in 20° of extension with fingers in the intrinsic plus position. The MCP joints are flexed with the interphalangeal (IP) joints held in full extension to prevent contracture from shortening of the MCP collateral ligaments and IP volar plates.

9.4.4 Metacarpal Fractures

Metacarpal fractures are classified based on anatomic location as head, neck, shaft, and base. Metacarpal head fractures are relatively uncommon but when they occur, they are often difficult to manage. A simple fracture pattern can be treated effectively with either closed reduction and percutaneous pinning (CRPP) or ORIF. Comminuted fractures can be treated similarly but have poorer outcomes.

Fractures of the metacarpal neck are common. A fracture of the fifth metacarpal neck is referred to as a "boxer's fracture" because of the typical mechanism, which is an axial load across a clenched fist. Metacarpal neck fractures generally assume an apex dorsal angulation deformity. They may also exhibit rotational deformity, which by itself merits reduction. Criteria for acceptable angulation varies but many hand surgeons use the 10–20–30–40 rule in which 10° is acceptable for the index finger, 20° for the long, 30° for the ring, and 40° for the small. If displacement is greater than the accepted degree for a particular finger, a closed reduction should be attempted. The Jahss maneuver is a commonly applied reduction technique that can be performed in the emergency department using a hematoma block for analgesia. The maneuver is performed by placing the MCP joint of the affected digit in 90° of flexion. A volar to dorsal force is then applied to the metacarpal head through the proximal phalanx so as to restore the normal alignment of the metacarpal neck [3]. Rotational deformity is also corrected while performing this maneuver. A plaster splint or cast should be applied to maintain the reduction with the MCP of the affected digit held in a 90° flexed position, which serves to maintain reduction as well as prevent the collateral ligaments from shortening. As the reduction is often difficult to maintain in a splint or cast, these fractures should be followed with serial X-rays and may require a repeat reduction or operative fixation (see Fig. 9.3).

MC shaft fractures are typically the result of either a crush injury or axial load. Apex dorsal angulation is the typical deformity due to the volar-directed vector of pull of the interosseous muscles. Most clinicians consider non-operative treatment

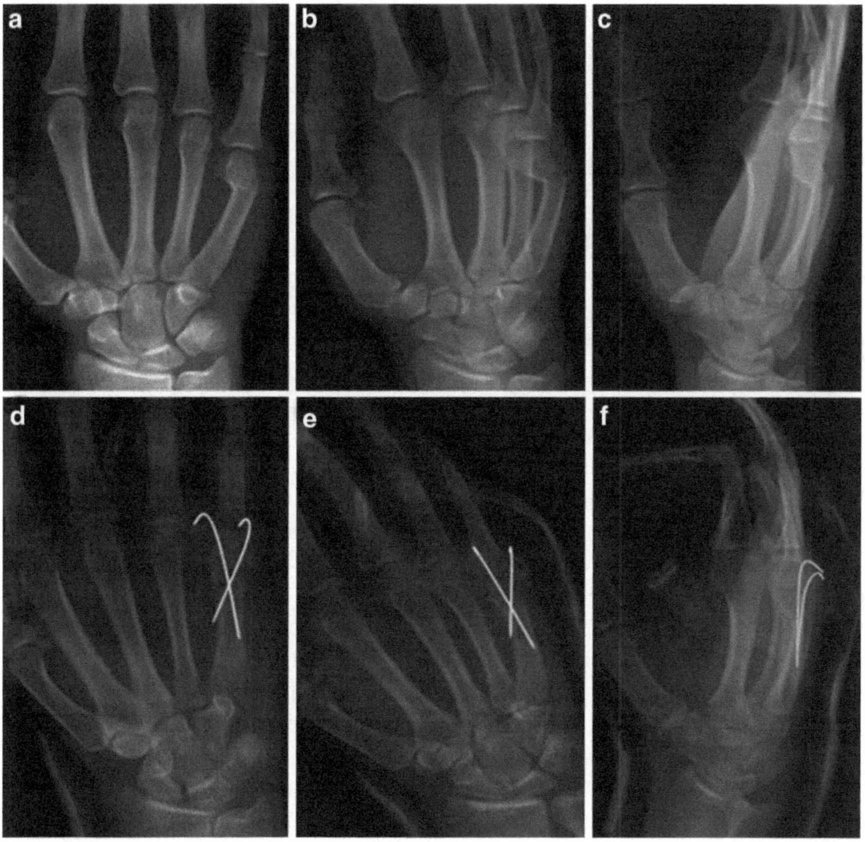

Fig. 9.3 Fifth metacarpal neck fracture. Preoperative X-rays of a fifth metacarpal neck fracture. (**a**) AP X-ray, (**b**) oblique X-ray, (**c**) lateral X-ray. Post-operative X-rays after fifth metacarpal closed reduction and percutaneous pinning. (**d**) AP X-ray, (**e**) oblique X-ray, (**f**) lateral X-ray (these images are courtesy of UPenn Orthopaedic Hand Service)

in a splint or cast if there is no significant rotational mal-alignment. In addition, the sagittal plane deformity should be less than 10° in the index and long finger metacarpals and less than 30° in the ring and small finger metacarpals. MC base fractures are less common than in the neck but can be more worrisome, particularly when intra-articular. They often involve the thumb or small finger. An intra-articular fracture at the base of the thumb MC, often referred to as a Bennett fracture, results from an axial load to a flexed thumb. Deformity and subluxation occurs as the abductor pollicis longus pulls the thumb MC shaft radially and dorsally while the volar oblique (beak) ligament remains attached to the volar fragment. As an aside, the eponym "Rolando fracture" is used when there is comminution at the thumb MC. Fractures at the base of the finger metacarpals may be associated with a carpometacarpal dislocation requiring surgical management. A "baby Bennett" fracture is the term used for an intra-articular fracture at the base of the small finger MC. In this scenario, the extensor carpi ulnaris tendon pulls the small finger MC shaft dorsally and ulnarly, which can impede appropriate fracture healing [3].

9.5 Operative Fixation

If a patient fails non-operative treatment, or if a fracture is deemed too unstable for definitive closed reduction and casting, surgical management may be considered. Guidelines, such as the LaFontaine criteria for distal radius fractures, may be helpful in determining which fractures may go on to failure with non-operative treatment modalities [4]. Ultimately, the risks and benefits of surgical intervention must be carefully weighed, especially in the geriatric patient.

Medical co-morbidities, functional status [5], and the patient's and family's expectations and input must be factored into the decision to proceed with surgery. It is important for the patient to have a clear understanding of the risks of surgery, including infection, neurovascular damage, compartment syndrome, stiffness, tendon attrition or rupture, and complex regional pain syndrome. In addition further procedures may be required for stiffness or removal of symptomatic hardware.

It is helpful for the orthopaedic surgeon and the patient's primary care physician/geriatrician/rheumatologist to communicate peri-operatively to optimize the patient for surgery. Extraordinary issues and salient past medical history are considered, and a long-term treatment plan is formulated, including management of osteoporosis [6]. Careful consideration must also be made with regard to concomitant injuries that may influence the treating surgeon's decision to pursue stable fixation for earlier and easier mobilization. Open fractures, fractures with associated soft tissue defects, and those fractures associated with neurovascular injury should be managed as special situations.

Orthopaedic upper extremity procedures are generally managed on an outpatient basis. The surgeon should communicate with the anesthesiologist regarding appropriate peri-operative pain control, which includes the type of anesthesia to be administered during surgery. The type of anesthesia is considered on a case-by-case basis depending on the co-morbidities as well as the location and extent of the surgical procedure. Options include general anesthesia, regional blockade, monitored anesthesia care (MAC), and local blocks—or a specific combination of the above. Procedures performed about the digits distally are amenable to local anesthesia whereas surgical treatment of the metacarpals and proximal is typically performed under regional blockade or general anesthesia. Once the appropriate anesthesia is administered, the surgeon will re-confirm surgical site, confirm appropriate prophylactic antibiotics, apply a pneumatic tourniquet based on the procedure, and proceed with surgery.

Upper extremity fractures may be managed non-operatively with closed reduction, casting, and splinting/taping. If a fracture is beyond the acceptable limits of angulation, rotation, or shortening, the surgeon may elect to pursue operative treatment. Surgical options include CRPP with Kirschner wires, ORIF with plates and screws, or external fixation with pins inserted proximal and distal to the fracture site and connected to bars outside the skin.

Distal radius fractures are one of the most common fractures, and the incidence is higher in the elderly. In the geriatric population, distal radius fractures may result from low-energy trauma, such as a fall on an outstretched hand, or as a "fragility fracture" related to poor bone mineral density. Surgical fixation, including plate fixation of distal radius fractures, is a viable and useful option in the elderly and osteoporotic population [7].

After initial closed reduction and splinting in the emergency room, the decision may be made to pursue operative fixation. Like carpal and phalangeal fractures, the distal radius may be reduced closed and stabilized with Kirschner wires, open reduced and fixed with plates and screws, or externally fixed with bars and pins [8].

Oftentimes, closed reduction and casting alone is not sufficient to prevent displacement of the fracture [9]. Osteoporotic bone presents unique challenges to the operating surgeon: the bone is not as strong as that seen in younger populations or those without osteoporosis, fixation constructs and implants must take into account poor bone stability, and healing of osteoporotic bone is less robust. Some have pointed to the need for osteoporosis to be independently considered when classifying fracture patterns [10].

Pre-operative imaging includes standard antero-posterior and lateral radiographs, supplemented by special radiographic views depending on the particular associated bones fractured and fracture pattern. Computed tomography (CT) scans may be a useful adjunct for severely comminuted fractures or those with articular compromise [11].

For ORIF, the distal radius may be approached from either side of the wrist, namely, the dorsal or volar aspects [12]. Each approach has advantages and disadvantages based on fracture pattern, degree of articular comminution, soft tissue injury, and preference and experience of the surgeon, and the respective implants used. Fluoroscopic guidance for confirmation of reduction and fixation is used intra-operatively.

There are several special considerations for osteoporotic fractures, or those with severe comminution. To minimize the need for reliance on bony support for implanted hardware, fixed-angle or "locked" plating constructs may be used. These plates rely on screw fixation to the plate, rather than screw purchase into bone. Therefore, the locked plate and screw construct can provide appropriate bony support, including subchondral support of the articular surface, in the face of poor bone quality. This greater purchase of fractured fragments in osteoporotic or highly comminuted fractures may allow for more stable fixation, thereby preventing displacement and allowing faster rehabilitation. Bone graft is more commonly needed to fill metaphyseal defects in patients with osteoporosis particularly when performing a dorsal approach. Autograft, allograft, or bone graft substitutes are considered. Other supplemental fixation methods in osteoporotic bone include hydroxyapatite-coated implants and screws and calcium phosphate bone cement augmentation [13].

Once adequate reduction and fixation of the fracture is performed, the wound is copiously irrigated with sterile saline. The wound is then closed in sequential fashion, and a sterile soft dressing is applied. While still under anesthesia, the patient is placed in a plaster splint – the type of splint chosen is based on fracture pattern and procedure performed – to immobilize the fracture until follow-up. The patient is then taken to the recovery room, and a careful neurovascular examination is performed.

9.6 Perioperative Management

Most patients are discharged to home after the procedure. Exceptions to outpatient care include extensive procedures requiring closer neurovascular monitoring or pain control, insufficient or unsafe patient home situation, or management of a polytrauma patient. The first 1–2 weeks after surgery, from the time the patient leaves the recovery room/hospital to the first post-operative clinic visit, is an important period.

The patient is instructed to keep the splint or dressing on and dry until follow-up. Pain is generally controlled initially with narcotic analgesia tapered to non-narcotic pain medications. Appropriate pain control must be balanced with the risks of over-sedation and polypharmacy drug interactions, especially in the elderly. In most cases, chemical deep venous thromboembolism prophylaxis is not prescribed, but this must be examined on a case-by-case basis and referenced to patient risk factors and the degree of immobility after the procedure. Most other home medications are restarted post-operatively per usual home regimen; certain anti-rheumatic drugs and blood thinners may be restarted according to their specific schedule. Pre-operative medical examination and recommendations aid the surgeon in timing, dosing, and appropriateness of home medications.

One of the most important factors in symptom control post-operatively is elevation of the operated extremity above the level of the heart. Reduction in swelling leads to improved pain control, easier range of motion of the digits, and overall comfort.

Depending on the procedure and stability of the fixation, gentle active range of motion of the un-involved joints is encouraged to avoid stiffness. It is important to encourage shoulder range of motion to prevent adhesive capsulitis following a wrist or hand injury. Digital range of motion exercises are performed soon after wrist surgery but may need to be limited initially for fractures of the digits. Specific protocols for advancing post-operative range of motion and therapy of the involved joint are based on the operative procedure and whether concomitant tendon transfers or soft tissue procedures are performed.

9.7 Rehabilitation

Rehabilitation is an important aspect of treating hand and wrist fractures, with the goals of avoiding complications and maximizing functional recovery from the injury. As discussed above in the Sect. 9.6, many patients are placed in a splint post-operatively and the range of motion at the fracture site is restricted to facilitate soft-tissue healing and resolution of swelling [12]. Sutures are typically removed between 7 and 14 days post-operatively. Sutures are retained longer for patients with extensive swelling or those taking medications that may limit wound healing. During the immediate post-operative period, acute edema management may include compression garments and elevation of the affected extremity, active/passive finger motion, icing, and retrograde massage [14]. More intensive rehabilitation is usually started post-immobilization.

Although immobilization is beneficial to fracture healing, immobilization results in muscle atrophy and joint stiffness which is then addressed during post-operative rehabilitation. Finger stiffness can be avoided by prompt referral to physiotherapy. To combat wrist stiffness in patients with a distal radius fracture, motion should be initiated as soon as bony healing is deemed adequate [8].

The length of immobilization and the pace of therapy is influenced by surgeon preference, fracture stability due to fixation method and inherent characteristics of the fracture pattern, and patient factors, including age, bone density, pain tolerance, and systemic disease [14]. For example, percutaneous pin fixation of a fracture is not stable enough to allow immediate motion, and patients treated with an external fixator will not be able to move the wrist early; however, distal radius fractures treated with fixed-angle volar plates may be stable enough for immediate wrist motion [15].

Both occupational therapists and physical therapists trained in hand rehabilitation may provide rehabilitation for hand and wrist fractures. A variety of modalities are at the disposal of the therapist to maximize a patient's functional recovery post-operatively. Heat packs, fluidotherapy, paraffin wax bath, and transcutaneous electrical nerve stimulation (TENS) will help decrease pain allowing the patient to progress their exercise protocol. Open wounds are treated with dressing changes, while healed wounds benefit from a scar management program with scar massage and compression dressings. Range of motion exercises often require active, active assistive and passive stretching with tendon glide exercises to ensure optimal range of motion. Various splints can be fabricated by the therapist ranging from static resting splints to dynamic or static progressive splints for stretching soft tissues. Continuous passive range of motion machines can be fitted and an assessment made for a therapist to visit in the home. Most importantly, the therapists can provide patient education and supervision of the exercise protocol ensuring that the patient is performing the appropriate home exercise program. Specific interventions are selected on an individual basis to meet the specific needs and goals of each patient.

A general protocol may involve controlled and progressive joint mobilization, initiated with a finger rehabilitation protocol and edema management, then progressing to finger or wrist motion based on healing and stability of the fracture. Although it is often thought that rehabilitation involves frequent visits to a hand therapist, rehabilitation exercises should continue to be performed at home. Krischak et al. [16] showed that a home exercise program using a booklet with guidance is a valid alternative to formal physical therapy in the postoperative rehabilitation of distal radius fractures.

Post-operative rehabilitation is essential for restoring functionality after a distal radius fracture. Finger motion exercises may be started immediately, and may include tendon gliding exercises and passive finger motion. Active motion of the uninvolved joints may also be started immediately post-operatively. Wrist motion is initiated at different times post-operatively once the cast or splint is removed, depending on the fracture site stability and the type of surgical fixation. In general, external fixation prevents wrist motion until the device is removed and therefore results in greater wrist stiffness initially, while plate fixation allows earlier loading of the fracture site. In addition, patient factors such as age, bone density, pain tolerance, and systemic disease may influence the pace of therapy and should be taken into account. Early callous begins forming around 4–6 weeks post-injury and this typically signals an advancement of some type in the therapy program, for example, initiation of active motion of the wrist, or decreasing splint wear to only in crowd situations and allowing normal lightweight use of the hand and wrist [11]. Once the fracture is clinically healed, rehabilitation is useful to improve ROM and for progressive strengthening. Forceful gripping is usually delayed until there is some fracture site healing. Strenuous activities including pushing, pulling, lifting, and twisting should be avoided for the first 3 months following surgery [12]. Patients are typically released to activities as tolerated by 3 months, although further improvements in strength and functional performance may be seen for up to a year or longer.

In summary, rehabilitation after operative fixation of hand and wrist fractures is an important component of functional recovery, and must be individualized based on the fracture type and fixation, patient characteristics, and surgeon preferences.

9.8 Prevention

Prevention of hand and wrist fractures is important. Patients who are at increased risk of falling have a higher risk of low-energy or fragility fractures of the hand and wrist. Survival rates following a distal radius fracture have been shown to be lower than individuals of similar age and gender [17]. Two potential methods of preventing these fractures are to decrease the risk of falling and the prevention and treatment of osteoporosis. Ambulatory assistive devices (i.e., cane or walker) may be helpful for a patient with impaired balance who is still able to ambulate. Increased stability while ambulating may decrease the risk of falling and thereby decrease the fracture rate.

Intervention by the orthopaedic team to address potential osteoporosis in patients with wrist and hand fractures resulting from low-energy trauma should include patient education, testing, treatment with supplements and pharmacotherapy when indicated, and referral as needed. After a patient suffers a fragility fracture, the risk of future fracture is increased 1.5- to 9.5-fold [18, 19]. By recognizing coexisting osteoporosis at the time of a fragility-type wrist fracture, the orthopaedic surgeon has an opportunity to help initiate treatment to try to prevent further fractures. Treatment for osteoporosis may involve pharmacologic treatment, including calcium and vitamin D supplements and bisphosphonates. Non-pharmacologic recommendations include fall prevention, hip protectors, and balance and exercise programs. Orthopaedic surgeons are in the unique position of often being the initial physician to evaluate a patient with undiagnosed osteoporosis. This provides the orthopaedist the opportunity for patient education and initiation of the diagnosis and treatment in order to reduce the risk of future fractures.

Acknowledgments There were no grants or external sources of funding utilized for this study. Authors report no conflicts of interest related to the subject matter.

References

1. Doyle J, Bott M. Surgical anatomy of the hand and upper extremity. Philadelphia: Lippincott Williams & Wilkins, 2003.
2. Hoppenfeld S, deBoer P. Surgical exposures in orthopaedics: the anatomic approach, 3rd ed. Philadelphia: Lippincott Williams & Wilkins, 2003.
3. Bucholz R, Heckman J, Court-Brown C, eds. Rockwood and Green's fractures in adults, 6th ed. Philadelphia: Lippincott Williams & Wilkins, 2005.
4. Lafontaine M, Hardy D, Delince P. Stability assessment of distal radius fractures. Injury. 1989;20(4):208–10.
5. Goldhahn J, Angst F, Simmen BR. What counts: outcome assessment after distal radius fractures in aged patients. J Orthop Trauma. 2008;22(8 Suppl):S126–30.
6. Bogoch ER, Elliot-Gibson V, Escott BG, Beaton DE. The osteoporosis needs of patients with wrist fracture. J Orthop Trauma. 2008;22(8 Suppl):S73–8.
7. Mudgal CS, Jupiter JB. Plate fixation of osteoporotic fractures of the distal radius. J Orthop Trauma. 2008;22(8 Suppl):S106–15.
8. Gehrmann SV, Windolf J, Kaufmann RA. Distal radius fracture management in elderly patients: a literature review. J Hand Surg Am. 2008;33(3):421–9.
9. Earnshaw SA, Aladin A, Surendran S, Moran CG. Closed reduction of colles fractures: comparison of manual manipulation and finger-trap traction: a prospective, randomized study. J Bone Joint Surg Am. 2002;84-A(3):354–8.
10. Kettler M, Kuhn V, Schieker M, Melone CP. Do we need to include osteoporosis in today's classification of distal radius fractures? J Orthop Trauma. 2008;22(8 Suppl):S79–82.
11. Henry MH. Distal radius fractures: current concepts. J Hand Surg Am. 2008;33(7):1215–27.
12. Nana AD, Joshi A, Lichtman DM. Plating of the distal radius. J Am Acad Orthop Surg. 2005;13(3):159–71.
13. Hoang-Kim A, Goldhahn J, Moroni A. Wrist fractures in osteoporotic patients. J Orthop Trauma. 2008;22(8 Suppl):S57–8.
14. Slutsky D, Herman M. Rehabilitation of distal radius fractures: a biomechanical guide. Hand Clin. 2005;21:455–68.
15. Henry M. Distal radius fractures: current concepts. J Hand Surg. 2008;33A:1215–27.
16. Krischak G, Krasteva A, Schneider F, Gulkin D, Gebhard F, Kramer M. Physiotherapy after volar plating of wrist fractures is effective using a home exercise program. Arch Phys Med Rehabil. 2009;90:537–44.
17. Rozenthal T, Branas C, Bozentka D, Beredjiklian P. Survival among elderly patients after fractures of the distal radius. J Hand Surg. 2002;27A(6):948–52.
18. Klotzbuecher C, Ross P, Landsman P, et al. Patients with prior fractures have an increased risk of future fractures: a summary of the literature and statistical synthesis. J Bone Miner Res. 2000;15:721–39.
19. Center J, Bliuc D, Nguyen T, et al. Risk of subsequent fracture after low-trauma fracture in men and women. JAMA. 2007;297:387–94.

Chapter 10
Fractures of the Shoulder and Elbow

J. Stuart Melvin, Karen Boselli, and G. Russell Huffman

Abstract Fractures of the shoulder and elbow are common in the elderly population. Osteopenia and osteoporosis put this population at risk for fractures from low-energy trauma. The majority of fractures of the shoulder and elbow in this population are best managed nonoperatively. However, surgical intervention with open or closed reduction with fixation, shoulder arthroplasty, or total elbow arthroplasty may offer more predictable and better functional outcomes for certain fracture patterns. Regardless of the treatment modality, the goal of treating these injuries is to provide stable fracture fixation or reconstruction allowing early mobilization and pain free upper extremity function.

Keywords Elderly • Insufficiency fracture • Osteoporosis • Proximal humerus fracture • Humeral shaft fracture • Distal humerus fracture • Locking plate

10.1 Proximal Humerus Fractures

10.1.1 Background and Epidemiology

Fractures of the proximal humerus are relatively rare fractures with an overall incidence of 4–5% of all fractures [1]. However, in patients older than 65 years old, these fractures are the third most common fracture after Colles fractures and fractures of the hip [2].

G.R. Huffman (✉)
Department of Orthopaedic Surgery, University of Pennsylvania,
3400 Spruce Street, 2 Silverstein Pavilion, Philadelphia, PA 19104, USA
e-mail: russell.huffman@uphs.upenn.edu

R.J. Pignolo et al. (eds.), *Fractures in the Elderly*, Aging Medicine,
DOI 10.1007/978-1-60327-467-8_10,

Most fractures of the proximal humerus occurring in elderly patients are associated with osteoporosis. There is a 2.5 times greater incidence of proximal humerus fractures in women than men, 87% of which are the result of a simple ground level fall [3, 4]. Additionally, an epidemiological study demonstrated the incidence followed a unimodal age distribution with most fractures being seen in patients over age 70 [5]. This is in contrast to the typical bimodal age distribution seen with most fractures in which there is a peak in young active males from high-energy trauma and a second peak in the elderly associated with insufficiency fractures. A recent study found that the risk of osteoporotic fracture is correlated with the *T*-scores derived from dual X-ray absorptiometry scans of the hip and spine. Each unit decrease in the hip and spine *T*-scores was associated with a 30% increase in the risk of fracture [6].

Proximal humerus fractures can lead to considerable morbidity and loss of shoulder function in the elderly and impair activities of daily living. Twenty to twenty-five percent of elderly patients (20–25%) who could shop, perform housework, and toilet independently will be unable to do so after healing of proximal humerus fractures treated nonoperatively. Ultimately, some previously independent elderly individuals will require domestic assistance or not be fit to return independently to home [5].

A fracture of the proximal humerus in the elderly should be considered in the broad context of the patient. One study found that osteoporosis and risk of falling were independently associated with proximal humerus fracture [7]. Another study found that suffering a proximal humerus fracture increases the risk of having a hip fracture by up to 16% [8]. Proximal humerus fractures in the elderly should be recognized as an insufficiency and fall prevention as well as osteoporosis treatment should be a routine part of the treatment of a proximal humerus fracture in this patient population.

10.1.2 Anatomy and Fracture Pattern

10.1.2.1 Anatomy

The glenohumeral joint is relatively free of bony restraint and has often been compared to a golf ball on a tee. This shallow ball and socket joint allows for tremendous range of motion. However, because of the lack of bony congruency, stability of the glenohumeral joint is dependent upon soft tissue restraints. At rest, negative intraarticular pressure plays the most important role. Throughout a functional range of motion, stability is conferred through the rotator cuff and the mechanism of concavity compression. At the extremes of motion, soft tissue restraints consisting of the glenohumeral capsuloligamentous structures provide stability and restraint to subluxation and dislocation [9–11].

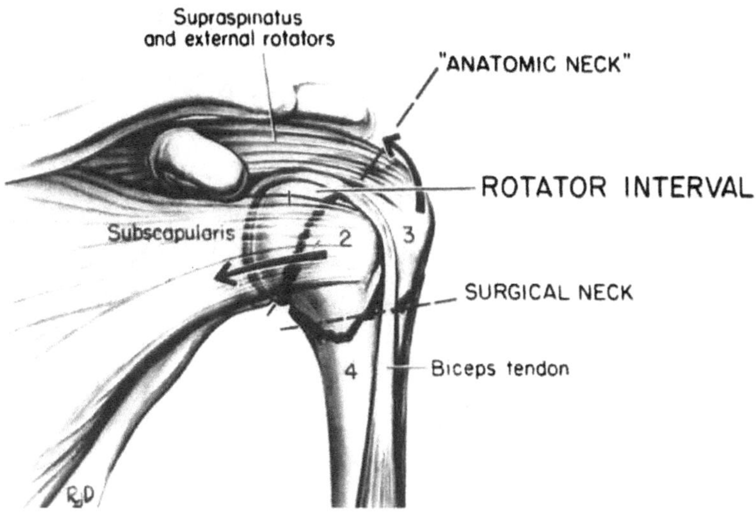

Fig. 10.1 Drawing illustrating the rotator interval and the four parts of the proximal humerus: *1* head, *2* lesser tuberosity, *3* greater tuberosity, *4* shaft (Reprinted with permission from Neer CS. Displaced proximal humeral fractures: 1. Classification and evaluation. J Bone Joint Surg 1970; 52A: 1077–1089)

The humerus is the largest bone in the upper extremity and articulates with the glenoid fossa of the scapula. The proximal humerus consists of a head, neck, and greater and lesser tuberosities (Fig. 10.1). The anatomic neck of the humerus is defined by a groove circumscribing the head. The surgical neck of the humerus is the portion of the proximal humeral metaphysis that is inferior to the greater and lesser tuberosities. The greater tuberosity is at the superolateral margin of the proximal humerus, while the lesser tuberosity projects anteriorly. The tendon of the long head of the biceps runs in the groove between the tuberosities.

The rotator cuff muscles actively elevate, abduct, and rotate the humeral head about the glenoid and are important stabilizers and depressors of the humeral head. Additionally, they cause displacement of fracture fragments. The supraspinatus, infraspinatus, and teres minor insert onto the greater tuberosity, while the subscapularis inserts onto the lesser tuberosity. The pectoralis major inserts lateral to the bicipital groove and often pulls the distal fragment medially. In the elderly, the tendons of the shoulder stabilizing muscles are often stronger than the bone of the proximal humerus.

The vascular anatomy to the humeral head is important in determining patient outcome and function after injury (Fig. 10.2). Disruption of the blood supply to the articular portion of the humerus, via the anterior and posterior humeral circumflex arteries, is associated with the severity of fracture and the amount of fracture displacement at time of injury. Development of avascular necrosis of the humeral head is directly correlated to poor functional outcome [12, 13].

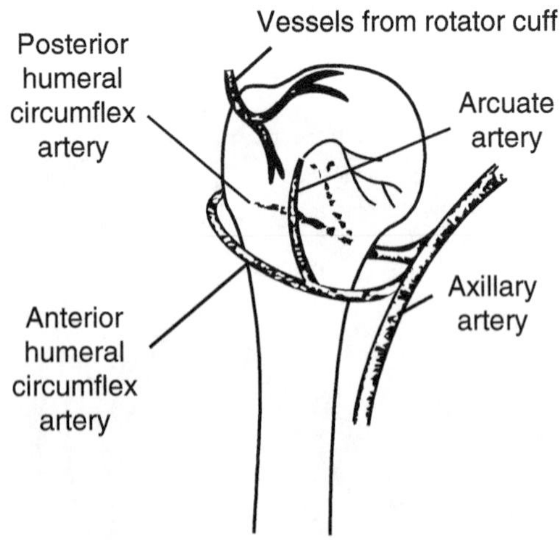

Fig. 10.2 Humeral head blood supply (© 1994 American Academy of Orthopaedic Surgeons Reprinted from the Journal of the American Academy of Orthopaedic Surgeons, 2(1), pp. 54–66 with permission)

10.1.2.2 Fracture Pattern

The most widely utilized fracture classification system is the Neer classification [14]. Neer based his classification on the prior observation made by Codman that nearly all proximal humerus fractures occurred along the lines of the closed growth plates. In Neer's classification, there are four possible parts including the humeral shaft, the humeral head, the greater tuberosity, and the lesser tuberosity (Fig. 10.3). In this classification scheme, the humeral shaft and head are divided at the surgical neck of the humerus. Neer defined a part as a fragment with at least 45° of angulation or greater than 1 cm of displacement. Parts with less than 45° of angulation or 1 cm of displacement are considered minimally displaced regardless of the number of fracture lines [14]. In the remainder of this chapter, the Neer classification system will be used in the description of fracture types.

10.1.3 Initial Presentation and Evaluation

Elderly patients with a proximal humerus fracture will typically present after a fall from standing. The cause of the fall should be investigated, as it may be the result of medical comorbidities. Upon presentation, the arm is often held closely to the chest wall by the opposite hand. The patient will complain of shoulder pain and there may be edema, ecchymosis, and tenderness to palpation of the shoulder with variable crepitus. It is important to fully evaluate the patient for associated trauma. Associated injuries may include ipsilateral upper extremity fractures, rib fractures, hemothorax, and pneumothorax. The neurovascular status must be

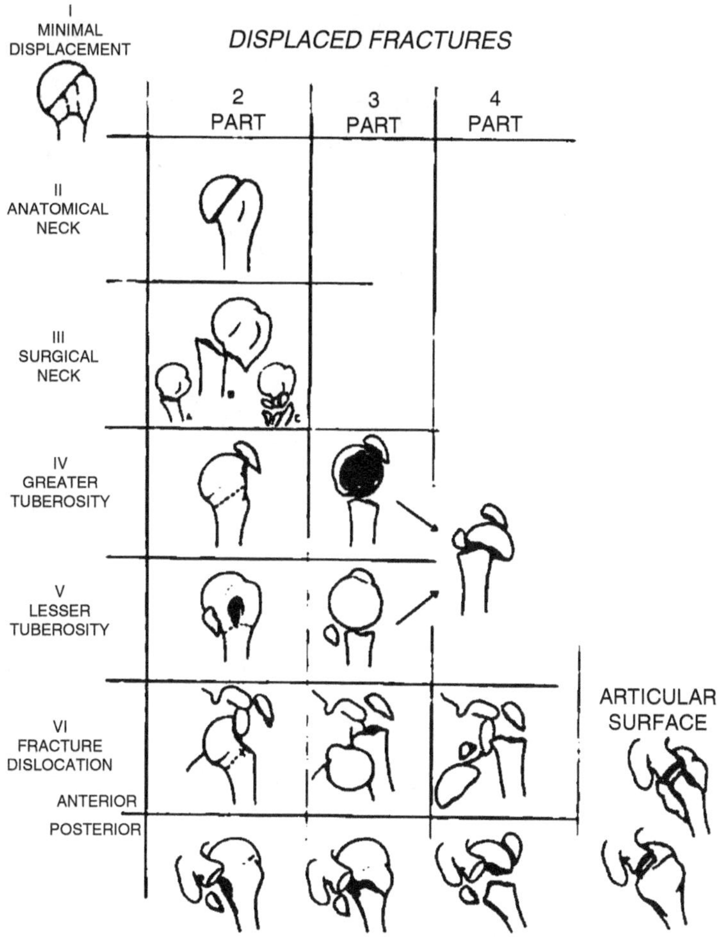

Fig. 10.3 The Neer four-part classification of proximal humerus fractures. A fracture is considered displaced if the fracture fragments are separated 1 cm or greater, or if angulation between the fracture fragments is more than 45° (Reprinted with permission from Neer CS. Displaced proximal humeral fractures: 1. Classification and evaluation. J Bone Joint Surg 1970; 52A:1077–1089)

carefully investigated. Injury to the axillary artery can occur and is more common with fracture dislocations.

Initial radiographic evaluation should include an AP, axillary lateral, and scapular Y view (Fig. 10.4). The axillary lateral can usually be performed with minimal abduction by having the arm supported by the physician. Computed tomography (CT) may be helpful to fully understand the fracture pattern of more complex and comminuted fractures. Magnetic resonance imaging (MRI) is also useful in determining the status of the rotator cuff in selected patients.

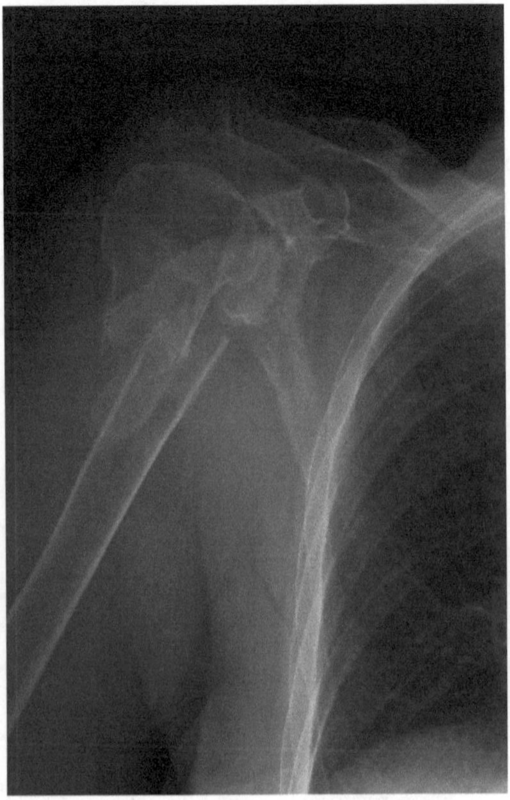

Fig. 10.4 Anterior–posterior radiograph of an osteoporotic fracture of the surgical neck

10.1.4 Nonoperative Treatment

The majority of proximal humerus fractures in the elderly can be managed nonoperatively. Nondisplaced or minimally displaced fractures comprise 49–85% of proximal humerus fractures and there is little controversy that these fractures, when they occur in isolation, should be managed nonoperatively [14, 15]. The only exception is a fracture of the greater tuberosity. Some evidence suggests that displacement of >5 mm can lead to significant functional impairment [16]. In the elderly, isolated two-part greater tuberosity fractures typically occur in the setting of an acute shoulder dislocation. MRI is warranted in instances in which the tuberosity is displaced less than 5 mm to ensure integrity of the rotator cuff. When displacement of greater than 5 mm is present, operative fixation ensures proper functioning of the supraspinatus and infraspinatus muscles and minimizes the incidence of impingement of the displaced tuberosity on the coracoacromial arch.

Nonoperative treatment with or without closed reduction should also be considered for displaced fractures as well. A study by Court-Brown et al. demonstrated that older patients actually did better in terms of shoulder function when displaced two-part surgical neck or valgus-impacted fractures were treated with sling immobilization compared to open reduction and internal fixation (ORIF) [5]. While these patients demonstrated objective functional limitations at one year postinjury, these deficits were not perceived to be significant by the patients. It was concluded that full glenohumeral motion or power is not required for elderly patients to return to routine activities. An additional study found no difference in outcome between elderly patients with three- or four-part fractures treated nonoperatively as compared to surgery [17]. However, these data predate the standard use of rigid fixation and immediate mobilization of displaced two- and three-part fractures with locked plate designs.

When nonoperative management is deemed appropriate, sling immobilization should be implemented for two weeks. Elbow, wrist, and hand range of motion is encouraged immediately. Radiographs should be performed weekly within the initial month after injury to evaluate for fracture displacement. In the absence of fracture displacement, gentle passive motion and pendulum exercises begin as tolerated at two weeks postinjury. Active motion can begin at six weeks or when early callus is noted on radiographs. The goals of nonoperative treatment include early mobilization, restoration of full passive motion, and eventual return to full function.

10.1.5 Operative Management

Current trends have favored operative treatment for most displaced two-, three-, and four-part fractures. However, any consideration of operative treatment in elderly patients must take into consideration the bone quality, as this may limit the surgical options. The quality of bone in the proximal humerus in some elderly patients may not be amenable to rigid internal fixation. Older age has been shown to be a primary predictor of implant failure. Additionally, cortical thickness of the proximal humeral diaphysis has been shown to be a predictor of bone mineral density as well as outcome of internal fixation. A combined cortical thickness of >4 mm as measured at two levels in the proximal humeral diaphysis is the minimum necessary for adequate screw purchase with standard internal fixation [18].

Biomechanical testing has shown superiority of locking plate designs over suture fixation, unlocked plate designs, and percutaneous pin fixation [19]. However, even with locked plates, fixation should be augmented with nonabsorbable suture secured to the plate.

Displaced two- or three-part fractures with inadequate bone quality may be effectively treated by tension banding with suture, locked plating or a combination of these techniques [20–23]. Anchoring the suture in the rotator cuff tendon provides stronger fixation than the osteoporotic bone. Our preference and the literature suggests that use of a locked plate augmented with suture fixation provides superior torsional and bending rigidity compared to an isolated tension band technique allowing earlier active motion [19, 21, 22].

Displaced two- or three-part fractures with adequate bone quality may be effectively treated by a number of methods. Closed reduction and percutaneous fixation with threaded pins or screws offers advantages in patients with bleeding disorders or other significant comorbidities. This method requires minimal surgical dissection and thus has less risk for further disruption of the blood supply to the humeral head (Fig. 10.5) [23]. However, fixation is less rigid, limiting early motion and second procedure for pin removal is usually required 4–6 weeks postoperatively. Open reduction and conventional plate and screw fixation can be considered for elderly patients with adequate bone stock. However, with the poor bone quality typical of this population, often it is difficult to obtain sufficient screw purchase to prevent screw loosening and pull out in the humeral head and metaphysis [24, 25]. Malreduction and rates of osteonecrosis as high as 35% have been associated with conventional plating techniques [16].

With advances in plate design, anatomically precontoured locking plates with suture eyelets are now readily available for proximal humerus fractures. Locking plate technology employs screws that lock into a threaded plate, thus creating a fixed angled construct. Stiffness and pull out strength of the locking plate are

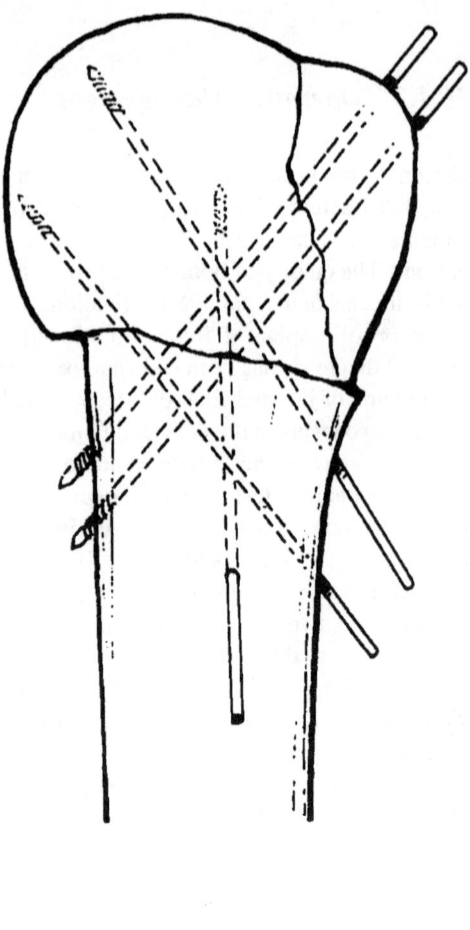

Fig. 10.5 Illustration of percutaneous pinning technique (Reprinted with permission from H Jaberg, JJ Warner, and RP Jakob J. Bone Joint Surg Am, April 1992; 74: 508–515)

related to the entire construct and not just the individual screw purchase [26, 27]. These plates are better able to resist cantilever bending forces and torsional forces [28]. Additionally, this technology does not rely on contact between the plate and bone, which reduces the amount of dissection and soft tissue stripping (Fig. 10.6).

Most three- and four-part fractures with severe osteopenia or comminution in the elderly are best treated with hemiarthroplasty (Fig. 10.7) [26, 29]. The exception is the valgus impacted four-part fracture that maintains medial cortical continuity, as this fracture has a significantly lower rate of osteonecrosis [23, 30]. An attempt at limited internal fixation with sutures or plate and suture fixation in situ is warranted for these fractures.

The goal of hemiarthroplasty is to restore the anatomic relationships of the tuberosities, the shaft, and humeral head. This can prove to be a difficult task in the elderly due to a lack of intraoperative anatomic reference points, poor bone quality, and fracture comminution at the surgical neck. It has been shown that hemiarthroplasty can reliably relieve pain generated from the proximal humerus, but functional outcome is much less predictable [29, 31–33]. Often patients are unable to regain function above shoulder height. This could be due to rotator cuff weakness, but is more commonly attributed to nonunion of the tuberosities or to nonanatomic

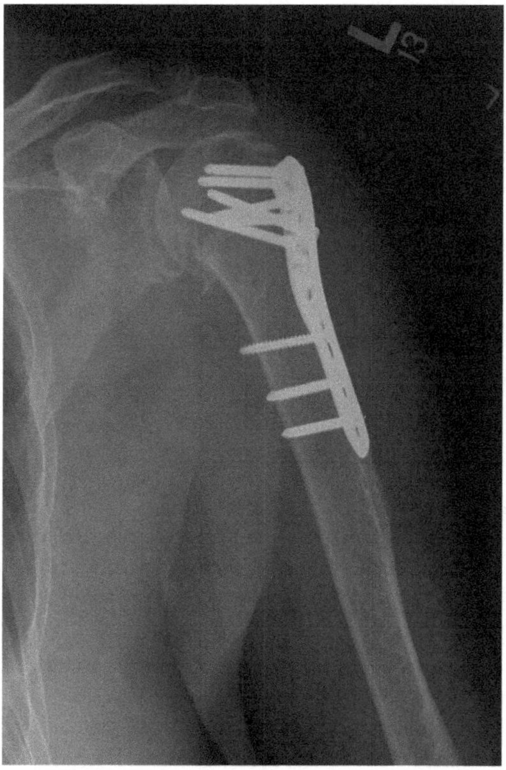

Fig. 10.6 Postoperative anterior–posterior radiograph of a proximal humerus locking plate

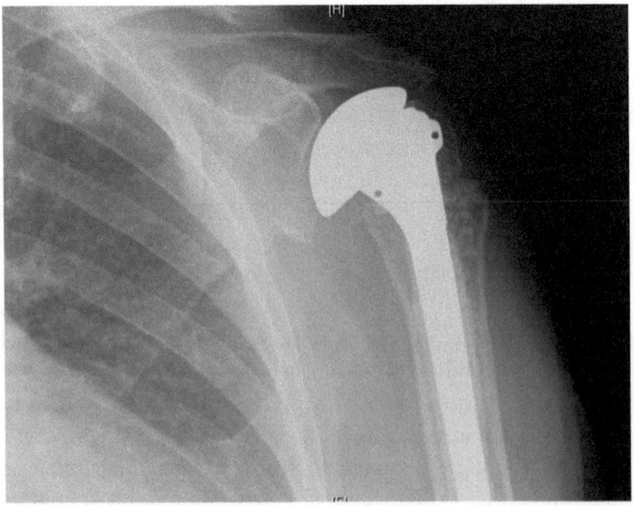

Fig. 10.7 Anterior–posterior radiograph depicting a hemiarthroplasty

tuberosity positioning [31, 34–37]. It is known that one of the most important predictors of a good functional outcome with hemiarthroplasty is anatomic healing of the greater tuberosity, as this restores rotator cuff function [31, 38].

Reverse total shoulder arthroplasty, in which the glenoid is converted into a spherical head and the head of the humerus into a socket, has been shown to have acceptable functional outcomes for degenerative arthritis in the presence of a profound rotator cuff deficiency [39]. This is currently being explored as an option for three- and four-part fractures in the elderly as it may provide better functional outcome in the presence of malunited or nonunited greater tuberosities for low-demand patients. Presently, the clearest roll for use of reverse implant designs in fracture patients is for patients with malunited proximal humerus fractures in which osteotomy of the tuberosities would be necessary.

10.1.6 Rehabilitation

For both operative and nonoperatively managed proximal humerus fractures in the elderly, formal physical therapy is important in helping to achieve restoration of motion and a return to full function. Prolonged immobilization should be avoided. For minimally displaced or stable fractures treated nonoperatively, rehabilitation should begin immediately. Surgically treated fractures may begin immediate passive motion under the supervision of a licensed physical therapist. A brief period of immobilization, not exceeding three weeks, may be appropriate for more complex, nondisplaced fractures treated nonoperatively. The goal of rehabilitation is to restore normal shoulder kinematics and allow restoration of pain-free shoulder function for activities of daily living. As pain and swelling improve, active assisted range of motion is initiated. During the final stages of therapy, active and resisted exercises are included and the sling is discarded. Additionally, fall prevention should be addressed throughout therapy and may include incorporation of an occupational therapist [40].

10.2 Fractures of the Humeral Shaft

10.2.1 Background and Epidemiology

Humeral shaft fractures are defined as fractures in which the major fracture line occurs distal to the insertion of the pectoralis major and proximal to the supracondylar ridge. It is estimated that these fractures comprise 3–5% of all fractures in adults [41]. Epidemiologic studies have clearly demonstrated the incidence has a bimodal distribution with a small peak in the third decade for men and much larger peak in the seventh decade for women [42, 43]. There appears to be a clear association between fractures of the humeral shaft and osteoporosis with an increasing incidence from the fifth decade onward. In the elderly, the most common mechanism is a fall from a standing. Osteoporosis evaluation and treatment as well as fall prevention are indicated in the treatment of elderly humeral shaft fractures.

The mobility of the glenohumeral joint and robust blood supply to the humeral diaphysis allow most of these fractures to be treated nonoperatively with functional bracing. Modest degrees of shortening and angular malalignment are well tolerated with little effect on upper extremity function. However, operative treatment is warranted for humeral shaft fractures that meet specific indications.

10.2.2 Anatomy and Fracture Pattern

10.2.2.1 Anatomy

The humeral shaft comprises the portion of the humerus distal to the pectoralis major insertion to the area immediately proximal to the supracondylar ridge. The proximal portion of the diaphysis is cylindrical and tapers to a triangular shape distally. The medullary canal also diminishes in diameter and ends just superior to the olecranon fossa. This abrupt tapering of the humeral canal differs from the canal of the femur and tibia in which the metaphysis widens. Unfamiliarity with this anatomy may lead to distraction of humeral shaft fractures during antegrade humeral nailing.

The humerus has an abundant vascular supply and is enveloped in soft tissue, which aids in healing. The medial and lateral muscular septa divide the arm into anterior and posterior compartments. The median nerve, musculocutaneous nerve, and brachial artery traverse the anterior compartment. The ulnar nerve begins proximally in the anterior compartment and passes through the medial intermuscular septum to enter the posterior compartment near the distal third of the humerus. The radial nerve begins in the posterior compartment and crosses the posterior aspect of the humerus 20 cm proximal to the medial epicondyle and 15 cm proximal to the lateral epicondyle in a region known as the spiral groove. The radial nerve then passes through the lateral intermuscular septum to enter the anterior compartment.

10.2.3 Classification

Classification of these fractures has historically been descriptive. The fracture is often described as open or closed, by the location within the humeral shaft (proximal, middle, or distal third) and overall character of the fracture pattern (transverse, oblique, spiral, comminuted).

10.2.4 Initial Presentation and Evaluation

Humeral shaft fractures in the elderly are often isolated injuries suffered after a fall from standing. The patient will present with arm pain, swelling, and often visible deformity. In the elderly patient, the cause of the fall will need to be investigated as it may have occurred during secondary medical comorbidities. Additionally, the patient should be fully assessed for associated injury and the skin over the humerus inspected for open fracture. A detailed neurovascular exam should be performed and documented, as injury to the radial nerve has been reported to occur in up to 18% of these fractures. Vascular injury is rare, but constitutes an emergency when present.

Radiographic evaluation should include AP and lateral view of the entire humerus, including the humeral head and elbow on a single radiograph (Fig. 10.8). In order to obtain the orthogonal views, the cassette or patient should be moved, as moving the arm will cause rotation of the distal fragment through the fracture site. Appropriate well-padded splinting or immobilization should be applied for immediate comfort until definitive treatment is rendered.

10.2.5 Nonoperative Management

Most humeral shaft fractures are successfully managed nonoperatively. The tremendous range of motion of the glenohumeral joint allows for functional

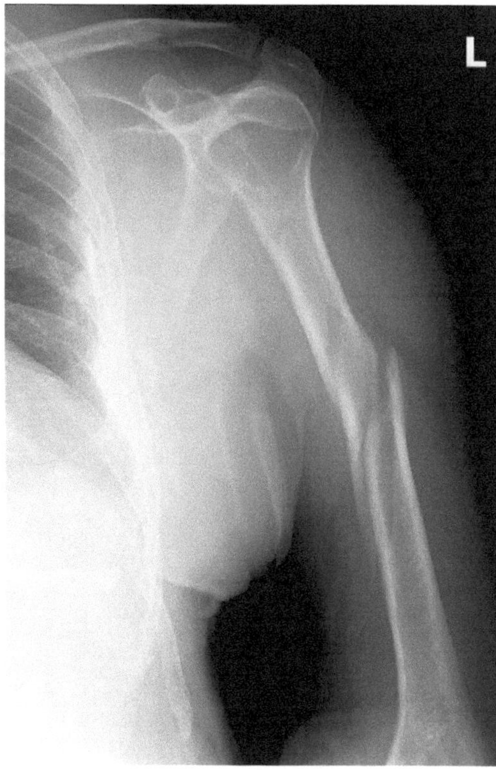

Fig. 10.8 Anterior–posterior radiograph of an osteoporotic humeral shaft fracture

compensation of moderate malunion and shortening. It is generally accepted that up to 3 cm of shortening and 20–30° of varus, anterior, or rotational deformity will result in an acceptable upper extremity function.

The current standard of care is the application of a functional brace with or without closed reduction once initial swelling has subsided. The timing of the application of the functional brace is somewhat controversial. Some prefer the initial application of a coaptation splint for more immediate immobilization until soft tissue swelling has subsided. Conversion to a functional brace then occurs 1–2 weeks after injury. Regardless of timing, early shoulder, elbow, wrist, and hand therapy should be instituted.

Functional bracing consists of a circumferential off-the-shelf orthosis secured with Velcro straps and a cuff and collar to support the forearm (Fig. 10.9) [44]. A sling should be avoided as it may contribute to varus angulation. The brace should extend as far proximally into the axilla as the patient's skin and neurovascular structures can tolerate. This is especially important for fractures of the proximal third of the shaft.

The functional brace works through three basic principles. The first is the hydraulic effect, in which circumferential compression helps to achieve reduction, restore

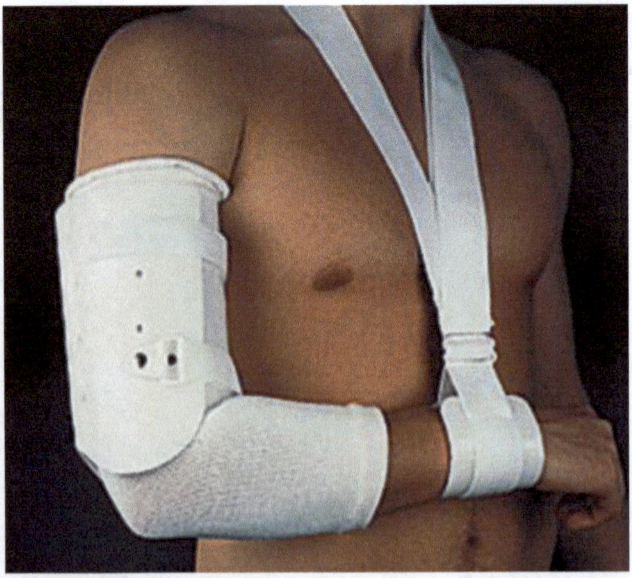

Fig. 10.9 Clinical photograph of a functional brace

humeral length, and confer stability. The second is that active muscle contraction within the brace will aid reduction. Lastly, the effect of gravity will counteract shortening and aid fracture reduction. A large series of patients treated with functional bracing found a 2% nonunion rate in closed fractures and a 6% nonunion rate in open fractures. This study also found that over 80% of patients healed with <16° of angulation and 98% of patients had minimal loss of shoulder motion [44].

10.2.6 Operative Treatment

While the majority of humeral shaft fractures are appropriately treated nonoperatively, there are humeral shaft fractures that are best treated operatively. The relative indications for operative intervention for humeral shaft fractures include segmental fractures, floating elbow injuries, transverse diaphyseal fractures, open fractures, nonunions, and polytraumatic injuries in which upper extremity weight bearing would facilitate early patient mobilization. In the elderly, the most common indications include pathologic fractures, associated trauma, or nonunion. Additionally, obesity, large breasts, and frail skin may make functional bracing technically impossible and would also be indications for surgery.

Plating of the humerus is the treatment of choice for most humeral shaft fractures when surgery is indicated (Fig. 10.10) [45–47]. Traditional plating techniques have achieved high union rates, low infection rates, and good shoulder and elbow function. Plating of the humerus allows immediate weight bearing and has been

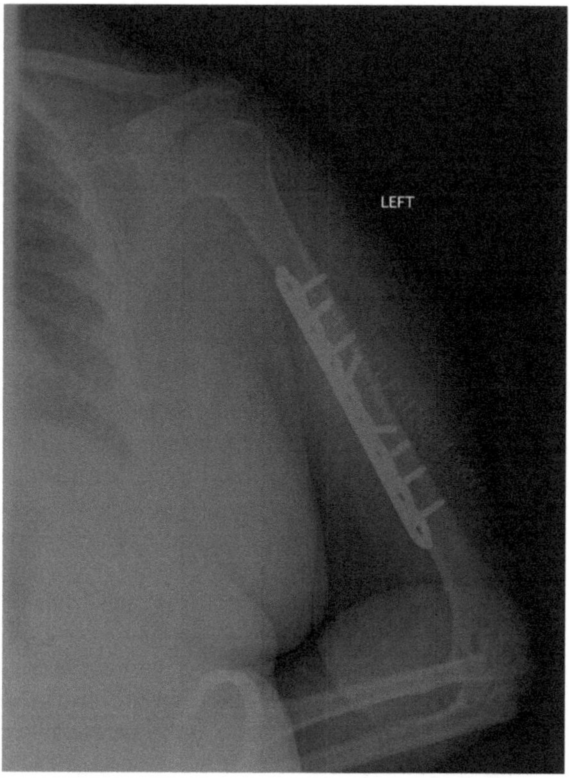

Fig. 10.10 Postoperative anterior–posterior radiograph of humeral shaft plate

shown to have a low infection rate when used in the treatment of open fractures [48]. In the elderly, screw purchase in osteoporotic bone may be compromised. Locking plates that create a fixed angled construct by the screw locking into the plate appear to provide better fixation and cause less devascularization [49]. The disadvantages of plating include the extensive exposure required, risk of injury to the radial nerve, and refracture after hardware removal.

In an attempt to reproduce the success of intramedullary fixation in the femur and tibia, intramedullary nails have been employed in the treatment of humeral shaft fractures. The theoretical advantages of intramedullary fixation in the humerus include limited dissection and load sharing by the implant across the fracture site. In practice, intramedullary fixation has not proven to be as successful as plating and has been associated with a number of complications including radial nerve injury and nonunion [50, 51]. Despite the overall inferior results of intramedullary nailing compared to plating, intramedullary fixation may be indicated for pathologic or impending pathologic fractures.

The most common complications of intramedullary nailing have been nonunion and shoulder pain [50–52]. Nonunion rates have been higher for intramedullary nailing for nearly all series reported. With the newer generation locked nails used today, fracture distraction, not inadequate fixation, is the most common cause of nonunion. Unlike the lower extremities, the humerus is not a weight-bearing bone and thus the normal compressive forces seen with weight bearing in the lower extremity are absent in the upper extremity. Additionally, the narrow distal intramedullary canal often allows the distal fragment to be distracted by the rod. Shoulder pain and functional loss have been another common and significant complication. The antegrade approach to IM nailing violates the rotator cuff insertion and may be the cause of pain and functional loss.

10.2.7 Rehabilitation

For nonoperative treatment, pendulum exercises for the shoulder as well as active and passive elbow, wrist, and hand range of motion exercises should be implemented immediately after application of the fracture brace. For those patients in which a coaptation splint is applied acutely, pendulum exercises will be delayed until the 1–2 week follow-up appointment at which time they will be advanced to a functional brace that allows these exercises. At 1–2 weeks postinjury, the patient should be instructed to remove the functional brace three times a day to perform pendulums, passive shoulder flexion, elbow, wrist and hand exercises, as well as bathing. The patient should remain nonweight bearing until the fracture heals, and active shoulder flexion and abduction are instituted after callus is noted radiographically. Patients with a radial nerve palsy should be fitted for a cock-up wrist splint [44].

After plate fixation of a humeral shaft fracture, active and passive range of motion exercises of the shoulder, elbow, wrist, and hand can begin immediately. The patient may weight bear with the operative extremity, but if using a crutch or walker for assistance with ambulation, an elbow platform may be more comfortable.

10.3 Distal Humerus Fractures

10.3.1 Background

Elbow injuries in the elderly can often lead to restriction of motion and chronic pain, accounting for significant disability. Fractures of the distal humerus are challenging injuries in any patient, and are especially difficult to manage in the elderly population. In patients with osteopenia, internal fixation is technically demanding due to the difficulty in obtaining secure fixation and the presence of fracture comminution. The surgeon must tailor the management of these fractures to meet the functional needs of the elderly patient.

10.3.2 Anatomy and Fracture Pattern

10.3.2.1 Anatomy

Understanding the bony anatomy of the distal humerus is critical, as the treatment of these injuries is based on the ability to restore the radiocapitellar, olecranon-trochlear, and proximal radioulnar articulations.

The cylindrical shaft of the humerus divides at the metaphysis into medial and lateral columns of bone, forming the supracondylar region of the elbow. Between these columns is a thin isthmus of bone constituting the coronoid fossa anteriorly and the olecranon fossa posteriorly. These fossae accommodate the coronoid and olecranon processes, respectively, during full flexion and extension of the elbow. The olecranon fossa is normally filled with fat [53].

The trochlea and capitellum, the articular surfaces of the distal humerus, lie at the base of the medial and lateral columns, respectively. The anatomy of the distal humerus, therefore, has often been described as a triangle, with the medial and lateral columns constituting the sides, and the articular surface as the base [53]. This relationship has also been likened to a spool of thread (the trochlea) being held between the thumb and index finger (the columns) [54]. The trochlea is larger in diameter medially than laterally and extends more distally than the capitellum in the coronal plane (Fig. 10.11).

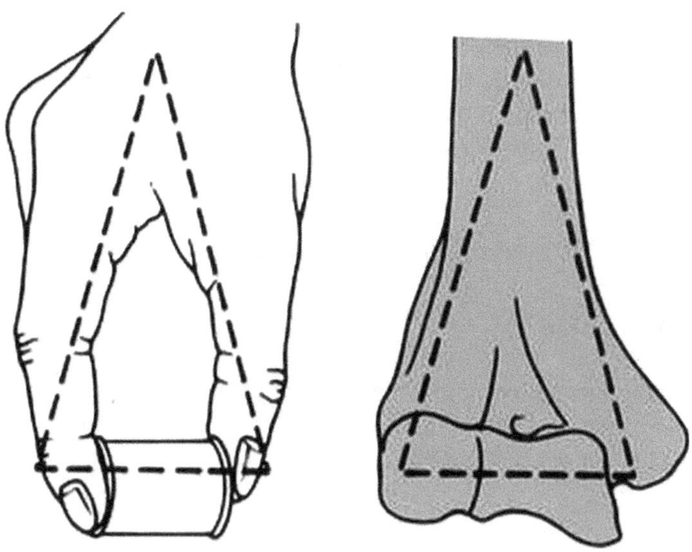

Fig. 10.11 Anatomy of the distal humerus. The trochlea is a central spool-shaped structure, bounded by the columns medially and laterally (This figure was published in Skeletal Trauma. Volume 2. Browner BD, Jupiter JB, Levine AM, et al. (eds.). Ch.42 Trauma to the Adult Elbow. pp. 1542. © Elsevier 2009)

Combined with internal rotation of the distal humeral articular surface 5–7° from the epicondylar axis and a valgus tilt angle of 6–8° of the humeral articular surface, the trochlear anatomy creates a valgus carrying angle of 11–17° of the elbow when fully extended. The distal humeral articular surface has a 30° anterior inclination in relation to the axis of the humeral shaft allowing full extension of the elbow and accommodating the large olecranon process, which articulates in the olecranon fossa posteriorly.

The distal aspect of the medial column is the medial epicondyle, which is the origin of the flexor-pronator mass and medial collateral ligament. The ulnar nerve courses posterior to the epicondyle, within the cubital tunnel. The distal aspect of the lateral column is the capitellum, which articulates with the radial head. This articulation helps to stabilize the elbow against varus and valgus stress, and provides a surface for forearm rotation [53].

10.3.3 Fracture Pattern

These fractures are typically classified descriptively as supracondylar (extraarticular) and intercondylar (intraarticular) fractures [54]. Intraarticular fractures are classified into subcategories including single column injuries, bicolumn injuries, capitellar fractures, and trochlear fractures. Extraarticular intracapsular injuries involve both columns of the humerus without disrupting the distal articular surface, and are most common in the pediatric population, but may rarely also be seen in the elderly [55].

Bicolumnar injuries are the most common type of fracture of the distal humerus, affecting all three parts of the distal humeral triangle. They are subdivided based on a descriptive classification of the fracture pattern. The most common patterns are T-pattern, Y-pattern, H-pattern, and λ-pattern (lambda) [54, 55].

10.3.4 Initial Presentation and Evaluation

10.3.4.1 Mechanism

Distal humeral fractures occur in a bimodal distribution. There is an early peak in young patients due to high-energy trauma, while the second peak occurs in the elderly due to low-energy falls [56].

10.3.5 History and Physical Examination

The initial assessment begins with a detailed history and physical examination. Hand dominance, occupation, and recreational activities as well as level of independence may determine treatment. The patient should be asked about pre-existing medical conditions that may have contributed to the injury as well as current medications.

It is also important to ask about the function of the joint prior to the injury and about any previous surgery to the extremity. Smoking history is important. As in any fracture in an elderly patient, a general functional assessment is necessary to guide treatment and set goals for rehabilitation.

The extremity should be examined for gross deformity and ecchymosis, and the skin assessed for open wounds. The entire limb needs to be palpated seeking concomitant injuries of the shoulder, wrist, or hand. The neurovascular status should be carefully assessed and documented. Particular attention is paid to examination of the motor and sensory integrity of the ulnar nerve.

10.3.5.1 Radiographs

Routine radiographs include a standard AP and lateral image of the elbow, with oblique images if warranted. If normal bony landmarks become distorted due to significant displacement or comminution of the fracture, images can be obtained while applying gentle traction to the extremity. This can often improve the general alignment and help to further characterize the fracture pattern [57]. Additionally, radiographs of the shoulder and wrist are obtained to exclude injury to adjacent joints. CT scan may be helpful in assessing the amount of comminution and in formulating the operative plan [58].

10.3.6 Nonoperative Management

Nonsurgical treatment has a limited role in management of these injuries, and is reserved for stable, nondisplaced fractures or elderly patients who have severe neurologic impairment, a nonfunctional extremity or high risk comorbidities.

10.3.7 Operative Management

Consideration should be given to ORIF for most of these fractures. The plan for fracture repair or reconstruction should follow the underlying principles of early surgical management (usually within 1–2 weeks), achievement of a rigid, stable construct, and immediate range of motion [53]. Patients with injuries not amenable to reconstruction may be candidates for total elbow arthroplasty (TEA).

When indicated, ORIF has been shown to give satisfactory results in the elderly patient (Fig. 10.12). John et al. studied 49 patients with a mean age of 80 years, at an average of 18 months after ORIF. Good or very good results were obtained in 85% of the patients, with 66% of patients reporting no pain. Arc of motion was 90° or greater in 85% of those studied. The authors concluded that old age alone is not a contraindication to ORIF of intraarticular distal humerus fractures [59]. A second study by Pereles et al. was a retrospective review of patients older than 60 years

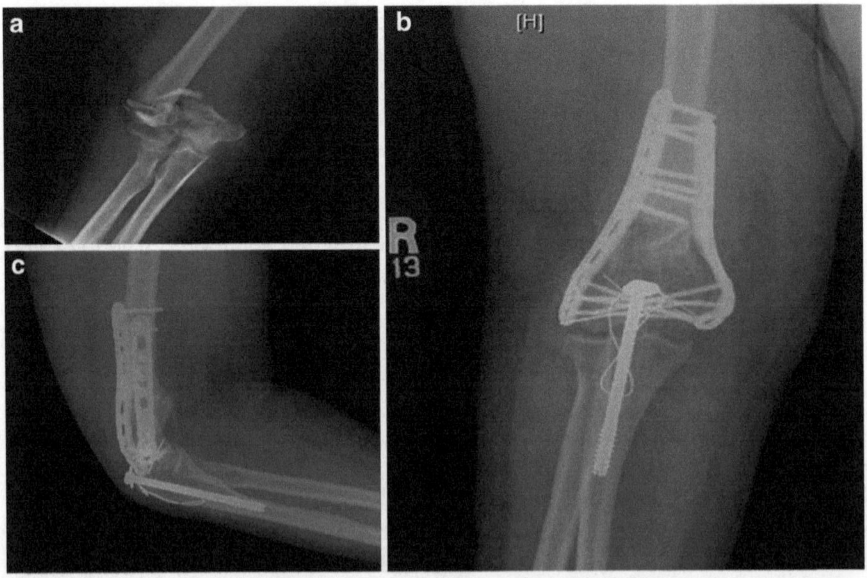

Fig. 10.12 Preoperative radiograph (**a**) of comminuted distal humerus fracture in a 72-year-old patient. Postoperative radiographs (**b**, **c**) demonstrate excellent healing, several months following open reduction and internal fixation (ORIF) with parallel plating and olecranon osteotomy

following ORIF of distal humeral fractures, which demonstrated an average arc of motion of 112°, good or excellent clinical results in all patients, and general health status (measured by SF-36) comparable to the published norms for patients of similar age in the United States [60].

In elderly patients with osteopenia or comminution of the joint surface, in whom a stable reconstruction cannot be achieved, TEA with a semiconstrained linked prosthesis may be preferable to ORIF (Fig. 10.13). In a multicenter, prospective randomized trial, TEA resulted in lower reoperation rates and more predictable functional results at two years [61] A retrospective study by Frankle et al. also compared TEA and ORIF for the treatment of intraarticular distal humerus fractures in women over age 65. Results in the TEA group were significantly better than those treated with ORIF. The authors concluded that TEA is a viable option for the primary management of distal humerus fractures in elderly women, especially those with associated comorbidities including rheumatoid arthritis, osteoporosis, and conditions requiring systemic steroid use. They further suggest that fractures with significant articular comminution should be managed with TEA, while those fractures with large articular fragments should be managed with attempted ORIF [62].

In general, treatment of distal humerus fractures in the elderly should take into account physiologic age, functionality, associated comorbidities, and fracture characteristics [62]. Use of a single posterior incision that deviates a full 2 cm away from the tip of the olecranon will minimize risk of skin breakdown and wound dehiscence while affording extensile exposure [61]. For reconstructable fractures, an

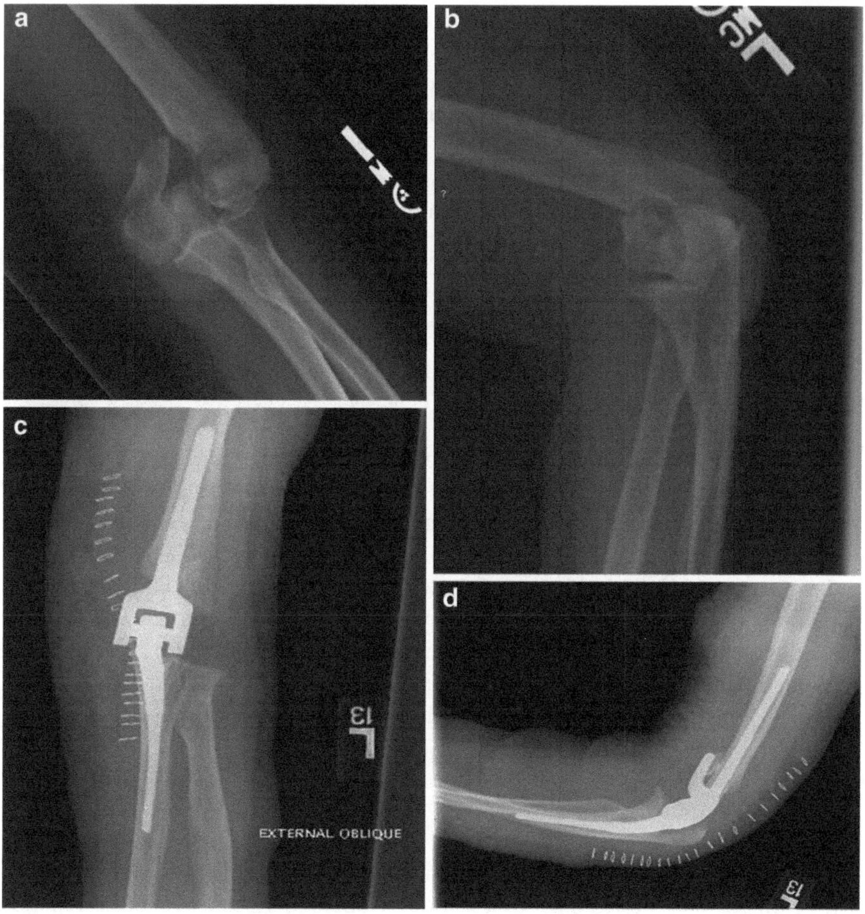

Fig. 10.13 Preoperative radiographs (**a**, **b**) of distal humerus fracture (with intraarticular extension) in an 88-year-old patient. Semiconstrained total elbow arthroplasty (**c**, **d**) was selected as the treatment of choice in this individual with low functional demands

olecrenon osteotomy facilitates exposure of the articular portion of the distal humerus. The ulnar nerve is routinely transposed subcutaneously in fracture fixation and TEA. However, hinged or static external fixation should be considered for temporary or definitive treatment in patients with severely contaminated open wounds or extensive soft tissue defects [63].

10.3.8 Rehabilitation

Rehabilitation is of critical importance in the elderly patient following a distal humerus fracture. Range of motion may start within 48 h of surgery. Active and active-assist exercises should be initiated during the hospital stay under the direction of an experienced physical therapist. The patient should also be educated on active range of motion of the shoulder, wrist, and fingers. A resting thermoplast extension splint is recommended for use between therapy sessions, especially at night. Daytime use of the splint can be weaned at 4–6 weeks, however, night use should be continued. Active strengthening exercises generally should not be initiated until radiographic union is seen and restoration of active motion has occurred [53].

10.3.9 Outcomes and Complications

10.3.9.1 Outcomes

In the elderly patient, subjective outcomes are important to assess, as objective measures such as time to union and range of motion may not be directly associated with patient satisfaction. Most patients can perform activities of daily living within a flexion-extension arc of 100° (range 30–130°), including 50° of both pronation and supination [64]. The elderly patient will easily meet most functional demands within this range and can comfortably tolerate the moderate limitations in motion following treatment of distal humeral injuries. Achievement of these goals has been facilitated with the development of precontoured anatomical plates, the use of parallel plate constructs, and rigid fixation allowing early range of motion.

10.3.9.2 Complications

Complications of distal humeral fractures include nonunion, infection, ulnar neuropathy, stiffness, and heterotopic ossification. Nonunion rates have been reported between 2 and 10%, and are frequently due to factors such as inadequate fixation, severe fracture comminution, or poor bone quality [65, 66]. Most patients require operative management of the nonunion due to significant pain and functional disability. Reported infection rates range from 0 to 9%, with management depending upon the time at which the infection presents, and the presence or absence of fracture union [65, 67]. Ulnar neuropathy is common following fractures of the distal humerus [65]. Stiffness and heterotopic ossification are more common in patients with polytruama, high-energy injuries, open fractures, and delays to definitive treatment [68].

10.4 Radial Head Fractures

10.4.1 Background and Epidemiology

The radial head was once considered to be an expendable structure, but is now recognized as an important bony stabilizer of the elbow [68].

Accounting for 33% of all elbow fractures, radial head injuries are relatively common, with their highest occurrence between ages 20 and 60. Women are twice as likely as men to sustain this injury. Although nondisplaced radial head fractures often occur in isolation, displaced fractures are frequently associated with other elbow injuries such as dislocations and ligamentous disruptions [69]. There may also be concomitant fractures of the coronoid process, olecranon, or capitellum. In the elderly patient who is more likely to suffer a comminuted radial head fracture with associated ligamentous injury, it is especially important to understand the role of the radial head as it relates to elbow stability.

10.4.2 Anatomy and Classification

10.4.2.1 Anatomy and Biomechanics

The head of the radius is a concave circular structure with a variable offset angle from the radial neck. It articulates with the spherical capitellum, however this articulation is minimally constrained due to the difference in radius of curvature between the two bony structures [69]. The radial head also articulates with the proximal ulna at the lesser sigmoid notch. Contact between the radius and ulna is maintained throughout pronation and supination, with the annular ligament stabilizing the proximal radioulnar articulation. Lateral ligamentous anatomy of the elbow is important as compromise of the lateral ulnar collateral ligament can lead to chronic elbow instability [70].

The radial head plays two roles in stability of the elbow. It is a secondary stabilizer against valgus forces and plays a primary role when the medial ulnar collateral ligament is incompetent [71]. The radial head also provides longitudinal stability, acting as a primary restraint to proximal migration of the radius. The soft tissues of the forearm, including the interosseus ligament and distal radioulnar joint, provide secondary longitudinal stability [68]. In a normal extremity, up to 60% of mechanical load at the wrist is transferred to the radial head via the interosseus ligament. Maximum force transmission at the radiocapitellar joint occurs during forearm pronation and elbow extension [72]. With an injured or excised radial head, normal load sharing at the radiocapitellar joint is disrupted, and all compressive loads at the elbow are transferred from the wrist through the ulna. This ultimately leads to proximal radial migration as well as increased contact pressure in the humeral trochlea. The latter may predispose the patient to arthritis [70].

10.4.2.2 Classification

Radial head injuries have traditionally been classified according to the Mason classification system [73]. Hotchkiss modified this scheme to include elbow dislocation (Table 10.1) [73]. Type I fractures are minimally displaced with no mechanical block to motion and can be managed nonoperatively. Type II fractures are displaced

Table 10.1 Mason classification of radial head fractures, as adapted by Hotchkiss

Mason classification	
Type I	Minimally displaced fracture, no mechanical block to forearm motion, intraarticular displacement <2 mm
Type II	Fracture displaced >2 mm or angulated, possible mechanical block to forearm rotation
Type III	Severely comminuted fracture, mechanical block to motion
Type IV	Radial fracture with associated elbow dislocation

more than 2 mm, with or without a mechanical block. These injuries are not significantly comminuted and should be treated operatively with ORIF. Type III fractures are so comminuted and displaced that internal fixation is not possible [73]. Type IV fractures have an associated elbow dislocation.

10.4.3 Initial Presentation and Evaluation

10.4.3.1 History and Physical Examination

Most commonly these fractures occur after a fall on an outstretched arm. In the elderly patient, the cause of the fall should be investigated. On physical examination, the radial head should be palpated for tenderness. Additionally, the interosseus ligament, distal radioulnar joint, and medial collateral ligament should be carefully assessed [69]. Associated forearm, shoulder, wrist, and hand injuries are common and should be anticipated.

In cases of isolated radial head fracture, range of motion at the elbow should be tested, noting any crepitus or mechanical blocks to flexion, extension, and rotation. If the patient cannot tolerate range of motion testing due to pain, the joint may be aspirated and local anesthetic injected for patient comfort. This will allow for an accurate assessment of any true mechanical block [69]. Elbow stability should be tested, including laxity to varus and valgus stress. In instances in which a terrible triad injury is suspected (a fractured radial head, an injury to the lateral ulnar collateral ligament, and a coronoid fracture), or in severely comminuted radial head fractures or open injuries, elbow stability is better assessed under sedation during operative management.

10.4.3.2 Radiographs

Routine AP, lateral, and oblique X-rays should be obtained. A radiocapitellar or "Greenspan" view can also be obtained if there is suspicion of injury to the radial head. This modified lateral view is taken with the X-ray bean angled 45° toward the radial head, allowing visualization of the radial head without overlap of the coronoid [74]. Nondisplaced radial head fractures can be quite subtle on a plain X-ray, and a posterior fat pad sign may be the only indication that an injury is present. In those patients with associated wrist tenderness, bilateral PA wrist X-rays in neutral rotation should be obtained to evaluate ulnar variance and assess for longitudinal radial instability. A side-to-side difference in ulnar variance may suggest disruption of the interosseus membrane and distal radioulnar joint. CT imaging may be helpful to further characterize the size of fracture fragments for pre-operative planning purposes and can also be helpful in identifying fractures not seen on plain film [69].

10.4.4 Management

Treatment of radial head fractures should take into account the patient's age, bone quality, associated injuries, and overall functional status. Especially in the elderly, management should focus on return to an activity level that allows the patient to independently participate in activities of daily living. The choice of treatment, as in all fractures in the elderly, should be guided by the patient's preoperative functional assessment.

10.4.4.1 Nonoperative Management

Nonoperative treatment is reserved for type I fractures. These injuries are nondisplaced or minimally displaced (<2 mm), with no mechanical block to motion [73]. A sling may initially be used for comfort, however, active motion should begin within one week to prevent stiffness. Follow-up radiographs should be obtained at 1–2 weeks to assess displacement.

Outcomes after nonoperative management of radial head fractures are generally favorable. Most studies report 85–95% good results for nondisplaced fractures treated with early motion, with a return to function within 6–12 weeks. Patients may be left with a mild residual flexion contracture, which is generally well tolerated in the elderly. Residual pain is uncommon [75].

10.4.4.2 Operative Management

The optimal surgical management of radial head fractures remains controversial. Operative treatment options include ORIF, radial head excision, and radial head replacement.

10.4.4.3 Open Reduction and Internal Fixation

Open reduction and internal fixation is indicated for type II injuries with adequate bone quality. It is also indicated for fractures that involve less than one-third of the radial head, but create a mechanical block to motion. Ring et al. performed a retrospective study to determine which fracture patterns are most amenable to treatment by ORIF. They concluded that ORIF is best reserved for minimally comminuted fractures, with three or fewer fracture fragments [73, 76]. King et al. noted that fractures may be more comminuted than suggested by plain radiographs, with intraoperative decision making required to determine feasibility of reconstruction. Excellent results were obtained for patients with anatomic reduction and rigid fixation, in whom early range of motion could be initiated. The authors suggest that for those in whom a stable anatomic reduction cannot be obtained, arthroplasty or radial head excision should be considered [77].

10.4.4.4 Excision

Radial head excision is often preferable to an unstable or incongruous internal fixation [76]. Prior to excision, however, the patient must carefully be evaluated for associated soft tissue injuries and concomitant fractures. When performed acutely, this procedure is contraindicated in patients with interosseus ligament injury, MCL injury, or elbow dislocation due to the risk of chronic valgus or longitudinal instability [78].

There are conflicting reports on outcomes following radial head excision [79, 80]. Some authors have reported delayed complications including pain, instability, proximal radial translation, decreased strength, arthrosis, and cubitus valgus [80]. In an elderly patient, however, radial head excision may remain a reasonable option for pain relief and early return to function.

10.4.5 Radial Head Replacement

Radial head replacement is indicated for displaced, comminuted fractures (type III) in which an anatomic reduction and stable internal fixation cannot be achieved. It is also indicated for fractures with associated ligamentous injury or elbow dislocation [73]. The radial head provides a secondary restraint to valgus instability and a primary restraint to longitudinal stability. Disruption of the medial ulnar collateral ligament combined with inability to rigidly and anatomically fix the radial head, thus, requires restoration of radiocapitellar contact to afford elbow stability. Historically, silicone implants have had high failure rates due to fragmentation and silicone synovitis [81]. Newer cobalt chrome implants are biomechanically superior and allow the surgeon to more closely replicate the native radial head (Fig. 10.14).

Good results with metallic radial head devices have been shown in multiple clinical series [82, 83]. Harrington et al. performed a long-term review of patients with metallic radial head replacement for radial head fractures and associated gross elbow instability [83]. Good or excellent functional results were reported in 16 of 20 patients. The authors concluded that radial head replacement is indicated for

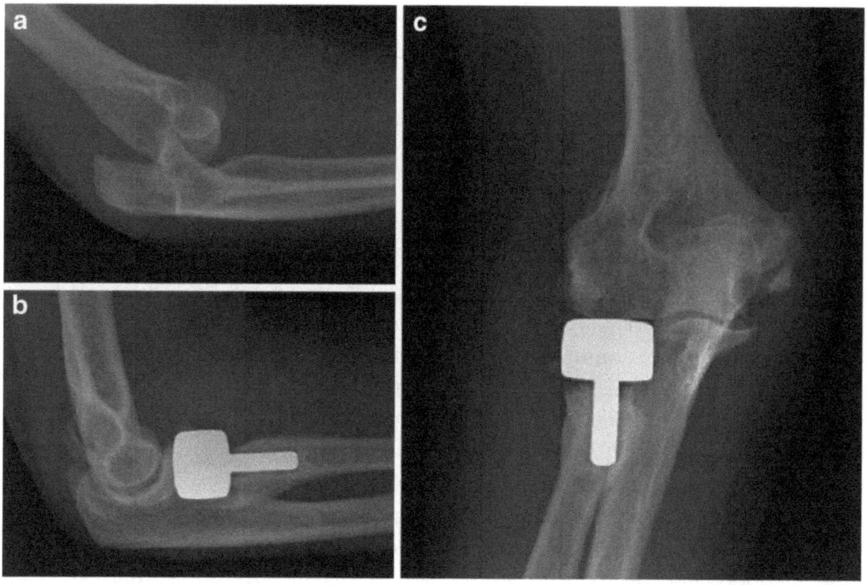

Fig. 10.14 Elbow dislocation and comminuted radial head fracture (**a**) managed with radial head replacement. Lateral radiographs (**b**) and AP [c) with the removal of the unreconstructable radial head fragments and the cobalt chrome replacement

patients with unreconstructable radial head fractures in the setting of a clinically unstable elbow. Knight et al. reviewed 31 comminuted fractures of the radial head, reporting similar results including reliable restoration of stability and prevention of proximal radial migration [83].

The best treatment for complicated radial head fractures with associated elbow or forearm instability is still controversial; clinical results of ORIF, excision, and arthroplasty are conflicting. Good to excellent outcomes have been shown with each modality of treatment, suggesting that the choice of management should be tailored to the individual patient based on functional demands, fracture pattern, and associated injuries.

10.4.6 Rehabilitation

Any concern about postoperative instability must be balanced against the need for early motion to prevent stiffness [68]. In general, early range of motion within a safe arc should be encouraged. For an isolated radial head fracture, motion should be initiated on the first postoperative day, with nighttime static extension splinting. For radial head fractures with associated elbow instability, primary ligamentous repair should be performed to allow early active range of motion. When a stable reconstruction is not possible, early motion may still be employed within the safe arc determined intraoperatively. Between therapy sessions, the elbow should be splinted at 90°, in either pronation or supination. Extension splinting should not be initiated until ligamentous healing has occurred several weeks after the repair [69].

10.4.7 Complications

Complications of radial head fractures include nerve injury, AVN, nonunion, malunion, osteoarthritis, stiffness, and instability. The risk of posterior interosseus nerve injury can be minimized by careful retractor placement around the radial head and pronation of the forearm during surgical approach [84]. Avascular necrosis is often asymptomatic, and frequently heals if stable fixation is present; late collapse is uncommon [70]. Nonunion, if asymptomatic, may also be managed expectantly in the elderly. Malunions in older patients may best be managed with radial head excision or replacement. Osteoarthritis after radial head fracture first develops in the radiocapitellar joint, followed by late arthrosis of the ulnohumeral joint; debridement, radial head replacement, radial head excision, and TEA are treatment options [69].

Stiffness most commonly presents with a loss of terminal extension, which may respond to passive stretching and static splinting. Those patients that fail nonoperative management may require a capsular release [85]. Valgus instability can be prevented by appropriate initial management of the radial head injury, avoiding radial head excision in the setting of medial ligamentous disruption.

10.5 Olecranon Fractures

10.5.1 Background

Proximal ulna injuries include olecranon fractures, olecranon fracture dislocations, Monteggia injuries, coronoid fractures, and elbow dislocations. These injuries important as they can compromise both the elbow and wrist articulations and lead to upper extremity dysfunction.

10.5.2 Anatomy and Fracture Patterns

10.5.2.1 Anatomy

The olecranon is a subcutaneous structure, making it vulnerable to direct trauma. Along with the coronoid process it forms the semilunar notch of the proximal ulna, which articulates with the trochlea of the distal humerus. This constrained articulation provides stability to the elbow joint, allowing motion in only one plane [70].

Adding to the inherent stability of the ulnohumeral articulation is a central longitudinal ridge in the semilunar notch, which interdigitates with a corresponding groove in the articular surface of the trochlea. Within the semilunar notch, there are distinct coronoid and olecranon areas in the articular surface, separated by a nonarticular transverse groove. This groove is located at the junction of the olecranon process with the metaphysis of the ulna, and is especially susceptible to fracture [86]. The triceps tendon has a broad insertion into the periosteum of the olecranon and proximal ulna posteriorly and covers the joint capsule with an expansion of fascia that extends medially and laterally [87, 88].

10.5.2.2 Classification

There is no universally accepted system for the classification of olecranon fractures. Morrey, however, proposed the Mayo classification scheme, which describes fractures based on three factors that influence treatment: stability, displacement, and comminution [89]. Type I fractures are nondisplaced, type II fractures are displaced and stable, and type III fractures are displaced and unstable.

10.5.3 Initial Presentation and Evaluation

10.5.3.1 Mechanism

Olecranon fractures can occur by direct or indirect trauma. A blunt trauma to the tip of the olecranon can fracture it directly, while a forceful contraction of the triceps in a partially flexed elbow may cause an indirect avulsion injury. The amount of displacement is dependent upon the magnitude of force applied to the joint [70]. On one end of the spectrum, nondisplaced injuries result from low-energy trauma. Conversely, high-energy injuries such as transolecranon fracture-dislocations lead to posterior olecranon displacement and to distal ulnar fragment and radial head displacement anterior to the humerus [87].

10.5.3.2 History and Physical Examination

Fractures of the olecranon are generally due to low-energy falls in the elderly. The patient should be evaluated for medical conditions that may have contributed to the fall, and the pre-injury function of the limb should be ascertained. The olecranon should be examined for a palpable sulcus at the fracture site and the entire extremity should be inspected for any open wounds. The neurovascular status of the limb should be documented, with particular attention to the ulnar nerve that is at risk following direct trauma. The hallmark of a true triceps mechanism disruption is an inability to extend the elbow actively against gravity; this sign may be difficult to elicit, however, due to pain and limited range of motion [70].

10.5.3.3 Radiographs

Initial radiographs should include AP and lateral views of the elbow. A true lateral is crucial to accurately assess the fracture. An oblique X-ray may aid in detection of coronoid process involvement. Repeat images should be obtained if necessary to obtain true orthogonal views [70]. The AP view will best demonstrate fractures in the sagittal plane, as well as any associated radial head or neck fracture.

10.5.4 Management

Prior to choosing a treatment strategy for the elderly patient, there are certain important considerations that may affect management. Soft tissue healing is crucial, and surgical intervention may need to be delayed if the patient will be at risk for skin breakdown following hardware placement. Nonoperative treatment, even of significantly displaced olecranon fractures, may be appropriate in patients with severe medical illnesses or cannot otherwise tolerate surgical intervention

The value of the Mayo classification is that it provides a framework for the management of olecranon injures (Fig. 10.15). The goals of surgery are maintaining the power of extension, restoring congruity of the articular surface, restoring stability of the elbow, preventing stiffness, and achieving stable fixation strong enough to allow protected ROM soon after surgery [89].

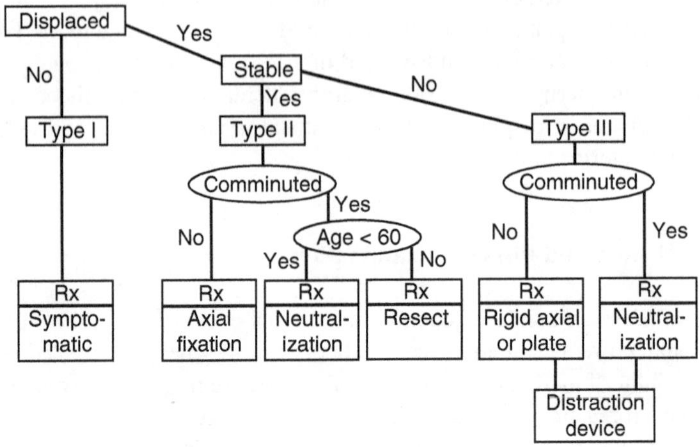

Fig. 10.15 Algorithm for management of olecranon fractures (Reprinted with permission from [88])

10.5.4.1 Type I Injuries

Stable, nondisplaced olecranon fractures can be immobilized in a long-arm cast with the elbow flexed between 45° and 90° and the forearm in neutral rotation [70]. If the elbow cannot be immobilized in flexion due to displacement of the fracture, an alternate treatment strategy needs to be employed [87]. The duration of immobilization varies amongst surgeons; however, 3–4 weeks of casting has been recommended, followed by protected range of motion until radiographic healing is demonstrated at 6–8 weeks [70]. Follow-up radiographs should be obtained one week after cast placement to ensure that fracture displacement has not occurred.

10.5.4.2 Type II Injuries

The most common olecranon fracture pattern is a noncomminuted, displaced, stable injury (type IIA) [89]. For these displaced fractures, ORIF is the treatment of choice. Type IIA fractures can reliably be stabilized with tension-band wiring, which is designed to convert the tensile distraction force of the triceps into a compressive force at the articular surface [89]. Intramedullary Kirschner wires or Steinmann pins are placed followed by a heavy figure of eight tension band wire (Fig. 10.16). Alternatively, a single 6.5-mm intramedullary screw with tension band augment may be used.

For comminuted type IIB injures, patients may best be treated by anatomic reduction and internal fixation with a plate and screws. For severely comminuted injuries, bone grafting may be necessary. The use of precountered plates augmented with sutures placed through the plate and into the triceps tendon, which typically has greater tensile strength than the surrounding osteoporotic metaphyseal bone, aids fixation, and allows immediate postoperative range of motion.

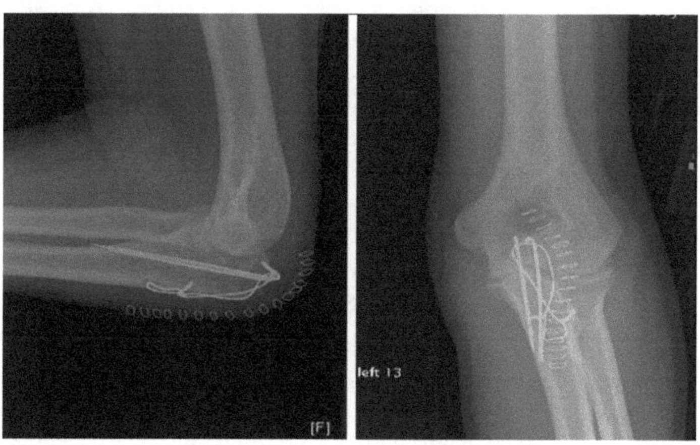

Fig. 10.16 The ORIF of noncomminuted olecranon fracture using a tension band technique

For the older patient with osteoporotic bone that may not be amenable to internal fixation, the comminuted fragment may be excised with advancement of the triceps to the remaining bone at the proximal ulna [88]. The triceps should be reattached immediately adjacent to the articular surface. Good functional results have been demonstrated after fragment excision and triceps advancement, especially in elderly patients. Gartsman et al. compared this technique to internal fixation, finding that the results for pain, function, range of motion, and elbow stability were similar for each group [90]. Furthermore, biomechanical testing demonstrated no significant difference in elbow extensor performance between the two groups. Nonetheless, the technique of olecranon resection should be reserved for low-demand patients who may have a contraindication to rigid internal fixation.

10.5.4.3 Type III Injuries

Given the associated instability of the forearm in type III fractures, these injuries are especially difficult to treat. Noncomminuted fractures can be stabilized with a plate and screw construct. Rigid internal fixation is imperative to provide stability to the displaced forearm [89]. Severely comminuted fractures are often associated injuries of the distal humerus, radial head, or radial and ulnar shafts. To the best of the surgeon's ability, the fracture should be rigidly fixed with plates, screws, and supplemental Kirschner wires. Bone grafting may be necessary, as may ulnar nerve dissection and transposition. A hinged external fixator may also be required to restore elbow stability [89].

10.5.5 Rehabilitation

The goal of operative management is fixation sufficiently stable to allow immediate postoperative range of motion. If there are no concerns for wound healing or patient compliance, active range of motion may begin on the first postoperative day [91]. A therapist should instruct the patient on gravity- and splint-assisted exercises. In older patients with tenuous fixation and comminuted fractures, a longer period of immobilization may be required. Hand exercises should be initiated immediately to minimize swelling and prevent stiffness [87]. Strengthening should be delayed until early healing is seen on radiographs, at 3–4 months.

10.5.6 Outcomes and Complications

Isolated closed fractures of the olecranon have favorable long-term results. However, there are few prospective studies in which validated outcome measures have been used to directly compare different methods of treatment [92]. A study by Karlsson et al. reviewed 73 patients with 19-year follow-up after olecranon fracture. Good or excellent results were reported in 96% of patients, regardless of fracture type (nondisplaced, displaced, or displaced comminuted). Although elbow flexion and extension were reduced, most patients had no subjective complaints. Radiographic signs of osteoarthritis were seen in 6% of patients; however, these degenerative changes did not correlate with a poor outcome [93].

Hardware prominence requiring removal is one of the most frequent complications following internal fixation of olecranon fractures, with reported incidence from 3 to 80%. This complication may be more common in elderly patients with poor bone stock and poor soft tissue coverage. Hardware removal, if necessary, should be delayed 12–18 months following surgery to minimize the risk of re-fracture unless skin integrity is compromised [87].

Additional complications after olecranon fractures include stiffness, nonunion, infection, ulnar neuropathy, and post-traumatic arthritis. Loss of motion is not typically problematic after isolated olecranon fractures, with an average postoperative flexion contracture of 10–15° [89]. Otherwise, capsular contractures generally respond to therapy and progressive splinting, and only infrequently require capsular contracture release [92].

Nonunion after simple olecranon fractures is unusual and is more often seen after fracture dislocations of the proximal ulna [94]. Infection rates range from 0 to 6%, with a higher frequency following open injuries. Severe arthrosis following olecranon fracture is uncommon, but may be more pronounced when an anatomic reduction (within 2 mm) cannot be obtained [95]. In the elderly patient with significant post-traumatic arthritis, semiconstrained TEA may be an option for pain relief and return of functional status.

10.6 Summary

Fractures of the shoulder and elbow are common in the elderly population and are typically due to low-energy trauma. Minimally displaced fractures in patients with limited functional capacity can often be managed nonoperatively, thus avoiding the surgical risks amongst patients with medical comorbidities. However, surgical intervention with open or closed reduction with fixation, shoulder arthroplasty, TEA, or radial head replacement may offer more predictable and better functional outcomes for certain fracture patterns. Regardless of the treatment modality, the goal of treating these injuries is to provide stable fracture fixation or reconstruction that allows early mobilization and pain free upper extremity function.

References

1. Horak J, Nilsson BE. Epidemiology of fracture of the upper end of the humerus. Clin Orthop Relat Res. 1975;112:250–253.
2. Baron JA, Barrett JA, Karagas MR. The epidemiology of peripheral fractures. Bone. 1996; 18(3 suppl):209S–213S.

3. Kannus P, Palvanen M, Niemi S, Parkkari J, Jarvinen M, Vuori I. Osteoporotic fractures of the proximal humerus in elderly Finnish persons: Sharp increase in 1970–1998 an alarming projections for the new millennium. Acta Orthop Scand. 2000;71:465–470.
4. Palvanen M, Kannus P, Neimi S, et al. Update in the epidemiology of proximal humeral fractures. Clin Orthop Relat Res. 2006;442:87–92.
5. Court-Brown CM, Garg A, McQueen MM. The translated two-part fracture of the proximal humerus. J Bone Joint Surg Br. 2001;83-B:799–804.
6. Abrahamsen B, Vestergaard P, Rud B, et al. Ten-year absolute risk of osteoporotic fractures according to BMD T score at menopause: The Danish Osteoporosis Prevention Study. J Bone Miner Res. 2006;21:796–800.
7. Lee SH, Dargent-Molina P, Breart G. Risk factors for fractures of the proximal humerus: Results from the EPIDOS prospective study. J Bone Miner Res. 2002;17:817–825.
8. Lauritzen J, Schwarz P, McNair P, Lund B, Turnsbol I. Radial and humeral fractures as predictors of subsequent fractures in women, and their seasonal variations. Osteoporos Int. 1993;3:133–137.
9. Bioleau P, Huten D, Pietu G, et al. L'arthroplastie prosthetique dans les fractures recentes complexes de l'extremite superieure de l'humerus: technique et inidications. Paris, Paris Expansion Scientifique Publications, 1999.
10. Kronberg M, Brwostom LA, Soderlund V. Retroversion of the humeral head in the normal shoulder and its relationship to the normal range of motion. Clin Orthop Relat Res. 1990; 153:113–117.
11. Iannotti JP, Gabriel JP, Schneck SL, et al. The normal glenohumeral relationships. An anatomical study of one hundred and forty shoulders. J Bone Joint Surg. 1992;74A:491–500.
12. Brooks CH, Revell WJ, Heatley FW. Vascularity of the humeral head after proximal humeral fractures: An anatomical cadaver study. J Bone Joint Surg Br. 1993;75:132–136.
13. Gerber C, Werner CM, Vienne P. Internal fixation of complex fractures of the proximal humerus. J Bone J Surg Br. 2004;86:848–855.
14. Neer CS. Displaced proximal humerus fractures: I. Classification and evaluation. J Bone Joint Surg Am. 1970;52:1077–1089.
15. Schlegel TF, Hawkins RJ. Displaced proximal humeral fractures: Evaluation and treatment. J Am Acad Orthop Surg. 1994;2:54–78.
16. Flatow EL, Cuomo F, Madey MG, et al. Open reduction and internal fixation of two-part displaced fractures of the greater tuberosity of the proximal part of the humerus. J Bone Joint Surg Am. 1991;73:1213–1218.
17. Zyto K, Ahrengart L, Sperber A, et al. Treatment of displaced proximal humeral fractures in elderly patients. J Bone Joint Surg Br. 1997;79:412–417.
18. Tingart MS, Apprelexa M, von Stechow D, et al. The cortical thickness of the proximal hueral diaphysis predicts bone mineral density of the proximal humerus. J Bone Joint Surg Br. 2003;85:611–617.
19. Chudik SC, Weinhold P, Dahners LE. Fixed-angle plate fixation in simulated fractures of the proximal humerus: A biomechanical study of a new device. J Shoulder Elbow Surg. 2003;12:578–588.
20. Hawkins RJ, Bell RH, Gurr K. The three-part fracture of the proximal part of the humerus: Operative treatment. J Bone Joint Surg Am. 1986;68:1410–1414.
21. Kwon BK, Goertzen DJ, O'Brien PJ, et al. Biomechanical evaluation of proximal humeral fracture fixation supplemented with calcium phosphate cement. J Bone Joint Surg Am. 2002;84:951–961.
22. Siffri PC, Peindl RD, Coley ER, et al. Biomechanical analysis of blade plate versus locking plate fixation for a proximal humerus fracture: Comparison using cadaveric and synthetic humeri. J Orthop Trauma. 2006;20:547–554.
23. Resch H, Povacz P, Frohlich R, Wambacher M. Percutaneous fixation of three- and four-part fractures of the proximal humerus. J Bone Joint Surg Br. 1997;79:295–300.
24. Egol KA, Kubiak EN, Fulkerson E, Kummer FJ, Koval KJ. Biomechanics of locked plates and screws. J Orthop Trauma. 2004;18:488–493.

25. Cornell CN. Internal fracture fixation in patients with osteoporosis. J Am Acad Orthop Surg. 2003;11:109–119.
26. Wijgman AJ, Roolker W, Patt TW, Raaymakers EL, Marti RK. Open reduction and internal fixation of three and four-part fractures of the proximal part of the humerus. J Bone Joint Surg Am. 2002;84:1919–1925.
27. Wagner M. General principles for the clinical use of the LCP. Injury. 2003;34(suppl 2): B31–42.
28. Haidukewych GJ. Innovations in locking plate technology. J Am Acad Orthop Surg. 2004;2: 205–212.
29. Zyto K, Wallace WA, Frostick SP, Preston BJ. Outcome after hemiarthroplasty for three- and four-part fractures of the proximal humerus. J Shoulder Elbow Surg. 1998;7:85–89.
30. Jakob RP, Miniaci A, Anson PS, et al. Four-part valgus impacted fractures of the proximal humerus. J Bone Joint Surg Br. 1991;73:295–298.
31. Mighell MA, Kolm GP, Collinge CA, Frankle MA. Outcomes of hemiarthroplasty for fractures of the proximal humerus. J Shoulder Elbow Surg. 2003;12:569–577.
32. Kralinger F, Schwaiger R, Wambacher M, et al. Outcome after primary hemiarthroplasty for fracture of the head of the humerus: A retrospective multicentre study of 167 patients. J Bone Joint Surg Br. 2004;86:217–219.
33. Christoforakis JJ, Kontakis GM, Katonis PG, Stergiopoulos K, Hadjipavlou AG. Shoulder hemiarthroplasty in the management of humeral head fractures. Acta Orthop Belg. 2004;70:214–218.
34. Demirhan M, Kilicoglu O, Altinel L, et al. Prognostic factors in prosthetic replacement for acute proximal humerus fractures. J Orthop Trauma. 2003;17:181–188.
35. Nyffeler RW, Sheikh R, Jacob HA, et al. Influence of humeral prosthesis height on biomechanics of glenohumeral abduction: An in vitro study. J Bone Joint Surg Am. 2004;86: 575–580.
36. Bono CM, Renard R, Levin RD, Levy AS. Effect of displacement of fractures of the greater tuberosity on the mechanics of the shoulder. J Bone J Surg Br. 2001;83:1056–1062.
37. Frankle MA, Greenwald DP, Marke BA, et al. Biomechanical effects of malposition of tuberosity fragments on the humeral prosthetic reconstruction for four-part proximal humerus fractures. J Shoulder Elbow Surg. 2001;10:321–326.
38. Prakash U, McGurty DW, Dent JA. Hemiarthroplasty for severe fractures of the proximal humerus. J Shoulder Elbow Surg. 2002;11:428–430.
39. Bufquin T, Hersan A, Hubert L, Massin P. Reverse shoulder arthroplasty for the treatment of three- and four-part fractures of the proximal humerus in the elderly. J Bone Joint Surgery Br. 2007;89B:516–520.
40. Hodgson S. Proximal humerus fracture rehabilitation. Clin Orthop Relat Res. 2006;442:131–138.
41. Brinker MR, O'Connor DP. The incidence of fractures and dislocations referred for orthopaedic services in a capitated population. J Bone Joint Surg Am. 2004;86:290–297.
42. Tytherleigh-Strong G, Walls N, McQueen MM. The epidemiology of humeral shaft fractures. J Bone Joint Surg Br. 1998;80B:249–253.
43. Ekholm R, Adami J, Tidermark J, Hansson K, Tornkvist H, Ponzer S. Fractures of the shaft of the humerus: An epidemiological study of 401 fractures. J Bone Joint Surg Br. 2006;88B: 1469–1473.
44. Sarmiento A, Zagorski JB, Zych GA, Latta LL, Capps CA. Functional bracing for the treatment of fractures of the humeral diaphysis. J Bone Joint Surg Am. 2000;82A:478–486.
45. Foster FJ, Dixon JL, Bach AW, et al. Internal fixations of fractures and nonunions of the humeral shaft. J Bone Joint Surg Am. 1985;67:857–864.
46. Mast JW, Spiegal PG, Harvey JP, et al. Fractures of the humeral shaft. Clin Orthop Relat Res. 1975;12:254–262.
47. McKee MD, Seiler J, Jupiter JB. The application of the limited contact dynamic compression plate in the upper extremity; an analysis of 114 cases. Injury. 1995;26:661–666.
48. Connolly S, Nair R, McKee MD, Waddell JP, Schemitsch EH. Immediate plate osteosynthesis of open fractures of the humeral shaft. Final Program of the Orthopaedic Trauma Association

Annual Meeting, October 22–24, 1999, Charlotte, NC. Rosemont, IL, Orthopaedic Trauma Association, 1999.
49. Hak DJ. Comparison of the AO locking plate with the standard limited-contact dynamic compression plate for fixation of osteoporotic humeral shaft fractures, Final Program of the Orthopaedic Trauma Association Annual Meeting, October 9–11, 2003, Salt Lake City, UT. Rosemont, IL, Orthopaedic Trauma Association, 2003.
50. Chapman JR, Henley MB, Agel J, et al. Randomized prospective study of humeral shaft fracture fixation: Intramedullary nails versus plates. J Orthop Trauma. 2000;14:162–166.
51. McCormack RG, Brien D, Buckley RE, et al. Fixation of fractures of the shaft of the humerus by dynamic compression plate or intramedullary nail: A prospective randomized trial. J Bone Joint Surg Br. 2000;82:336–339.
52. Rarragos AF, Schemitxch ED, McKee MD. Complications of intramedullary nailing for fractures of the humeral shaft: A review. J Orthop Trauma. 1999;13:258–267.
53. Barei DP, Hanel DP. Fractures of the distal humerus. In Green DP, Hotchkiss RN, Pederson WC, et al., Eds. *Green's operative hand surgery 5th Edition* Vol. 1. Philadelphia, PA: Elsevier, Inc: 2005: 809–843.
54. Jupiter JB, Mehne DK. Fractures of the distal humerus. Orthopedics. 1992;15(7):825–833.
55. Mehne DK, Matta J. Bicolumn fractures of the adult humerus. In 53rd Annual Meeting of the American Academy of Orthopaedic Surgeons, New Orleans, 1986.
56. Palvanen M, Niemi S, Parkkari J, et al. Osteoporotic fractures of the distal humerus in elderly women. Ann Intern Med. 2003;139(3):235.
57. Zayer M, Mathiesen TI. Relevancy of radiographic features in elbow fractures. Acta Radiol. 1997;38(3):363–367.
58. Jupiter JB, Barnes KA, Goodman LJ, et al. Multiplane fracture of the distal humerus. J Orthop Trauma. 1993;7(3):216–220.
59. John H, Rosso R, Neff U, et al. Operative treatment of distal humeral fractures in the elderly. J Bone J Surg Br. 1994;76(5):793–796.
60. Pereles TR, Koval KJ, Gallagher M, Rosen H. Open reduction and internal fixation of the distal humerus: Functional outcome in the elderly. J Trauma. 1997;43(4):578–584.
61. Mckee MD, Veillette CJ, Hall JA, et al. A multicenter, prospective, randomized, controlled trial of open reduction-internal fixation versus total elbow arthroplasty for displaced intra-articular distal humeral fractures in elderly patients. J Shoulder Elbow Surg. 2009;18:3–12.
62. Frankle MA, Herscovici D Jr, DiPasquale TG, et al. A comparison of open reduction and internal fixation and primary total elbow arthroplasty in the treatment of intraarticular distal humerus fractures in women older than age 65. J Orthop Trauma. 2003;17(7):473–480.
63. Anglen J. Distal humerus fractures. J Am Acad Orthop Surg. 2005;12:291–297.
64. Morrey BF, Askew LJ, Chao EY. A biomechanical study of normal functional elbow motion. J Bone Joint Surg Am. 1981;63(6):872–877.
65. Helfet DL, Schmeling GJ. Bicondylar intraarticular fractures of the distal humerus in adults. Clin Orthop Relat Res. 1993;(292):26–36.
66. Jupiter JB. Complex fractures of the distal part of the humerus and associated complications. Instr Course Lect. 1995;44:187–198.
67. Gofton WT, Macdermid JC, Patterson SD, et al. Functional outcome of AO Type C distal humeral fractures. J Hand Surg Am. 2003;28(2):294–308.
68. Tejwani NC, Mehta H. Fractures of the radial head and neck: Current concepts in management. JAAOS. 2007;15(7):380–387.
69. King GJ. Fractures of the head of the radius. In Green DP, Hotchkiss RN, Pederson WC, et al., Eds. *Green's operative hand surgery 5th Edition* Vol. 1. Philadelphia, PA: Elsevier, Inc: 2005: 845–887.
70. Mezera K, Hotchkiss RN. Fractures and dislocations of the elbow. In Bucholz RW, Heckman JD, Eds. *Rockwood and Green's fractures in adults 5th Edition* Vol. 1. Philadelphia, PA: Lippincott, Williams, & Wilkins: 2002: 921–952.
71. Morrey BF, Tanaka S, An KN. Valgus stability of the elbow: A definition of primary and secondary constraints. Clin Orthop Relat Res. 1991;265:187–195.

72. Morrey BF, An KN, Stormont TJ. Force transmission through the radial head. J Bone Joint Surg Am. 1988;70(2):250–256.
73. Hotchkiss RN. Displaced fractures of the radial head: Internal fixation or excision? JAAOS. 1997;5:1–10.
74. Greenspan A, Norman A, Rosen H. Radial head-capitellum view in elbow trauma: Clinical application and radiographic-anatomic correlation. Am J Roentgenol. 1984;143(2):355–359.
75. Mason ML. Some observations on fractures of the head of the radius with a review of one hundred cases. Br J Surg. 1954;42(172):123–132.
76. Ring D, Quintero J, Jupiter JB. Open reduction and internal fixation of fractures of the radial head. J Bone Joint Surg Am. 2002;84-A(10):1811–1815.
77. King GJ, Evans DC, Kellam JF. Open reduction and internal fixation of radial head fractures. J Orthop Trauma. 1991;5(1):21–28.
78. Adler JB, Shaftan GW. Radial head fractures, is excision necessary? J Trauma. 1962;4: 115–136.
79. Herbertsson P, Josefsson PO, Hasserius R, et al. Fractures of the radial head and neck treated with radial head excision. J Bone Joint Surg Am. 2004;86:1925–1930.
80. Ikeda M, Oka Y. Function after early radial head resection for fracture: A retrospective evaluation of 15 patients followed for 3–18 years. Acta Orthop Scand. 2000;71(2):191–194.
81. Morrey BF, Askew L, Chao EY. Silastic prosthetic replacement for the radial head. J Bone Joint Surg Am. 1981;63(3):454–458.
82. Harrington IJ, Sekyi-Otu A, Barrington TW, et al. The functional outcome with metallic radial head implants in the treatment of unstable elbow fractures: A long-term review. J Trauma. 2001;50:46–52.
83. Knight DJ, Rymaszewski LA, Amis AA, et al. Primary replacement of the fracture radial head with a metal prosthesis. J Bone J Surg Br. 1993;75(4):572–576.
84. Diliberti T, Botte MJ, Abrams RA. Anatomical considerations regarding the posterior interosseus nerve during posterolateral approaches to the proximal part of the radius. J Bone Joint Surg Am. 2000;82(6):809–813.
85. King GJ, Faber KJ. Posttraumatic elbow stiffness. Orthop Clin North Am. 2000;31(1): 129–143.
86. Morrey BF. Anatomy of the elbow joint. In Morrey BF (Ed.) *The elbow and its disorders 2nd Edition.* Philadelphia, PA: WB Saunders: 1993: 16–52.
87. Ring D, Jupiter JB. Fractures of the proximal ulna. In Green DP, Hotchkiss RN, Pederson WC, et al., Eds. *Green's operative hand surgery 5th Edition* Vol. 1. Philadelphia, PA: Elsevier, Inc: 2005: 889–906.
88. Morrey BF. Current concepts in the treatment of fractures of the radial head, the olecranon, and the coronoid. J Bone Joint Surg Am. 1995;77(2):316–327.
89. Cabanela ME, Morrey BF. Fractures of the proximal ulna and olecranon. In Morrey BF (Ed.) *The elbow and its disorders 2nd Edition.* Philadelphia, PA: WB Saunders: 1993: 405–428.
90. Gartsman GM, Sculco TP, Otis TC. Operative treatment of olecranon fractures. Excision or open reduction with internal fixation. J Bone Joint Surg Am. 1981;63(5):718–721.
91. Wolfgang G, Burke F, Bush D, et al. Surgical treatment of displaced olecranon fractures by tension band wiring technique. Clin Orthop Relat Res. 1987;224:192–204.
92. Hak DJ, Golladay GJ. Olecranon fractures: Treatment options. J Am Acad Orthop Surg. 2000;8(4):266–275.
93. Karlsson MK, Hasserius R, Karlsson C, et al. Fractures of the olecranon: A 15- to 25-year followup of 73 patients. Clin Orthop Relat Res. 2002;403:205–212.
94. Helm RH, Hornby R, Miller SW. The complications of surgical treatment of displaced fractures of the olecranon. Injury. 1987;18:48–50.
95. Murphy DF, Greene WB, Dameron TB Jr Displaced olecranon fractures in adults: Clinical evaluation. Clin Orthop Relat Res. 1987;224:215–223.

Chapter 11
Vertebral Compression Fractures

Ejovi Ughwanogho and Nader M. Hebela

Abstract Vertebral compression fractures (VCFs) are the most common fragility fractures that affect the elderly population accounting for over 70,000 hospital admissions annually in the United States. Osteoporosis is a significant risk factor for VCFs which affects white females at a disproportionately greater rate than any other demographic group. Quantitative microarchitectural changes in the cancellous and cortical bone in the vertebral body result in qualitative changes to the vertebral endplate biomechanical properties leading to failure of the anterior column and subsequent compression fractures. While the majority of fractures are asymptomatic, pain with routine activities is a common presenting symptom. Non-steroidal medications, bracing, and low-dose narcotic medications are usually effective in treating most patients who have symptomatic VCFs. Percutaneous injection of polymethylmethacrylate has shown some promise in relieving pain from VCF, although recent studies have questioned these findings. Preventative care with vitamin D, calcium supplementation, and bone mineral density studies can significantly decrease the risk of developing osteoporosis and subsequently VCFs.

Keywords Vertebral compression fractures • Vertebroplasty • Kyphoplasty • Anterior column fracture

11.1 Introduction

The World Health Organization defines osteoporosis as bone mineral density (BMD) 2.5 standard deviations below the average BMD of a young adult using dual-energy X-ray absorptiometry. The primary clinical consequence of osteoporosis is fragility

N.M. Hebela (✉)
Department of Orthopaedic Surgery, University of Pennsylvania School of Medicine, Penn Presbyterian Medical Center, 1 Cupp Pavilion, 51 N 39th Street, Philadelphia, PA 19104, USA
e-mail: nader.hebela@uphs.upenn.edu

R.J. Pignolo et al. (eds.), *Fractures in the Elderly*, Aging Medicine,
DOI 10.1007/978-1-60327-467-8_11,

fractures. Osteoporotic vertebral compression fractures (VCFs) are the most common fragility fractures.

A VCF is an insufficiency fracture involving the anterior column of vertebrae. The precise incidence and prevalence of osteoporotic VCFs is poorly defined in the literature because of the disparate definitions that exist among clinicians. In addition, a significant number of VCFs are not diagnosed because of the often subclinical nature of these fractures [1, 2]. Current evidence suggests VCF is the most common fragility fracture in the United States whose incidence has been estimated at approximately 700,000 yearly. Of these patients, 10% will be hospitalized [3]. Approximately 25% of postmenopausal females have a VCF in their lifetime, with white females constituting the majority of these patients. The life-time risk of clinical vertebral fracture has been estimated to be approximately 16% and 5% in white females and white males, respectively [4].

The risk factors of osteoporotic vertebra compression fractures include age, female gender, low BMD, a sedentary lifestyle, and a history of fragility fractures [5]. Of these, a history of fragility fractures has been shown to have the strongest correlation with the development of additional VCFs. The increased risk of a new fracture in patients with a pre-existing VCF has been documented in the literature. Ross et al. reported a fivefold increment in the incidence of a new vertebral fracture in patients with a baseline vertebral fracture, when compared with those without prior fractures [6].

11.2 Biomechanics/Anatomy

The vertebral body is a cylindrical mass of cancellous bone enclosed in a cortical shell. The concave superior and inferior surfaces of the vertebral body are the vertebral endplates. Posterior to the vertebral body is the neural arch, consisting of two pedicles, two laminae, and transverse, articular, and spinous processes. The size of each vertebra progressively increases from thoracic to lumbar vertebrae. This is a mechanical adaptation to the increasing compressive load to which each vertebra is subjected [7].

The architectural structure of the vertebral cancellous core consists of vertical trabecular columns supporting both endplates. Between these columns are horizontal struts of trabecular bone. The cancellous core bears the majority of axial load on the vertebrae and failure occurs when its strength is exceeded by normal physiologic or traumatic loads. In the osteopenic vertebra, a reduction in the number and size of the vertical and horizontal trabecular columns weakens the vertebral body (Fig. 11.1). Failure is often a result of cyclic physiologic insults as opposed to a single traumatic event [7, 8].

When correlated with vertebral strength, the load applied to the spine from normal activities can be used to calculate a "factor of risk" [9]. Hayes et al. describe this risk as the likelihood of a vertebral fracture occurring while performing a given activity. A value greater than 1 indicates a high likelihood of fracture. Routine activities such as bending, lifting of weights, and arising from a seated position have all been associated with VCFs. The factor of risk of these activities has

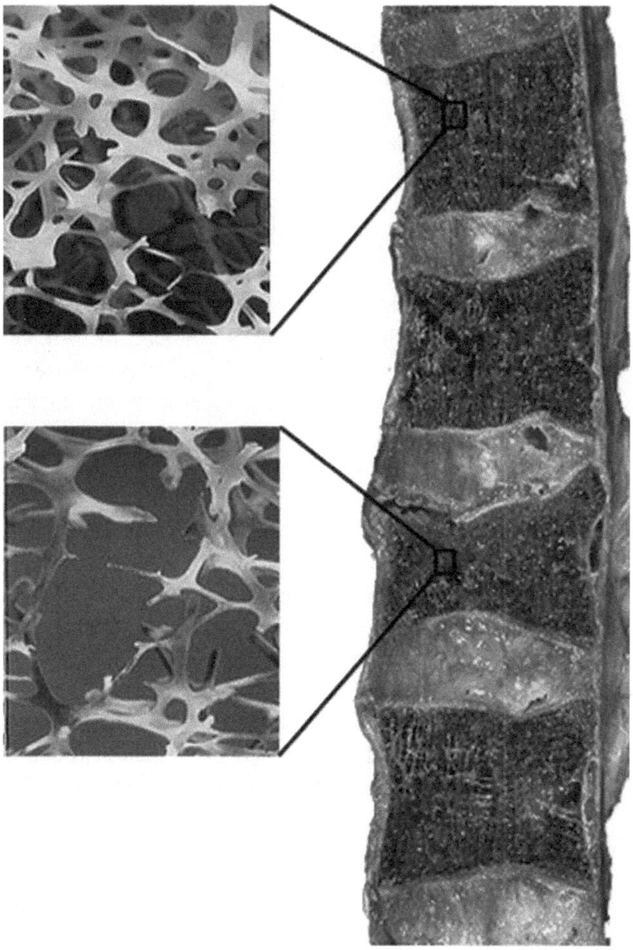

Fig. 11.1 Vertebral compression fractures are due to a quantitative reduction in normal quality bone and changes in the microarchitecture of the cancellous trabeculae

been estimated as 1.5, 2.5, and 1.4, respectively, in a patient with BMD of 0.3 which corresponds to a T-score > 5; a state of severe osteoporosis. These values suggest that in the markedly osteoporotic spine, most everyday activities pose a significant risk of fracture [8, 9].

11.3 Pathogenesis

Classically, BMD has been used as an index of bone strength. Current data however suggest BMD alone correlates poorly with the increased risk of additional vertebral fractures in patients with pre-existing fractures. Other factors, not reflected by BMD, may account for this observation and include the qualitative properties of the vertebra, spinal curvature, and spondylotic changes between the vertebrae [10, 11].

In the normal vertebral body, there are an increased number of trabeculae with greater average thickness in the central region subjacent to intervertebral discs [7]. In contrast, bone mass is eccentrically distributed in the vertebrae that suffer fragility fractures. In these vertebrae, there is lower bone density, lower trabecular thickness, and lower trabecular numbers in the anterior column [12, 13]. In addition, these vertebra have increased trabecular spacing, lower osteocyte density, and reduced cortical thickness [11].

Abnormal spinal anatomy and alignment also correlates to the increased risk of fracture in people with VCFs. Individuals with VCFs tend to have smaller vertebral cross-sectional area than those without VCFs. Furthermore, those with vertebral fractures also have shorter distance between the erector spinae muscle and vertebral bodies, which become more pronounced in the flexed and kyphotic spine. Gilsanz et al. demonstrated that the combination of this shortened lever arm and reduced vertebral cross-sectional area increases the mechanical load on the vertebrae by 8% in the erect stance, and 15% in the flexed stance [13, 14]. The increment in vertebral loading observed in these patients accelerates spodylotic changes.

Degenerative disc disease results in peripheral dissipation of normal axial loads. Consequently, the central regions of the vertebrae become stress-shielded and bone resorption is accelerated [15]. More force is required to actively move vertebra with interposed degenerated disk, further increasing the load on the involved vertebral endplate. The increased loading imparted on an already osteopenic vertebrae increases the risk of fracture [16]. Sornay-Rendu demonstrated a significant correlation with decreased disk space and increased incidence of VCFs [17].

11.4 Clinical Presentation

Osteoporotic VCFs are often asymptomatic at presentation and may be incidental findings on routine chest radiographs. When symptomatic, patients primarily complain of back pain with onset correlating with a relatively atraumatic event such as bending, arising from a seated position, or lifting a heavy object. Pain is often exacerbated by coughing, sneezing, defecation, and relieved by bed rest. The pain may last for several weeks. Because vertebral fractures are usually stable, neurological symptoms are infrequent. When present, patients may report pain radiating anteriorly along the costal distribution of the affected spinal nerve. Cord compression is rare and should suggest a more ominous diagnosis such as tumor or infection [18, 19].

On examination, focal tenderness to palpation at the involved vertebrae is often present. In addition, focal kyphosis, loss of lumbar lordosis, and loss of height may also be noted in patients with multiple compression fractures. Early satiety and reduction in exercise tolerance are late sequelae of VCFs and are secondary to the reduction in abdominal and thoracic cavity associated with multiple vertebral fractures [3, 18].

11.5 Radiology

The plain radiograph is the primary imaging modality for the evaluation of VCFs. In a lateral view, loss of anterior body height relative to the posterior height is typically indicative of a compression fracture (Fig. 11.2).

Accurate radiographic assessment of VCF is important because of the increased morbidity associated with multiple VCFs. As indicated above, a VCF, even when asymptomatic, increases the risk of additional VCFs (10), so the benefits of prevention are significant. The semi-quantitative approach has been proposed as a method of evaluating vertebral fragility fractures. In this approach, vertebral fractures are graded by visual deformity and assigned a grade based on the severity of the deformity (Table 11.1). A normal score (grade 0) is assigned when there is no observed deformity. A grade 1 fracture denotes a 20–25% reduction in height, and 10–20% reduction in projected vertebral area; grade 2 fracture suggests a 26–40% reduction in height and a 21–40% reduction in projected vertebral area. A severely deformed or grade 3 fracture pattern describes a fracture with >40% reduction in vertebral height and projected vertebral area. The involved vertebra is also compared to adjacent vertebrae or normal expected variants for alteration in shape. In the experienced hand, this combination of qualitative and quantitative analyses optimizes the sensitivity and specificity of the semi-quantitative method [20].

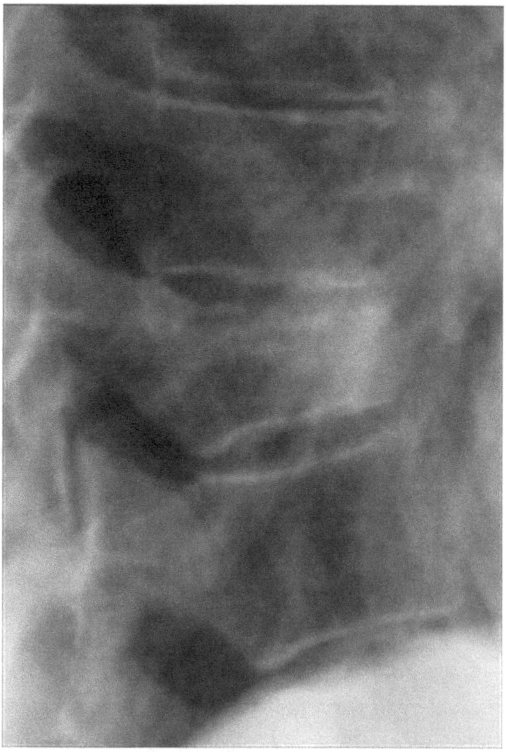

Fig. 11.2 Lateral X-ray showing loss of anterior column height indicative of a vertebral compression fracture

Table 11.1 Semi-quantitative grading scale

Grade 0	No observed deformity
Grade 1	20–25% reduction in height and 10–20% reduction in projected vertebral area
Grade 2	26–40% reduction in height and 21–40% reduction in projected vertebral area
Grade 3	>40% reduction in vertebral height and projected vertebral area

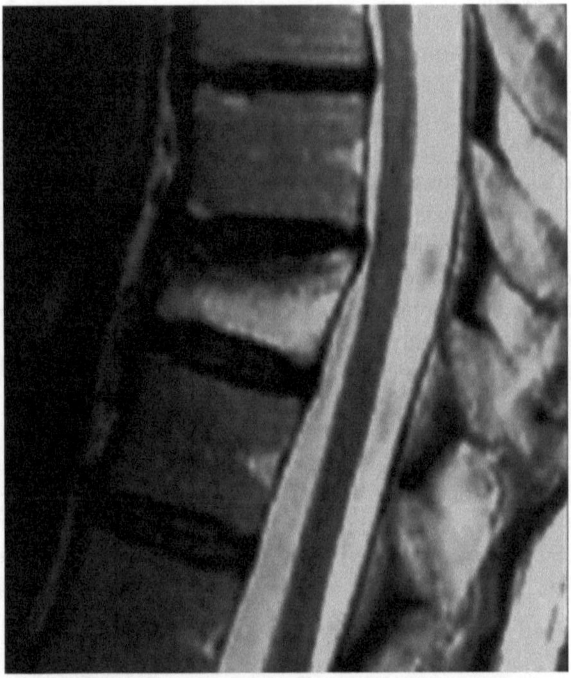

Fig. 11.3 MRI T2-weighted image with increase in edema, loss of anterior vertebral body height. There is no evidence of heterogeneous signal in the bone marrow and no evidence of epidural extension

Magnetic resonance imaging (MRI) is an important modality in the evaluation of VCFs. MRIs can detect occult fractures, determine the acuity of known fractures, and also delineate other potential causes of back pain such as tumor and infection. High signal intensity in the vertebral body on T2-weighted images and STIR images is indicative of fracture edema (Fig. 11.3). Increased signal in the posterior elements, heterogenous signal within the bone marrow, epidural extension, and involvement of paraspinal soft tissues are suggestive of infection or tumor (Fig. 11.4).

CT scan is not routinely used in the diagnosis of VCF. However, in patients at risk of VCF undergoing routine abdominal/thoracic CT scans for other reasons, sagittal reconstruction of the thoracolumbar spine may be of diagnostic utility. Bauer et al., in a cadaveric study, showed a 90% (compared to 82% for lateral

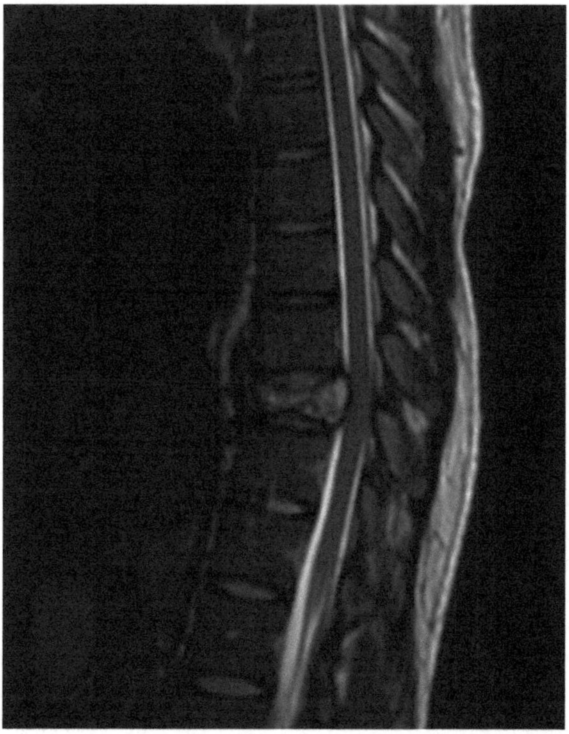

Fig. 11.4 MRI evidence of vertebral fracture likely not due to osteoporosis. Heterogenous signal and epidural extension are suggestive of a tumor or infection. Open biopsy revealed an aneurysmal bone cyst

radiographs) sensitivity in the detection of VCF using sagittal reconstructions of thin cut (<3 mm) CT scans [21].

11.6 Management

Initial management of symptomatic acute VCFs involves rest and adequate analgesia to ensure early mobilization. Prolonged immobilization can result in further diminution of an already osteopenic bone mass [19]. Furthermore, systemic complications associated with prolonged bed rest in the elderly, skin break down, poor pulmonary toilet, and thromboembolic disease exacerbates their prognosis. Rigid thoracolumbar orthoses are rarely well tolerated in the elderly patient with VCF, but semi-rigid braces or lumbar corsets can offer patients an effective means for pain control. The majority of patients with VCFs respond well to these non-operative measures.

Several pharmacological options have been explored in the treatment of the symptomatic acute VCF. Parental administration of bisphosphonates and intranasal/

subcutaneous administration of calcitonin has shown some efficacy in the alleviation of pain in patients presenting with VCFs [22–24].

Individuals diagnosed with a VCF should be treated for osteoporosis without further diagnostic work-up. A few agents have shown efficacy in the reduction of the risk of vertebral fractures in osteoporotic patients: anti-resorptive agents such as bisphosphonates, selective estrogen receptor modulators (SERMs), calcitonin, and anabolic agents such as parathyroid hormone analogs (Table 11.2).

Oral bisphosphonates are commonly used for the management of osteoporosis. Though not readily absorbed, the bisphosphonates are concentrated in bone and bind to hydroxyapatite. Here, they slow bone resorption by inhibiting osteoclast activity.

The efficacy of three bisphosphonates, etidronate, alendronate, and risedronate in the prevention of VCFs has been demonstrated. Storm et al. showed a 60% reduction in the incidence of vertebral fractures in patients who were started on etidronate [24]. Use of alendronate was shown to reduce the risk of vertebral fractures by 48% and 45% in two studies [25, 26]. Likewise, Reginster et al. showed a 49% reduction in the incidence of VCFs in patients taking risedronate [27]. Weekly formulations of alendronate and risedronate have increased the convenience of their use and patient compliance. The most significant complication of bisphosphonate therapy, esophagitis, can be limited by the use of lower dosages [19].

SERMs have also been shown to be effective in the prevention of VCFs. Raloxifene is the most commonly used agent in this class. It has selective estrogen receptor antagonist activity in the breast and endometrium, but agonist activities in the bone. The MORE study, a multicenter, randomized, blinded, placebo-controlled trial involving 7,705 women age 31–80, showed a 30–50% reduction in the incidence of VCF in patients treated with raloxifene [28].

Table 11.2 Selected pharmacological options for management of vertebral compression fractures

Drug class	Mechanism	Indications	Examples
Bisphosphonates	Anti-resorptive. Induces osteoclast apoptosis	Prevention and treatment of postmenopausal osteoporosis	Etidronate, alendronate, risedronate
SERMs	Anti-resorptive. Increases bone mass	Prevention and treatment of postmenopausal osteoporosis	Raloxifene
Synthetic parathyroid hormone	Stimulates new bone formation by enhancing osteocyte viability, increasing calcium absorption, decreases urinary calcium excretion	Treatment of postmenopausal osteoporosis	Teriparitide
Calcitonin	Decreases release of skeletal calcium, phosphorus, hydroxyproline	Treatment of acute vertebral compression fractures. Prevention and treatment of osteoporosis	Calcitonin

Tetraparalide, a synthetic parathyroid hormone, is the only anabolic agent currently used clinically in the prevention of osteoporosis. It maintains osteoclast viability and has been shown to decrease the incidence of osteoporosis [29].

Calcium and vitamin D are nutritional supplements that help improve BMD and help guard against the complications associated with osteoporosis. Calcium and vitamin D have been shown to improve bone density. Calcium and vitamin D deficiencies are common in people with osteoporosis. Although they have not demonstrated efficacy in the reduction of subsequent VCFs [8], they play an important role in the prevention of osteoporosis.

Until recently, hormone replacement therapy (HRT) was a mainstay in the management of patients with osteoporosis. However, the risk associated with the use of HRT such as breast cancer, cerebrovascular, and cardiovascular events outweighs its benefits in this setting [30].

11.7 Surgical management

Two percutaneous procedures have been described and are commonly performed as surgical treatment options for VCFs. Vertebroplasty involves fluoroscopically guided infusion of polymethylmethacrylate into the fractured vertebrae. This results in impaction of the surrounding cancellous bone and stabilization of the fracture (Fig. 11.5). Kyphoplasty, a modification of vertebroplasty, requires inflation of a balloon within the vertebral body to create a void in the collapsed body prior to infusion of cement. Proponents of kyphoplasty have suggested several advantages of this procedure over a vertebroplasty: (1) The impacted rim of cancellous bone created by

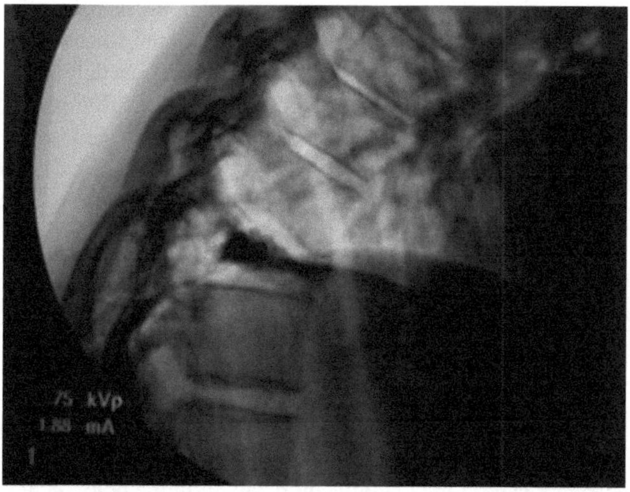

Fig. 11.5 Percutaneous, fluoroscopic guidance of cement into the vertebral body may help to stabilize the bone and decrease pain

the balloon limits the egress of cement from the vertebra; (2) because a cavity is created by the balloon prior to infusion of the cement, less infusion pressure is needed for the cement therefore reducing the risk of extravasation; and (3) the exact volume needed to fill the vertebral cavity can be estimated from the amount of air needed to fill the balloon. These technical differences have been purported to reduce the risk of cement extravasation [31, 32].

Early studies reported significant pain relief after percutaneous vertebral augmentation [33–36]. However, a majority of these studies were non-randomized trials without controls. Recent prospective randomized controlled studies have questioned the efficacy of this popular procedure. Buchbinder et al. [37], in a blinded randomized controlled trial involving 78 participants, found no beneficial effects of vertebroplasty over a sham procedure at the 1 week, then 1-, 3-, and 6-month intervals after surgery. Their findings were corroborated by Kallmes et al. in a similar study with 131 participants. They found no significant difference in pain scores immediately after surgery, at 1 month and at 3 months after surgery [38]. Both studies however showed subsidence of pain and improvement of function over time in both treatment arms. Rousing et al., in a randomized, non-placebo-controlled trial, recently showed relative pain reduction and improved VAS scores after the first month in patients undergoing vertebroplasty versus those managed conservatively. There was no difference in both groups at the 3-month and 12-month interval. They recommended vertebral augmentation in patients with significant pain who are unable to tolerate conservative treatment [39].

A few limitations of these studies have been expressed by several authors [40–42]. A consistent concern among critics is the potential for selection bias given the low enrollment rates of both studies. Another common criticism was the relatively small sample sizes of both studies and the absence of subgroup analysis which may delineate sub-populations that can benefit from vertebral augmentation. Finally some have suggested that the sham treatment used in these studies, especially the injection of a local anesthetic, may have therapeutic effects exceeding the placebo effect.

Open stabilization of vertebral compression is seldom indicated but should be considered for patients with neurological deficits and significant deformity. Traditional surgical management involves anterior decompression through a retroperitoneal or thoracic approach. The involved segments are reconstructed with structural grafts. When combined with posterior stabilization, fusion rate is optimized. Because these patients are osteopenic, adequate hardware fixation into the vertebra becomes difficult. Techniques such as polymethylmethacrylate augmentation, use of pedicle screws, and sublaminar hooks have been used to enhance stability [31].

11.8 Conclusion

Vertebral compression fractures are the most common fragility fractures in the elderly population. They are caused by a significant decrease in the bony architecture of the cancellous and cortical bone of the vertebral bodies. As a result of these quantitative changes in bone, routine activities of daily living can lead to VCFs. Treatment options include both non-operative and operative management, although further studies are needed to help establish the long-term efficacy of surgical intervention.

References

1. Cummings SR, Melton LJ. Epidemiology and outcomes of osteoporotic fractures. *Lancet.* 2002;359(9319):1761–1767.
2. Cooper C, Atkinson EJ, O'Fallon WM, Melton LJ, 3rd. Incidence of clinically diagnosed vertebral fractures: a population-based study in Rochester, Minnesota, 1985–1989. *J Bone Miner Res.* 1992;7(2):221–227.
3. Kim DH, Vaccaro AR. Osteoporotic compression fractures of the spine; current options and considerations for treatment. *Spine J.* 2006;6(5):479–487.
4. Melton LJ, 3rd. Epidemiology of spinal osteoporosis. *Spine (Phila Pa 1976).* 1997;22 (24 Suppl):2S–11S.
5. Albrand G, Munoz F, Sornay-Rendu E, DuBoeuf F, Delmas PD. Independent predictors of all osteoporosis-related fractures in healthy postmenopausal women: the OFELY study. *Bone.* 2003;32(1):78–85.
6. Ross PD, Davis JW, Epstein RS, Wasnich RD. Pre-existing fractures and bone mass predict vertebral fracture incidence in women. *Ann Intern Med.* 1991;114(11):919–923.
7. White AAI, Panjabi MM. Physical properties and functional biomechanics of the spine. In: White AAI, Panjabi MM (eds) Clinical Biomechanics of the Spine, 2nd ed. Philadelphia: Lippincott; 1990:28–45.
8. Myers ER, Wilson SE. Biomechanics of osteoporosis and vertebral fracture. *Spine (Phila Pa 1976).* 1997;22(24 Suppl):25S–31S.
9. Hayes WC, Piazza SJ, Zysset PK. Biomechanics of fracture risk prediction of the hip and spine by quantitative computed tomography. *Radiol Clin North Am.* 1991;29(1):1–18.
10. Lunt M, O'Neill TW, Felsenberg D, et al. Characteristics of a prevalent vertebral deformity predict subsequent vertebral fracture: results from the European Prospective Osteoporosis Study (EPOS). *Bone.* 2003;33(4):505–513.
11. Briggs AM, Greig AM, Wark JD. The vertebral fracture cascade in osteoporosis: a review of aetiopathogenesis. *Osteoporos Int.* 2007;18(5):575–584.
12. Ciarelli TE, Fyhrie DP, Parfitt AM. Effects of vertebral bone fragility and bone formation rate on the mineralization levels of cancellous bone from white females. *Bone.* 2003;32(3):311–315.
13. Gilsanz V, Loro ML, Roe TF, Sayre J, Gilsanz R, Schulz EE. Vertebral size in elderly women with osteoporosis. Mechanical implications and relationship to fractures. *J Clin Invest.* 1995;95(5):2332–2337.
14. Tveit P, Daggfeldt K, Hetland S, Thorstensson A. Erector spinae lever arm length variations with changes in spinal curvature. *Spine (Phila Pa 1976).* 1994;19(2):199–204.
15. Pollintine P, Dolan P, Tobias JH, Adams MA. Intervertebral disc degeneration can lead to "stress-shielding" of the anterior vertebral body: a cause of osteoporotic vertebral fracture? *Spine (Phila Pa 1976).* 2004;29(7):774–782.
16. Adams MA, Pollintine P, Tobias JH, Wakley GK, Dolan P. Intervertebral disc degeneration can predispose to anterior vertebral fractures in the thoracolumbar spine. *J Bone Miner Res.* 2006;21(9):1409–1416.
17. Sornay-Rendu E, Boutroy S, Munoz F, Delmas PD. Alterations of cortical and trabecular architecture are associated with fractures in postmenopausal women, partially independent of decreased BMD measured by DXA: the OFELY study. *J Bone Miner Res.* 2007;22(3):425–433.
18. Glaser DL, Kaplan FS. Osteoporosis. Definition and clinical presentation. *Spine (Phila Pa 1976).* 1997;22(24 Suppl):12S–16S.

19. Francis RM, Baillie SP, Chuck AJ, et al. Acute and long-term management of patients with vertebral fractures. *Q J Med*. 2004;97(2):63–74.
20. Genant HK, Jergas M. Assessment of prevalent and incident vertebral fractures in osteoporosis research. *Osteoporos Int*. 2003;14(Suppl 3):S43–S55.
21. Bauer JS, Muller D, Ambekar A, et al. Detection of osteoporotic vertebral fractures using multidetector CT. *Osteoporos Int*. 2006;17(4):608–615.
22. Maksymowych WP. Managing acute osteoporotic vertebral fractures with calcitonin. *Can Fam Physician*. 1998;44:2160–2166.
23. Lyritis GP, Tsakalakos N, Magiasis B, Karachalios T, Yiatzides A, Tsekoura M. Analgesic effect of salmon calcitonin in osteoporotic vertebral fractures: a double-blind placebo-controlled clinical study. *Calcif Tissue Int*. 1991;49(6):369–372.
24. Storm T, Thamsborg G, Steiniche T, Genant HK, Sorensen OH. Effect of intermittent cyclical etidronate therapy on bone mass and fracture rate in women with postmenopausal osteoporosis. *N Engl J Med*. 1990;322(18):1265–1271.
25. Liberman UA, Weiss SR, Broll J, et al. Effect of oral alendronate on bone mineral density and the incidence of fractures in postmenopausal osteoporosis. The Alendronate Phase III Osteoporosis Treatment Study Group. *N Engl J Med*. 1995;333(22):1437–1443.
26. Hochberg MC, Thompson DE, Black DM, et al. Effect of alendronate on the age-specific incidence of symptomatic osteoporotic fractures. *J Bone Miner Res*. 2005;20(6):971–976.
27. Reginster J, Minne HW, Sorensen OH, et al. Randomized trial of the effects of risedronate on vertebral fractures in women with established postmenopausal osteoporosis. Vertebral Efficacy with Risedronate Therapy (VERT) Study Group. *Osteoporos Int*. 2000;11(1):83–91.
28. Cummings SR, Eckert S, Krueger KA, et al. The effect of raloxifene on risk of breast cancer in postmenopausal women: results from the MORE randomized trial. Multiple Outcomes of Raloxifene Evaluation. *JAMA*. 1999;281(23):2189–2197.
29. Neer RM, Arnaud CD, Zanchetta JR, et al. Effect of parathyroid hormone (1–34) on fractures and bone mineral density in postmenopausal women with osteoporosis. *N Engl J Med*. 2001;344(19):1434–1441.
30. Lippuner K. Medical treatment of vertebral osteoporosis. *Eur Spine J*. 2003;12 Suppl 2:S132–141.
31. Shen M, Kim Y. Osteoporotic vertebral compression fractures: a review of current surgical management techniques. *Am J Orthop (Belle Mead NJ)*. 2007;36(5):241–248.
32. Eck JC, Nachtigall D, Humphreys SC, Hodges SD. Comparison of vertebroplasty and balloon kyphoplasty for treatment of vertebral compression fractures: a meta-analysis of the literature. *Spine J*. 2008;8(3):488–497.
33. Jensen ME, Evans AJ, Mathis JM, Kallmes DF, Cloft HJ, Dion JE. Percutaneous polymethylmethacrylate vertebroplasty in the treatment of osteoporotic vertebral body compression fractures: technical aspects. *AJNR Am J Neuroradiol*. 1997;18(10):1897–1904.
34. Martin JB, Jean B, Sugiu K, et al. Vertebroplasty: clinical experience and follow-up results. *Bone*. 1999;25(2 Suppl):11S–15S.
35. Layton KF, Thielen KR, Koch CA, et al. Vertebroplasty, first 1000 levels of a single center: evaluation of the outcomes and complications. *AJNR Am J Neuroradiol*. 2007;28(4):683–689.
36. Deramond H, Depriester C, Galibert P, Le Gars D. Percutaneous vertebroplasty with polymethylmethacrylate. Technique, indications, and results. *Radiol Clin North Am*. 1998;36(3):533–546.
37. Buchbinder R, Osborne RH, Ebeling PR, et al. A randomized trial of vertebroplasty for painful osteoporotic vertebral fractures. *N Engl J Med*. 2009;361(6):557–568.
38. Kallmes DF, Comstock BA, Heagerty PJ, et al. A randomized trial of vertebroplasty for osteoporotic spinal fractures. *N Engl J Med*. 2009;361(6):569–579.
39. Rousing R, Hansen KL, Andersen MO, Jespersen SM, Thomsen K, Lauritsen JM. Twelve-months follow-up in forty-nine patients with acute/semiacute osteoporotic vertebral fractures treated conservatively or with percutaneous vertebroplasty: a clinical randomized study. *Spine (Phila Pa 1976)*. 2010;35(5):478–482.

40. Bono CM, Heggeness M, Mick C, Resnick D, Watters WC, 3rd. North American Spine Society: Newly released vertebroplasty randomized controlled trials: a tale of two trials. *Spine J.* 2010;10(3):238–240.
41. Bolster MB. Consternation and questions about two vertebroplasty trials. *Cleve Clin J Med.* 2010;77(1):12–16.
42. Orr RD. Vertebroplasty, cognitive dissonance, and evidence-based medicine: what do we do when the 'evidence' says we are wrong? *Cleve Clin J Med.* 2010;77(1):8–11.

Chapter 12
Hip Fractures

Andrew F. Kuntz, Albert O. Gee, Jaimo Ahn, and Samir Mehta

Abstract Geriatric hip fracture patients represent an increasingly elderly, frail, and medically complex patient class. Hip fractures represent one of the most serious medical problems in the elderly population, and are often life-altering, if not life-ending. Surgical treatment is the current standard of care for hip fractures. Multiple surgical options exist for the treatment of the different types of hip fractures. In order to reduce morbidity and mortality associated with this type of injury, it is imperative to focus on both surgical treatment as well as the management of all coexisting medical issues. A multidisciplinary approach to treatment that incorporates orthopedic, geriatric, rehabilitation, endocrine, and social work services will help increase the potential for successful patient outcomes after this devastating injury.

Keywords Femoral neck • Intertrochanteric • Pertrochanteric • Fracture • Elderly

12.1 Epidemiology

The term "hip fracture" usually refers to two distinct fracture types involving the proximal end of the femur: femoral neck fractures and intertrochanteric region fractures. Intertrochanteric fractures travel between the greater and lesser trochanters of the femur, typically from superiorly and laterally to inferiorly and medially. The term "pertrochanteric" is used to describe an intertrochanteric fracture that extends below the level of the lesser trochanter. Subtrochanteric fractures are sometimes included in this terminology as well, even though these fractures represent proximal femur fractures. Femoral neck and intertrochanteric fractures comprise the vast majority of geriatric hip fractures, and these two fracture types will be discussed primarily in this chapter.

S. Mehta (✉)
Orthopedic Trauma and Fracture Service, Department of Orthopaedic Surgery, Hospital of the University of Pennsylvania, Silverstein 2, 3400 Spruce Street, Philadelphia, PA 19104, USA
e-mail: samir.mehta@uphs.upenn.edu

R.J. Pignolo et al. (eds.), *Fractures in the Elderly*, Aging Medicine,
DOI 10.1007/978-1-60327-467-8_12,

Currently, 329,000 elderly patients sustain a hip fracture each year in the United States [1]. Hip fractures can generally be divided into two broad categories – fractures involving the femoral neck and fractures of the intertrochanteric region. As the elderly population increases, the number of hip fractures is expected to rise to 500,000 per year by the year 2040 [2]. Geriatric hip fractures are usually due to abnormally weak bone, often the result of osteoporosis. As such, 80% of hip fractures occur in women [3]. Femoral neck fractures account for roughly 50% of all hip fractures. These fractures have a peak occurrence during the eighth decade in both males and females. Intertrochanteric fractures typically occur in older patients with more medical comorbidities than do femoral neck fractures [4]. The annual incidence of intertrochanteric fractures is 63 per 100,000 in females and 34 per 100,000 in males [2]. Overall, the incidence of hip fractures increases with increasing age – people over the age of 85 having 10–15 times the rate of hip fractures than those of age 60–65 [5, 6]. Greater than 95% of hip fractures among adults older than 65 years of age are due to a low-energy fall (e.g., fall from standing) [7]. The overall mortality rate after hip fracture ranges from 20 to 30% at 1 year [8–10].

12.2 Evaluation

Examination of the geriatric patient with a hip fracture should begin with a thorough history and physical examination. Evaluation for other potentially life-threatening injuries such as intracranial hemorrhage should be based on clinical suspicion, keeping in mind that similar to hip fractures, these injuries can occur after relatively low-energy trauma in the geriatric population [11]. Additionally, other orthopedic injuries including ipsilateral upper extremity injuries are not uncommon, making a complete musculoskeletal examination a necessity. In patients who have a high-energy mechanism, a thorough trauma evaluation is a necessity, following Advanced Trauma Life Support protocol. As part of the resuscitation, geriatric physiological response to increased fluid balance should be taken into account.

Elderly patients presenting with a hip fracture will most often complain of groin and thigh pain after a low-energy fall and the inability to bear weight on the injured leg. In addition to determining all medical comorbidities, the history should explore the pre-injury ambulatory status of the patient. Medical comorbidities and ambulatory status play a significant role in surgical treatment options and patient outcomes.

Physical examination of the patient with a displaced hip fracture most commonly reveals the injured leg shortened and externally rotated. Those patients with minimally displaced fractures will present without obvious lower extremity deformity but will complain of groin pain with hip rotation and resisted flexion. The skin should be evaluated for any lacerations or abrasions that may indicate an open fracture, although this is uncommon. As with all fractures, the neurovascular status of the affected extremity must be thoroughly examined and followed over time. Occasionally, a foot-drop may be noticed prior to surgical intervention, rather than as a result of it. Specifically, the terminal branches of the femoral artery and the femoral and sciatic nerves must be evaluated in the affected lower extremity. The remaining extremities should be examined to detect other musculoskeletal injuries and assess neurovascular competence.

Plain radiographs of the affected hip should be taken in the anteroposterior (AP) and cross-table lateral projections. An AP view of the pelvis is also necessary to adequately evaluate the fracture and to compare leg lengths. Occasionally, patients complaining of groin pain, thigh pain, and difficulty bearing weight, may have normal appearing plain radiographs. In this situation, additional imaging is indicated to rule out an occult hip fracture. MRI is the imaging modality of choice as it provides a prompt diagnosis and has the ability to rule out other conditions which may be the cause of pain, including osteonecrosis, stress fracture, and tumor. Bone scan is another method of diagnosing an occult hip fracture, especially for patients in which MRI is either contraindicated or cannot be tolerated. However, there remains controversy as to whether bone scans can detect femoral neck fractures before 72 h in osteoporotic patients [12, 13]. CT scan of the hip is also a potential diagnostic modality to detect fractures which are indiscernible on plain radiographs. However, a CT scan cannot be used to definitively rule out an occult hip fracture since non-displaced fractures can be missed.

Standard preoperative laboratory tests should include a complete blood count, full blood chemistry panel, coagulation panel, and a type and screen for anticipated perioperative blood transfusions. Patients should have a standard preoperative chest radiograph as well as an electrocardiogram. A urinalysis is typically obtained prior to the placement of a surgical implant in order to rule out an occult urinary tract infection. In addition, there should be some consideration to obtain baseline nutrition labs, calcium and Vitamin D levels, and an evaluation of thyroid function. The involvement of a geriatrician or internal medicine specialist is important in managing patients' multiple comorbidities, optimizing their preoperative status, and managing postoperative medical issues.

12.3 Fracture Pattern

Fractures of the femoral neck are often classified by the Garden classification. This system divides these fractures into four patterns that are commonly encountered clinically. Stage I fractures are incomplete fractures or valgus-impacted femoral neck fractures. These fractures take on a slight valgus malalignment with impaction of the femoral head onto the neck. Often, in this fracture type, the trabeculae along the inferior neck remain undisturbed making these fractures difficult to diagnose on plain radiographs. Stage II fractures are complete fractures through the femoral neck that are very slightly displaced with varus malalignment. Stage III fractures are partially displaced from the normal anatomic alignment, and stage IV represents complete displacement of the two fracture fragments with no continuity between them. For practical purposes, most orthopedic surgeons will group stages I and II together as non-displaced femoral neck fractures and stages III and IV as displaced fractures, because the degree of displacement is positively correlated to the risk of osteonecrosis of the femoral head [14]. Classifying femoral neck fracture into this simpler binary grading scheme simplifies the choice of surgical treatment.

Intertrochanteric femur fractures in geriatric patients are typically the result of a low-energy mechanism. However, due to poor bone quality, the fracture patterns observed in the geriatric population can often mimic high-energy fracture patterns observed in the younger patient population. In general, these fractures are classified broadly as stable versus unstable. Those that are termed stable represent fractures in which there is no comminution of the medial aspect of the intertrochanteric region (proximal to and including the lesser trochanter). This ensures good cortical contact between fracture fragments medially which is an important region biomechanically for weight-bearing. The stability of the fracture will therefore dictate treatment. In unstable fracture patterns, the posteromedial cortex in the area of the lesser trochanter and calcar region is comminuted. As a result these fracture patterns tend to fail into varus angulation despite initial operative anatomic reduction. Reverse obliquity fractures are also inherently unstable because of the tendency for the femoral shaft to displace medially, especially with certain types of fixation options.

12.4 Treatment options

12.4.1 Non-operative Treatment

Non-operative management is rarely indicated in the treatment of hip fractures. Historically, non-operative management was considered an option for stable, valgus-impacted, non-displaced femoral neck fractures. However, one recent study revealed a non-union rate of 39% [15]. Currently, non-operative management of femoral neck and intertrochanteric fractures is reserved for the non-ambulatory, demented patient with minimal pain from the hip fracture and significant medical comorbidities that preclude surgery.

In the limited subset of patients treated non-operatively, a course of bed rest is indicated to minimize fracture displacement and promote healing. Skeletal traction may also be used to improve fracture alignment, restore fracture length, reduce deformity, and decrease muscle spasms. In the general population, non-operative management of lower extremity fractures with skeletal traction is associated with fracture malunion, limb shortening, skin and respiratory complications, and prolonged hospitalization. In the elderly population, the morbidity of prolonged bed rest is even greater, resulting in severe deconditioning, frequent pulmonary complications, and decubitus ulcers. Given the generally poor results associated with non-operative treatment and the improvements in surgical treatment options, anesthetic techniques, and postoperative management, surgical treatment of hip fractures in the elderly population has become the standard of care.

12.4.2 Operative treatment

The general goal of surgical management of hip fractures is to restore functional anatomy in a way that will allow for early mobilization and rehabilitation while promoting fracture healing. Prior to pursuing operative treatment, the surgeon and patient must define the goals of surgery. The patient's age, pre-existing medical comorbidities, current medical condition, and previous level of function must be considered in conjunction with the patient's desires and the risks associated with surgery. Surgical treatment of the various types of hip fractures differs significantly. This is due to variations in the anatomy, biomechanics, and healing potential that exist between femoral neck and pertrochanteric hip fractures. As such, surgical treatment of these two types of hip fractures will be addressed independently in the subsequent sections.

Regardless of the type of hip fracture, several studies have demonstrated the importance of early surgical intervention. Zuckerman et al. showed that there was an increase in the 1-year mortality rate in patients that did not undergo operative treatment within 2 days of injury [16], Another more recent prospective series of 2,660 elderly patients revealed similar findings [17]. In this study, healthy patients that underwent surgery within 4 days of fracture had no difference in mortality rate at 1-year follow-up from patients that had operative treatment within 24 h. However, when surgery for patients without medical comorbidities was delayed 4 days or more after presentation, the 90-day and 1-year mortality rate was increased. For patients with an acute medical comorbidity that resulted in a surgical delay of more than 24 h, the 30-day mortality was 2.5 times greater than in patients without comorbidities that delayed surgery. Both of these studies reinforce the importance of early surgical intervention in the treatment of hip fractures, highlighting significantly increased mortality when the delay in surgery was due to an acute medical comorbidity.

Despite the need for acute surgical intervention, patients with hip fractures are often cared for on a medical or surgical inpatient service for a period of time prior to operative treatment. During the preoperative period, some surgeons have advocated the use of skin traction to maintain limb length and fracture alignment. Similar to skeletal traction, skin traction relies on the use of a pulley to connect weight to a soft boot attached to the affected extremity, and can be used as a non-invasive method for maintaining fracture alignment and limb length. However, there are no data to support the notion that skin traction maintains or improves fracture position. Additionally, there is concern for soft tissue breakdown due to mechanical shearing at the site of the traction boot as well as an increased risk for decubitus ulcers due to less frequent turning. A randomized prospective trial investigating the effects of skin traction in patients with hip and proximal femur fractures revealed no differences in terms of preoperative pain, anesthesia required for surgery, or surgical ease as reported by the surgeon [18]. Likewise, there was no difference in the frequency of pressure sores between groups. Similar results were reported in a later study investigating the effects of skin traction in patients with hip fractures only [19]. This study also showed no difference in union rates or fracture alignment at 4 months follow-up. Overall, no benefit has been confirmed for the routine use of temporary skin traction prior to hip fracture surgery.

12.4.2.1 Operative Treatment of Femoral Neck Fractures

When determining the surgical treatment of choice for a femoral neck fracture in an elderly patient, the degree of fracture displacement is critical. In addition to fracture configuration, bone quality, the patient's medical comorbidities, activity level, and cognitive status must all be considered when determining the best treatment option. Overall, in situ screw fixation is favored for non-displaced or stable fractures with a low tendency for displacement. Typically, femoral neck fractures with a more vertical component exhibit greater shear forces across the fracture site, resulting in a higher potential for displacement. Fractures with this configuration may therefore be more suitably treated with a fixed-angle device, such as a blade plate or dynamic hip screw (DHS) [20]. Internal fixation is commonly the treatment of choice in the young patient (<65 years old), regardless of whether the fracture is displaced or not, as this treatment allows for preservation of native bone.

In the geriatric patient with a displaced femoral neck fracture, hip arthroplasty is typically performed. In geriatric patients that have concomitant dementia, hemiarthroplasty allows for immediate postoperative weight-bearing with a relatively low chance of dislocation. Total hip arthroplasty is more commonly reserved for the active, ambulatory elder with good cognitive function, as this group of patients will place higher demands on the hip while adhering to the standard hip precautions. Total hip arthoplasty should also be considered in patients with concomitant acetabular arthritis from degenerative changes, rheumatoid arthritis, or Paget's disease.

A recent survey of American and European orthopedic surgeons revealed a preference for internal fixation in the patient less than 60 years old with a femoral neck fracture [21]. This same group preferred arthroplasty for the geriatric patient over 80 with the same fracture. A considerable difference in opinion existed for the treatment of choice for the elderly patient between 60 and 80 years of age with a femoral neck fracture. When considering costs associated with each of these treatment methods, total hip arthroplasty was more cost-effective than hemiarthroplasty or internal fixation when taking into account complications and revision surgery [22].

Percutaneous Screw Fixation

Percutaneous screw fixation of femoral neck fractures offers a minimally invasive, relatively efficient method of fracture stabilization. The procedure involves placement of multiple screws into the femoral neck under fluoroscopic guidance through small skin incisions over the lateral thigh. The screws begin in the lateral femoral cortex, cross the fracture site, and terminate in the subchondral bone of the femoral head (Fig. 12.1).

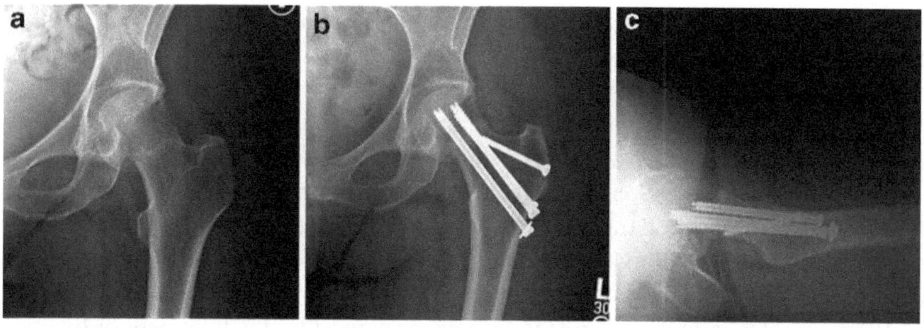

Fig. 12.1 (**a**) Anteroposterior (AP) radiograph showing a non-displaced femoral neck fracture. Postoperative radiographs in the AP (**b**) and lateral (**c**) projections, respectively, show percutaneous pin fixation

Screw placement is important and typically involves the use of an inverted triangle construct, with two parallel screws placed superiorly in the femoral neck and a third screw in the middle of the inferior aspect of the femoral neck. Other constructs involving two screws placed vertically or four screws in a diamond configuration have been described. Four-screw constructs are typically reserved for more unstable fracture patterns. A biomechanical comparison of several two- and three-screw constructs revealed superior mechanical properties with the inverted triangle construct [23]. It has been shown that in osteoporotic bone, the most caudal screw should be placed as close to the calcar region as possible to help minimize the risk of inferior displacement of the femoral neck.

Femoral neck fractures treated with open reduction and internal fixation in patients under the age 65 are associated with a non-union rate of approximately 5% and femoral head osteonecrosis in roughly 25% of cases [24]. In contrast, a meta-analysis comparing surgical treatment options for femoral neck fractures revealed non-unions to be the most common complication following internal fixation in a group with a median age of 77. In this cohort, non-union occurred in one-third of all cases [25]. Overall, only 25% of patients who develop osteonecrosis will require further surgery, compared to 75% of patients with non-united fractures. Another significant complication following screw fixation can result from improper placement of the screws. When the starting position of the screws is below the level of the lesser trochanter on the lateral femoral cortex, the mechanical environment of the proximal femur is altered, a stress rise is created, and an intertrochanteric or subtrochanteric fracture may propagate around the implanted screws.

Arthroplasty

Arthroplasty following femoral neck fracture is another potential treatment for the elderly patient. Hip replacement can be used to treat displaced or non-displaced fractures with a predictably low complication rate [11]. Additionally, the durability of current implants and advances in surgical techniques allow for immediate postoperative weight-bearing and rehabilitation. There are many options pertaining to hip arthroplasty that must be considered. Specifically, the orthopedic surgeon must decide between a total joint arthroplasty, or replacement of the femoral head and neck as well as the acetabular lining, and a hemiarthroplasty, or replacement of the femoral head and neck alone (Fig. 12.2).

Hemiarthroplasty has long been the choice of many orthopedic surgeons for the treatment of femoral neck fractures in the geriatric population. The fractured portion of the femoral neck is removed and replaced with a metal prosthesis, substituting for the femoral head and neck.

Both unipolar and bipolar prostheses have been used for the treatment of femoral neck fractures. In the short term, there is no advantage of one type of implant versus the other, aside from cost (the unipolar device is cheaper) [26]. However, one study showed that after 7-year follow-up, there was a lower incidence of revision surgery in patients who had initially undergone bipolar hemiarthroplasty [25].

Hemiarthroplasty prostheses can be fixed into the host femoral canal using either cemented or cementless technique. Several studies have demonstrated improved outcomes following cemented hemiarthroplasty in the geriatric population [11, 25]. The use of cement improves bony fixation in the osteoporotic host bone, which has a relatively poor ability to provide solid prosthesis fixation without cement supplementation. However, the use of cement does not come without the potential for complication. Cementing has been demonstrated to increase the risk of intraoperative medical complications and death, likely due to embolization of the bone marrow contents during cement placement and the cardiopulmonary impact of

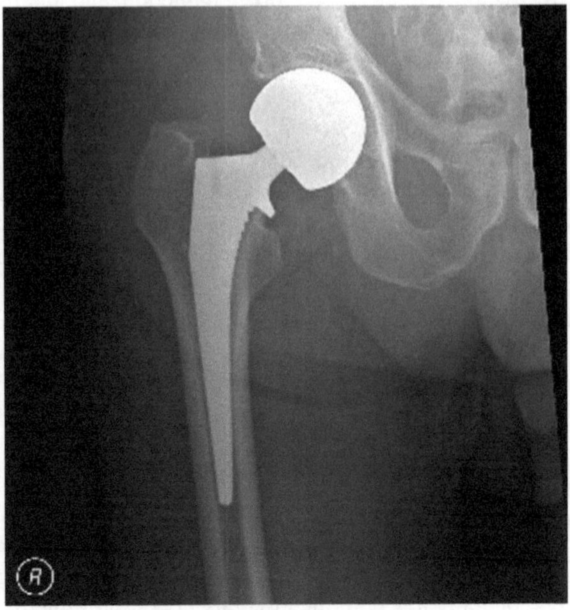

Fig. 12.2 A right hip hemiarthroplasty seen on an AP radiograph

cement monomer release during implantation. Newer cementing techniques have helped to minimize these complications. However, the rate of intra-operative sudden death during arthroplasty for a femoral neck fracture is 1 in 500 [27, 28]. Certainly, the use of cement must be based on the patient's perceived functional demands as well as overall health and the coexistence of medical problems. In most cases, the use of an uncemented unipolar prosthesis is reserved for the extremely low-demand patient with multiple medical comorbidities [4].

Historically, only the geriatric patient with a femoral neck fracture and concurrent, pre-existing hip arthritis was considered for total hip arthroplasty. As the survivorship after hip fractures continues to increase and complications decrease, total hip arthroplasty is becoming a common treatment for the healthy, active geriatric femoral neck fracture patient. Compared with internal fixation and hemiarthroplasty, total hip arthroplasty for femoral neck fracture results in better pain relief and functional outcome, without an increased risk of morbidity or mortality [29–31]. The best outcomes in published series of total hip arthroplasty after femoral neck fracture occurred in healthy patients with normal cognitive function. A randomized study comparing total hip arthroplasty to internal fixation in patients over 70 years of age with minimal cognitive deficits who lived and ambulated independently prior to fracture revealed that patients who underwent total hip arthroplasty had a 4% complication rate and a 4% reoperation rate compared to 42% and 47%, respectively, in the internal fixation group [32]. Interestingly, mortality rate, hip function, and the ability to perform activities of daily living were the same at 4 years regardless of the type of treatment. The most common complication following total hip arthroplasty was dislocation. All joint replacement procedures also carry the risk of infection, implant subsidence, deep vein thrombosis, and periprosthetic fracture.

12.4.2.2 Operative Treatment of Intertrochanteric Fractures

Multiple surgical options exist for the treatment of intertrochanteric hip fractures. Similar to femoral neck fractures, operative treatment is the standard of care except in the situation of severe medical comorbidity. Currently, the sliding hip screw and the intramedullary hip screw are the most commonly used surgical constructs. Although used much less commonly, external fixation is another surgical treatment option. Overall, the goal of treatment is to provide stable fracture fixation to promote healing while allowing the patient to begin early mobilization and weight-bearing. Surgical fixation of an intertrochanteric fracture is not different from any other geriatric hip fracture – the surgeon must consider not only fracture pattern but also the patient's age, medical condition, and pre-injury functional status.

Sliding Hip Screw

Also commonly referred to as a compression hip screw, sliding hip screws (SHS) allow for controlled, dynamic compression at the fracture site. This device simultaneously maintains alignment and enhances compression at the fracture site. Sliding hip screws are placed through a lateral incision over the proximal femur. Screw fixation is used to secure the plate portion of the construct to the femoral shaft (Fig. 12.3a, b). The hip screw itself is inserted through the femoral neck and into the subchondral bone of the femoral head. Care must be taken to center the hip screw within the femoral head and advance the screw firmly into the subchondral bone. Screw cut-out, a situation in which the mechanical forces placed on the hip and implant cause the hip screw to lever out of the bone, is usually due to improper placement or poor reduction and occurs in 2.5% of cases [33]. Screw cut-out is the most common mechanism of implant failure, accounting for 84% of all SHS failures [34].

The use of a compression hip screw is associated with an 88% union rate at 6 months [35]. In terms of functional outcomes, this same study found that 70% of patients treated with a compression hip screw required ambulatory aid 6 months after surgery, compared to only 38% pre-injury. Similarly, Medoff and Maes found only 50% of patients to be walking independently at the time of hospital discharge following compression hip screw treatment [36]. Another study found that only 21% of patients treated with a compression hip screw regained pre-injury function and independence [37].

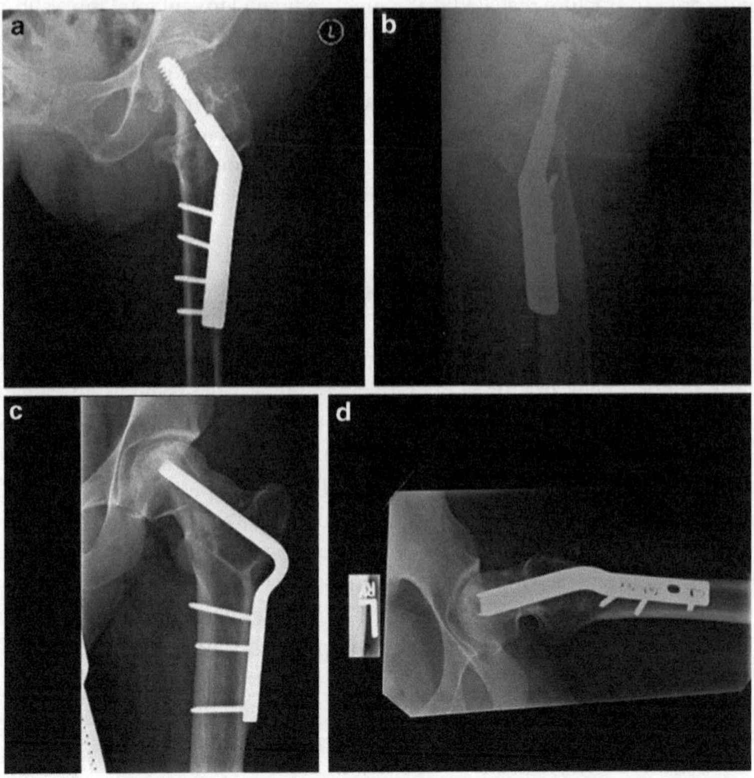

Fig. 12.3 AP and lateral radiographs of an intertrochanteric fracture treated with a dynamic hip screw (**a**, **b**) and a fixed-angle blade plate (**c**, **d**)

Intramedullary Hip Screw

Intramedullary hip screws offer a relatively new alternative for surgical fixation of intertrochanteric fractures. Also referred to as a cephalomedullary nail, this construct makes use of a single, large diameter lag screw traversing the femoral shaft and neck into the femoral head (Fig. 12.4a–c). However, instead of a lateral side plate, the hip screw is fixed to an intramedullary nail. The intramedullary rod is placed in an antegrade fashion, inserted at the tip of the greater trochanter and passed distally into the femoral shaft. In theory, the use of an intramedullary implant reduces deforming forces at the fracture site by decreasing the lever arm from the hip screw to its point of fixation. However, computer modeling and biomechanical testing have not supported this theory [38, 39]. Another potential advantage of this implant is the ability to perform a closed reduction and fixation as opposed to the open reduction required for the compression hip screw. Just as with the compression hip screw, intramedullary hip screws are also subject to cut-out (Fig. 12.4d–f). Additionally, thigh pain and femoral shaft fracture are not uncommon with intramedullary hip screw use [33].

When compared, sliding hip screws and intramedullary hip screws have similar rates of screw cut-out, blood loss during surgery, length of hospital stay, wound complications, and all-cause mortality [35, 37, 40]. Another prospective study by Bridle et al. reported similar findings with the exceptions of a lower cut-out rate,

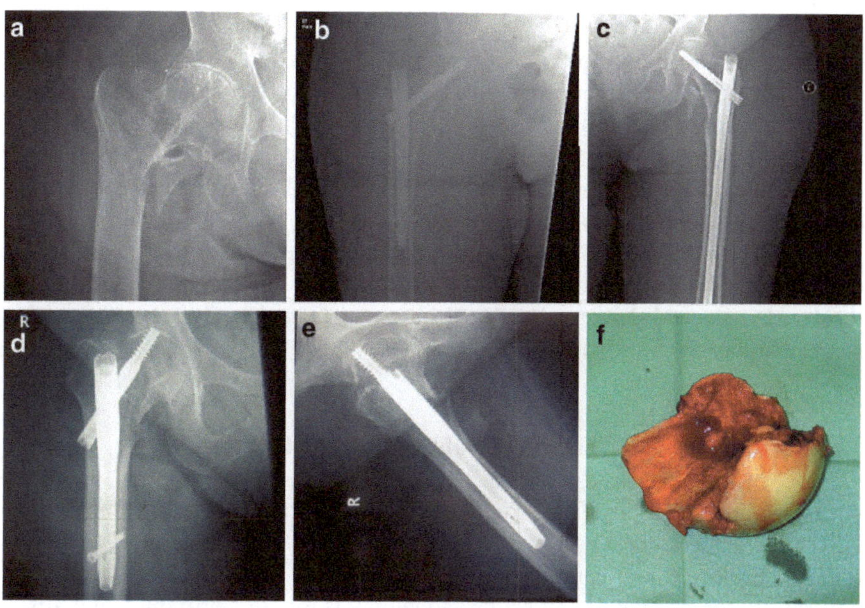

Fig. 12.4 (**a**) AP radiograph demonstrating an intertrochanteric fracture. Postoperative AP radiographs of a short (**b**) and long (**c**) intramedullary hip screw. The most common catastrophic complication of hip screw placement is screw cut-out, seen here on AP and lateral hip radiographs (**d, e**). The patient was treated with a hip arthroplasty and the retrieved femoral head is shown (**f**)

but higher incidence of femoral fracture with intramedullary hip screw use [41]. In this study, there was no difference in mobility postoperatively while other studies have reported improved mobility following the use of an intramedullary device [42]. In comparison with the sliding hip screw, intramedullary implants are also significantly more expensive.

Blade Plate

A proximal femoral blade plate is a fixed angle device that can be used for the treatment of femoral neck, intertrochanteric, and subtrochanteric fractures (Fig. 12.3c, d). Blade plates have been replaced with compression hip screws and intramedullary devices due to the technically challenging aspects of blade plate insertion. However, it does represent a viable option for revision and non-union situations, in particular those patients with a steep fracture angle. One study comparing a 95° fixed angle blade plate with an intramedullary device in 39 elderly patients revealed increased surgery time, blood loss, and length of hospital stay with blade plate use [43]. The authors concluded that based on their results, routine use of blade plates was not recommended.

External Fixation

Although not commonly performed, external fixation can be used for definitive treatment of intertrochanteric fracture. Historically, this technique was associated with poor fixation due to pin loosening. However, with the use of hydroxyapatite-coated pins, acceptable results can be achieved. In a prospective, randomized study comparing external fixation to a sliding hip screw for the treatment of pertrochanteric fractures, Moroni et al. reported satisfactory reduction and healing in both groups [44]. In this study of 40 patients without dementia, all over 65 years of age, only patients who were independent ambulators prior to injury were studied. The results also showed decreased surgical time and lower requirement for revision surgery in the external fixation group.

12.4.2.3 Operative Treatment of Subtrochanteric Fractures

As mentioned previously, subtrochanteric femur fractures are often grouped with hip fractures due to their anatomic location and similar surgical treatment options. Subtrochanteric fractures are extracapsular and subject to significant deforming forces due to muscular attachments on the proximal and distal aspects of the femur. As such, these fractures can be difficult to reduce and the treatment of choice is surgical fixation. Commonly used surgical techniques include the intramedullary hip screw, blade plate, or sliding hip screw, as previously discussed.

12.5 Functional Rehabilitation

Despite advances in the areas of fracture fixation techniques with newer and improved implant design and technology, outcomes after hip fracture treatment are less than expected. The morbidity and mortality associated with geriatric hip fractures has been found to be dependent on a number of factors which can be divided into three categories: (1) premorbid patient factors, (2) perioperative management, and (3) postoperative care [45].

Premorbid patient factors, including age, sex, medical and psychiatric comorbidities, and pre-injury level of function, have been shown to significantly affect both mortality and morbidity after treatment of hip fractures. Increased patient age has been correlated with increased mortality as well as decreased potential for return to pre-injury functional level. The patient's gender has also been linked to outcomes after hip fracture. Men have been found to be more likely to return to pre-injury ambulation levels after hip fracture, but are also more likely to die compared to women within 1 year after sustaining a hip fracture. An increasing number of comorbid medical conditions as well as pre-existing dementia have been associated with an increased mortality, decreased likelihood of returning to pre-injury ambulation status, and an increased likelihood of institutionalization after discharge from the acute hospital stay. Both pre-injury ambulation status as well as pre-injury living environment (home versus nursing-home) have also been shown to correlate with patient outcomes after hip fractures. In the case of ambulatory status, Koval and colleagues found that patients who had poor ambulatory abilities pre-injury were more likely to regain that same level of function after treatment [45]. Specifically, patients who used a cane or walker to ambulate prior to their hip fracture were more likely to get back to that level of ambulation than those patients who did not require such assistive devices.

Due to the importance of all these patient factors on treatment outcomes, perioperative management should be aimed at addressing those issues over which the physician has some measure of control. Several studies have shown the importance of identifying medical comorbidities preoperatively and correcting any active medical conditions prior to surgical treatment. This is most important in patients with cardiopulmonary problems as well as electrolyte imbalances [46, 47]. As discussed previously, timing of surgery is also an important factor in mortality, with early surgery the goal unless contraindicated due to acute medical comorbidities.

After surgery, regardless of type of fracture or type of surgery performed, all patients should undergo a regimented and rigorous rehabilitation process. Patients should be allowed to weight-bear as tolerated on the injured extremity without concern for displacing or disrupting the surgical fixation. It was found by Koval et al. that patients after hip fracture surgery (both femoral neck and intertrochanteric hip fractures), who were allowed to weight-bear as tolerated, self-limited the amount of weight placed on their extremity. They found no radiographic evidence to support fracture displacement or loss of fixation when allowing patients to weight-bear as tolerated [48].

The rehabilitation process after surgery should be a multidisciplinary effort involving orthopedists, geriatricians, rehabilitation specialists, physiotherapists, and occupational therapists. The recommended protocol consists of early standing and progression to ambulation. The first postoperative day should involve standing and unrestricted weight-bearing on both lower extremities with the use of an assist device (walker, cane, crutches). As walking ability improves, over the course of the next several postoperative days, the assist device should be adjusted by the physical therapist. Unfortunately, several recent reviews, including two Cochrane reviews, have provided mixed results regarding definitive improvements in morbidity and mortality with aggressive rehabilitation [49–51]. Fall prevention programs, which will be discussed later, should also be initiated as part of the rehabilitation process during the early postoperative period.

An important part of the medical care of postoperative hip fracture patients is aggressive management of osteoporosis. This should begin with assessment and treatment of any vitamin D and/or calcium deficiencies. Treatment of osteoporosis should be initiated with a bisphosphonate. Zoledronic acid given within 90 days after surgical treatment has been shown to reduce the risk of further fragility fractures by 35% and reduce mortality risk in geriatric patients after a hip fracture [52].

Nutrition is another area that can be addressed both pre- and postoperatively. Patterson et al. found protein depletion in patients with hip fractures to be associated with a higher complication rate as well as a decrease in 1-year survival [53]. These authors postulated that a multidisciplinary approach, involving nutritionists, visiting nurses and home physical therapists, would help identify patients at risk for malnutrition. Using this approach, proper patient nutrition could be addressed in an attempt to further minimize morbidity and mortality.

Several authors have reported the importance of a multidisciplinary approach to care for geriatric patients with hip fractures in improving outcomes. Considering the complex medical and social nature of these patients, care that integrates orthopedic surgery, geriatric medicine, and physical and occupational therapy is best suited to attain successful outcomes. Zuckerman et al. found fewer postoperative complications, fewer intensive-care unit transfers, and improved ability to walk and fewer nursing home discharges when they compared their interdisciplinary hospital program to historical controls [54]. Fisher et al. corroborated this in a recent study in which they found a reduction in in-hospital mortality as well as in the rate of rehospitalization within 6 months when patients were managed jointly by both orthopedic surgeons and geriatricians. Importantly, they found an increase in anti-osteoporotic treatment for secondary prevention when compared with historical control groups [55].

12.6 Prevention

Since simple falls account for 95% of elderly hip fractures, falls prevention is paramount to reducing the incidence of these injuries. Effective falls prevention requires a multidimensional approach that incorporates both patient and environmental elements. These elements include patient education, community-based fall prevention programs, home modifications to minimize potential hazards, and nursing home interventions to prevent falls [3].

From the healthcare provider's perspective, patient-related factors that increase the risk of hip fracture following a fall can be addressed in order to improve prevention of these injuries. This includes treating osteoporosis, minimizing the risk of stroke and cardiovascular diseases, and medical management of diabetes and hyperlipidemia. Medications such as hormone replacement therapy, which has been shown to protect against osteoporotic hip fractures, may be considered in the proper patient. Other medications which negatively affect balance, such as benzodiazepines, should be minimized or eliminated as these have been shown to increase hip fracture incidence in older women. In addition to medication and medical issues, visual impairment has also been associated with increased fall risk [3]. As such, patients should receive regular eye care.

Lifestyle factors have also been implicated in hip fracture risk. Counseling on reducing or eliminating high alcohol and caffeine consumption, and tobacco cessation should be provided when appropriate. In such settings, these interventions represent other important opportunities where the primary care physician can have an impact on hip fracture risk reduction. Promoting regular exercise and activities to improve balance and strength has also been shown to reduce fall risks in the elderly [56].

Hip protectors have also been tried and tested for the prevention of hip fractures in the elderly. These devices consist of plastic or foam shields which are designed to be inserted into special underwear to protect the greater trochanters from direct impact when the person falls to the side. Although the theory behind the protectors may be sound, the evidence for efficacy has been absent. A recent Cochrane review of 15 trials using the hip protector showed no reduction in hip fracture incidence for elderly people living at home. There was previously some evidence to support the use of hip protectors in nursing home situations where the risk of falls is quite high, but new data have made this fact less certain as well [57].

12.7 Conclusion

Geriatric hip fractures are devastating injuries with high rates of associated morbidity and mortality. The rate of hip fractures continues to rise as the proportion of elderly individuals in the general population increases. Unfortunately, multiple prevention strategies and medical treatments have been unsuccessful in reducing the rate of occurrence of these injuries. An integrated, multidisciplinary approach incorporating timely surgical management, comprehensive medical treatment and aggressive postoperative rehabilitation, and social work services provides these patients the best possible chance at functional recovery.

References

1. Robbins J, Aragaki AK, Kooperberg C, Watts N, Wactawski-Wende J, Jackson RD, LeBoff MS, Lewis CE, Chen Z, Stefanick ML, Cauley J: Factors associated with 5-year risk of hip fracture in postmenopausal women. JAMA 2007; 298(20):2389–98.
2. Cummings SR, Rubin SM, Black D: The future of hip fractures in the United States. Numbers, costs, and potential effects of postmenopausal estrogen. Clin Orthop Relat Res 1990; (252):163–6.
3. Stevens JA, Olson S: Reducing falls and resulting hip fractures among older women. MMWR Recomm Rep 2000; 49(RR-2):3–12.
4. Haidukewych GJ, Jones CB: Hip fractures in the geriatric population, in Orthopaedic Knowledge Update: Trauma 3. Edited by Tornetta P 3rd, Baumgaertner M. Chicago, IL, American Academy of Orthopaedic Surgeons, 2005, pp 479–92.
5. Samelson EJ, Zhang Y, Kiel DP, Hannan MT, Felson DT: Effect of birth cohort on risk of hip fracture: age-specific incidence rates in the Framingham Study. Am J Public Health 2002; 92(5):858–62.
6. Scott JC: Osteoporosis and hip fractures. Rheum Dis Clin North Am 1990; 16(3):717–40.
7. Grisso JA, Kelsey JL, Strom BL, Chiu GY, Maislin G, O'Brien LA, Hoffman S, Kaplan F: Risk factors for falls as a cause of hip fracture in women. The Northeast Hip Fracture Study Group. N Engl J Med 1991; 324(19):1326–31.
8. Roberts SE, Goldacre MJ: Time trends and demography of mortality after fractured neck of femur in an English population, 1968-98: database study. BMJ 2003; 327(7418):771–5.
9. Goldacre MJ, Roberts SE, Yeates D: Mortality after admission to hospital with fractured neck of femur: database study. BMJ 2002; 325(7369):868–9.
10. Miller CW: Survival and ambulation following hip fracture. J Bone Joint Surg Am 1978; 60(7):930–4.
11. Haidukewych GJ, Israel TA, Berry DJ: Long-term survivorship of cemented bipolar hemiarthroplasty for fracture of the femoral neck. Clin Orthop Relat Res 2002; (403):118–26.
12. Rizzo PF, Gould ES, Lyden JP, Asnis SE: Diagnosis of occult fractures about the hip. Magnetic resonance imaging compared with bone-scanning. J Bone Joint Surg Am 1993; 75(3):395–401.
13. Rubin SJ, Marquardt JD, Gottlieb RH, Meyers SP, Totterman SM, O'Mara RE: Magnetic resonance imaging: a cost-effective alternative to bone scintigraphy in the evaluation of patients with suspected hip fractures. Skeletal Radiol 1998; 27(4):199–204.
14. Bachiller FG, Caballer AP, Portal LF: Avascular necrosis of the femoral head after femoral neck fracture. Clin Orthop Relat Res 2002; (399):87–109.
15. Tanaka J, Seki N, Tokimura F, Hayashi Y: Conservative treatment of Garden stage I femoral neck fracture in elderly patients. Arch Orthop Trauma Surg 2002; 122(1):24–8.
16. Zuckerman JD, Skovron ML, Koval KJ, Aharonoff G, Frankel VH: Postoperative complications and mortality associated with operative delay in older patients who have a fracture of the hip. J Bone Joint Surg Am 1995; 77(10):1551–6.
17. Moran CG, Wenn RT, Sikand M, Taylor AM: Early mortality after hip fracture: is delay before surgery important? J Bone Joint Surg Am 2005; 87(3):483–9.
18. Anderson GH, Harper WM, Connolly CD, Badham J, Goodrich N, Gregg PJ: Preoperative skin traction for fractures of the proximal femur. A randomised prospective trial. J Bone Joint Surg Br 1993; 75(5):794–6.
19. Jerre R, Doshe A, Karlsson J: Preoperative skin traction in patients with hip fractures is not useful. Clin Orthop Relat Res 2000; (378):169–73.
20. Hammer AJ: Nonunion of subcapital femoral neck fractures. J Orthop Trauma 1992; 6(1):73–7.
21. Bhandari M, Devereaux PJ, Tornetta P 3rd, Swiontkowski MF, Berry DJ, Haidukewych G, Schemitsch EH, Hanson BP, Koval K, Dirschl D, Leece P, Keel M, Petrisor B, Heetveld M, Guyatt GH: Operative management of displaced femoral neck fractures in elderly patients. An international survey. J Bone Joint Surg Am 2005; 87(9):2122–30.

22. Iorio R, Healy WL, Lemos DW, Appleby D, Lucchesi CA, Saleh KJ: Displaced femoral neck fractures in the elderly: outcomes and cost effectiveness. Clin Orthop Relat Res 2001; (383):229–42.
23. Selvan VT, Oakley MJ, Rangan A, Al-Lami MK: Optimum configuration of cannulated hip screws for the fixation of intracapsular hip fractures: a biomechanical study. Injury 2004; 35(2):136–41.
24. Asnis SE, Wanek-Sgaglione L: Intracapsular fractures of the femoral neck. Results of cannulated screw fixation. J Bone Joint Surg Am 1994; 76(12):1793–803.
25. Lu-Yao GL, Keller RB, Littenberg B, Wennberg JE: Outcomes after displaced fractures of the femoral neck. A meta-analysis of one hundred and six published reports. J Bone Joint Surg Am 1994; 76(1):15–25.
26. Ong BC, Maurer SG, Aharonoff GB, Zuckerman JD, Koval KJ: Unipolar versus bipolar hemiarthroplasty: functional outcome after femoral neck fracture at a minimum of thirty-six months of follow-up. J Orthop Trauma 2002; 16(5):317–22.
27. Parvizi J, Holiday AD, Ereth MH, Lewallen DG: The Frank Stinchfield Award. Sudden death during primary hip arthroplasty. Clin Orthop Relat Res 1999; (369):39–48.
28. Pitto RP, Blunk J, Kossler M: Transesophageal echocardiography and clinical features of fat embolism during cemented total hip arthroplasty. A randomized study in patients with a femoral neck fracture. Arch Orthop Trauma Surg 2000; 120(1–2):53–8.
29. Keating JF, Grant A, Masson M, Scott NW, Forbes JF: Randomized comparison of reduction and fixation, bipolar hemiarthroplasty, and total hip arthroplasty. Treatment of displaced intracapsular hip fractures in healthy older patients. J Bone Joint Surg Am 2006; 88(2):249–60.
30. Rogmark C, Carlsson A, Johnell O, Sernbo I: A prospective randomised trial of internal fixation versus arthroplasty for displaced fractures of the neck of the femur. Functional outcome for 450 patients at two years. J Bone Joint Surg Br 2002; 84(2):183–8.
31. Tidermark J, Ponzer S, Svensson O, Soderqvist A, Tornkvist H: Internal fixation compared with total hip replacement for displaced femoral neck fractures in the elderly. A randomised, controlled trial. J Bone Joint Surg Br 2003; 85(3):380–8.
32. Blomfeldt R, Tornkvist H, Ponzer S, Soderqvist A, Tidermark J: Comparison of internal fixation with total hip replacement for displaced femoral neck fractures. Randomized, controlled trial performed at four years. J Bone Joint Surg Am 2005; 87(8):1680–8.
33. Parker MJ, Pryor GA: Gamma versus DHS nailing for extracapsular femoral fractures. Meta-analysis of ten randomised trials. Int Orthop 1996; 20(3):163–8.
34. Baumgaertner MR, Curtin SL, Lindskog DM, Keggi JM: The value of the tip-apex distance in predicting failure of fixation of peritrochanteric fractures of the hip. J Bone Joint Surg Am 1995; 77(7):1058–64.
35. Ahrengart L, Tornkvist H, Fornander P, Thorngren KG, Pasanen L, Wahlstrom P, Honkonen S, Lindgren U: A randomized study of the compression hip screw and Gamma nail in 426 fractures. Clin Orthop Relat Res 2002; (401):209–22.
36. Medoff RJ, Maes K: A new device for the fixation of unstable pertrochanteric fractures of the hip. J Bone Joint Surg Am 1991; 73(8):1192–9.
37. Adams CI, Robinson CM, Court-Brown CM, McQueen MM: Prospective randomized controlled trial of an intramedullary nail versus dynamic screw and plate for intertrochanteric fractures of the femur. J Orthop Trauma 2001; 15(6):394–400.
38. Curtis MJ, Jinnah RH, Wilson V, Cunningham BW: Proximal femoral fractures: a biomechanical study to compare intramedullary and extramedullary fixation. Injury 1994; 25(2):99–104.
39. Sim E, Freimuller W, Reiter TJ: Finite element analysis of the stress distributions in the proximal end of the femur after stabilization of a pertrochanteric model fracture: a comparison of two implants. Injury 1995; 26(7):445–9.
40. Baumgaertner MR, Curtin SL, Lindskog DM: Intramedullary versus extramedullary fixation for the treatment of intertrochanteric hip fractures. Clin Orthop Relat Res 1998; (348):87–94.
41. Bridle SH, Patel AD, Bircher M, Calvert PT: Fixation of intertrochanteric fractures of the femur. A randomised prospective comparison of the gamma nail and the dynamic hip screw. J Bone Joint Surg Br 1991; 73(2):330–4.

42. Hardy DC, Descamps PY, Krallis P, Fabeck L, Smets P, Bertens CL, Delince PE: Use of an intramedullary hip-screw compared with a compression hip-screw with a plate for intertrochanteric femoral fractures. A prospective, randomized study of one hundred patients. J Bone Joint Surg Am 1998; 80(5):618–30.
43. Sadowski C, Lubbeke A, Saudan M, Riand N, Stern R, Hoffmeyer P: Treatment of reverse oblique and transverse intertrochanteric fractures with use of an intramedullary nail or a 95 degrees screw-plate: a prospective, randomized study. J Bone Joint Surg Am 2002; 84-A(3):372–81.
44. Moroni A, Faldini C, Pegreffi F, Hoang-Kim A, Vannini F, Giannini S: Dynamic hip screw compared with external fixation for treatment of osteoporotic pertrochanteric fractures. A prospective, randomized study. J Bone Joint Surg Am 2005; 87(4):753–9.
45. Koval KJ, Zuckerman JD: Functional recovery after fracture of the hip. J Bone Joint Surg Am 1994; 76(5):751–8.
46. Galasko CS, Rushton S, Sylvester BS, Steingold RF, Noble J, Boston DA: The significance of peak expiratory flow rate in assessing prognosis of elderly patients undergoing operations on the hip. Injury 1985; 16(6):398–401.
47. Schultz RJ, Whitfield GF, LaMura JJ, Raciti A, Krishnamurthy S: The role of physiologic monitoring in patients with fractures of the hip. J Trauma 1985; 25(4):309–16.
48. Koval KJ, Sala DA, Kummer FJ, Zuckerman JD: Postoperative weight-bearing after a fracture of the femoral neck or an intertrochanteric fracture. J Bone Joint Surg Am 1998; 80(3):352–6.
49. Halbert J, Crotty M, Whitehead C, Cameron I, Kurrle S, Graham S, Handoll H, Finnegan T, Jones T, Foley A, Shanahan M: Multi-disciplinary rehabilitation after hip fracture is associated with improved outcome: a systematic review. J Rehabil Med 2007; 39(7):507–12.
50. Cameron ID, Handoll HH, Finnegan TP, Madhok R, Langhorne P: Co-ordinated multidisciplinary approaches for inpatient rehabilitation of older patients with proximal femoral fractures. Cochrane Database Syst Rev 2001; (3):CD000106.
51. Handoll HH, Sherrington C: Mobilisation strategies after hip fracture surgery in adults. Cochrane Database Syst Rev 2007; (1):CD001704.
52. Lyles KW, Colon-Emeric CS, Magaziner JS, Adachi JD, Pieper CF, Mautalen C, Hyldstrup L, Recknor C, Nordsletten L, Moore KA, Lavecchia C, Zhang J, Mesenbrink P, Hodgson PK, Abrams K, Orloff JJ, Horowitz Z, Eriksen EF, Boonen S: Zoledronic acid and clinical fractures and mortality after hip fracture. N Engl J Med 2007; 357(18):1799–809.
53. Patterson BM, Cornell CN, Carbone B, Levine B, Chapman D: Protein depletion and metabolic stress in elderly patients who have a fracture of the hip. J Bone Joint Surg Am 1992; 74(2):251–60.
54. Zuckerman JD, Sakales SR, Fabian DR, Frankel VH: Hip fractures in geriatric patients. Results of an interdisciplinary hospital care program. Clin Orthop Relat Res 1992; (274):213–25.
55. Fisher AA, Davis MW, Rubenach SE, Sivakumaran S, Smith PN, Budge MM: Outcomes for older patients with hip fractures: the impact of orthopedic and geriatric medicine cocare. J Orthop Trauma 2006; 20(3):172–8; discussion 179–80.
56. Benetos IS, Babis GC, Zoubos AB, Benetou V, Soucacos PN: Factors affecting the risk of hip fractures. Injury 2007; 38(7):735–44.
57. Parker MJ, Gillespie WJ, Gillespie LD: Hip protectors for preventing hip fractures in older people. Cochrane Database Syst Rev 2005; (3):CD001255.

Chapter 13
Fractures of the Distal Femur

Jesse T. Torbert and John L. Esterhai

Abstract Fragility fractures of the distal femur pose a challenge for stable internal fixation and good functional outcomes. Among those challenges are frailty of the elderly patient, high degree of osteoporosis, instability of the fracture patterns, short distal femur segment, and amount of comminution. Mortality at 1 year has been reported as high as 30%. Morbidity includes significant decreases in function, quality of life as well as medical and surgical complications. Medical stabilization and optimization are extremely important in this frail population. Non-surgical management is reserved for minimally displaced fractures in the patient who will likely not tolerate the risks of anesthesia or surgical intervention. Surgical treatment, which is the favored treatment, is necessary to prevent prolonged immobilization and its sequelae. Surgical treatment options include antegrade or retrograde intramedullary nailing, standard lateral plating, the use of fixed angle devices, and total knee arthroplasty. Rehabilitation is necessary and includes early range of motion, strengthening, mobilization, gait training if possible, and prevention of common medical complications.

Keywords Fracture • Supracondylar • Distal femur • Elderly • Fragility • Osteoporotic • Internal fixation • Arthroplasty • Outcomes

13.1 Introduction

The management of elderly patients with distal femur fractures often presents a challenge. The frailty of the elderly patient, high degree of osteoporosis, instability of the fracture patterns, short distal femur segment in which to place internal fixation, and the amount of comminution even in low-energy fractures make stable internal

J.L. Esterhai (✉)
Department of Orthopaedic Surgery, Hospital of the University of Pennsylvania,
2 Silverstein, 3400 Spruce Street, Philadelphia, PA 19104, USA
e-mail: John.Esterhai@uphs.upenn.edu

R.J. Pignolo et al. (eds.), *Fractures in the Elderly*, Aging Medicine,
DOI 10.1007/978-1-60327-467-8_13,

fixation and good functional outcomes a challenge to achieve. Mortality at 1 year as high as 30% has been reported [1], along with significant decrease in function and quality of life [2]. Earliest attempts at surgical fracture fixation resulted in poor outcomes, and many of these fractures were treated non-operatively, usually with less than satisfactory results [3]. The improvement in surgical technique and instrumentation eventually resulted in better operative outcomes [4]. The risk of surgery must be weighed against the risks of prolonged immobilization and casting. Today, with less invasive surgical approaches, improved fixation techniques, and the trend toward early mobilization, the benefits of surgical intervention usually outweigh the risks. Surgical treatment is vitally important to prevent prolonged immobilization and the resulting increase in complications. Optimal medical management is necessary to allow surgery to take place and to minimize poor outcomes.

13.2 Epidemiology

Of all femoral fractures, approximately 4–7% are of the distal femur [5]. Historically, there has been a bimodal distribution, consisting of young patients with high-energy trauma and elderly patients with low-energy falls. Nevertheless, active seniors can sustain high-energy fractures as well. Approximately 85% of distal femoral fragility fractures occur in patients over 50 years old [6]. The incidence of supracondylar or distal femoral fracture adjacent to a total knee arthroplasty is approximately 1%.

13.3 Pre-operative Assessment

Pre-operative assessment of the geriatric patient with a distal femur fracture requires a thorough history, review of systems, physical exam, radiologic exam, and medical assessment.

13.3.1 History

The medical history obtained in the setting of a fragility fracture can significantly impact the pre-operative medical workup, surgical treatment, post-operative treatment, and post-hospital placement. As a result, a detailed history of the events leading to the fracture is essential. It is especially important to determine whether the fracture was due to a syncopal episode, a disturbance in sense of balance, intoxication, or simply secondary to tripping on an uneven sidewalk. The pre-injury ambulatory status of the patient (community ambulator, household ambulator, wheelchair bound, or bed bound) and details regarding walking aids may affect the treatment plan. The past medical history should include details about general health status, previous falls and fractures, osteoporosis, previous strokes, diabetes, cardiopulmonary disease, and skin ulcerations. Past surgical history is important to obtain; details regarding previous surgeries including fracture fixation, knee and hip replacement, and other surgeries affecting the involved limb such as femoral popliteal arterial bypass grafting should be obtained. Social history including types of medications used, drinking and smoking history, marital status, living arrangements, and support systems are all relevant in patients who may not be able to care for themselves post-operatively.

13.3.2 Physical Examination

In addition to the complete physical exam performed for pre-operative geriatric patients, the physical exam for an acute fracture of the distal femur should include a neurologic and vascular exam of the involved leg, assessment of the surrounding skin to rule out an open fracture and ensure future surgical incisions will not be compromised as well as a search for additional injuries. Common injuries in geriatric patients after falls include those of the spine, wrist, hip, and ankle.

13.3.3 Radiographic Imaging

AP and lateral X-rays of the femur alone often are not adequate for the assessment of distal femur fractures. Dedicated AP, lateral, and oblique X-rays of the knee better define complex fracture patterns often found in osteoporotic patients. A plain X-ray centered on the proximal femur should be included in order to rule out a hip fracture, a finding which would influence the type of internal fixation planned. When significant comminution exists, the appropriate length of the femur is difficult to determine and full length X-rays of the contralateral femur may be valuable. CT scans are not routinely necessary; however, if there is any question regarding the interpretation of the X-rays or if the fracture involves the joint surface, CT with sagittal and coronal reconstructions is useful. CT better delineates fracture patterns and articular involvement. Nork et al. [7] found that 38% of supracondylar–intercondylar distal femoral fractures had an associated coronal plane fracture, many of which were undiagnosed on radiographs and discovered on CT imaging.

Distal femoral fractures can be categorized using the AO classification. Type A fractures are extra-articular fractures which do not involve the joint surface of the knee (Fig. 13.1a). Type B fractures are unicondylar fractures and extend into the joint surface (Fig. 13.1b). Type C fractures involve both condyles and extend into the joint surface (Fig. 13.1c). The complete OA classification with illustrations can be found on the Orthopaedic Trauma Association (OTA) website [8] or in the *Journal of Orthopaedic Trauma* [9].

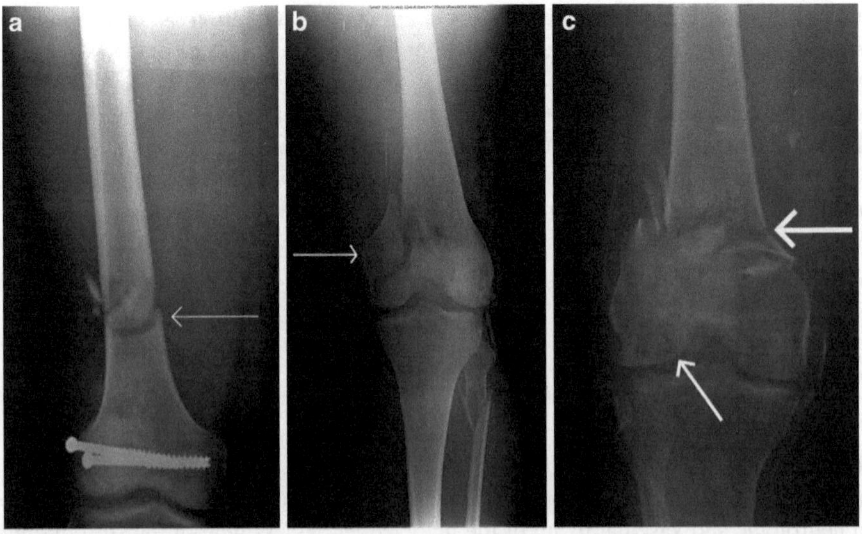

Fig. 13.1 (**a**) The OTA type A distal femur fracture is shown by the *arrow*. This fracture occurred in a patient who had fractured and underwent fixation of their lateral femoral condyle several months earlier. (**b**) This OTA type B distal femur fracture involves the medial condyle and extends into the joint surface. (**c**) The OTA type C distal femur fracture above, which involves the joint surface and leaves both condyles separate from the shaft, is demonstrated by the *two arrows* (these images are courtesy of UPenn Orthopaedic Trauma Service)

13.3.4 Medical Assessment

Surgical intervention for a distal femoral fracture requires a well-resuscitated patient without life-threatening injuries. Surgical risk stratification and medical optimization are often required in the elderly patient. Pertinent pre-operative laboratory tests and studies such as chest radiographs and electrocardiograms should be available for the medical or geriatric consultant. To further optimize or assess surgical risk, the medical consultant may suggest an additional workup, such as a cardiac stress test or echocardiogram. Therefore, medical consultation should be requested and performed as early as possible to avoid delays in surgical care.

13.4 Treatment

The earliest attempts at surgical fracture fixation resulted in poor outcomes, and many of these fractures were treated non-operatively, usually with less than satisfactory results [3]. The improvement in surgical technique and instrumentation eventually resulted in better operative outcomes [4]. Today, with less invasive surgical approaches, improved fixation techniques, the trend toward early patient mobilization, and improved outcomes associated with operative treatment, distal femur factures are rarely treated non-operatively.

13.4.1 Non-operative Treatment

Skeletal traction with a traction pin inserted in the proximal tibia or distal femur can be utilized as temporary immobilization and pain relief or as a definitive treatment for patients in whom operative intervention is contraindicated due to severe medical comorbidities. Traction may be applied for approximately 6 weeks, with range of motion started at 3–4 weeks, and a functional brace used after traction. Casting is also an option. However, non-operative treatment and the resulting immobilization can result in significant morbidity and mortality. In one randomized control trial of operative versus non-operative treatment in 42 elderly patients with distal femur fractures, the rate of deep vein thrombosis (DVT), urinary tract infection (UTI), decubitus ulcer formation, chest infection, malunion, and delayed union was roughly three times higher in the non-operative group [10]. In the operative group, two patients died: one after 3 weeks from myocardial infarction, and one after 4 weeks from pulmonary embolism (PE). In the non-operative group, one patient died after 4 weeks secondary to pneumonia. In a systematic review of distal femoral fractures [11], operative treatment resulted in a 32% reduction in the risk of poor results compared to non-operative management.

13.4.2 Operative Treatment

13.4.2.1 Indications and Goals

Given the complications of non-operative treatment, nearly all supracondylar femur fractures should be treated operatively. The goals of treatment are to obtain precise reduction of the articular surface if it is disrupted, preserve the soft-tissue envelope around the fracture, achieve stable internal fixation, initiate early range of motion and mobility, and restore length, alignment, and rotation.

13.4.2.2 Antegrade Intramedullary Nailing

Antegrade intramedullary (IM) nailing is typically reserved for extra-articular fractures due to the risk of further displacement in intra-articular fractures. The use of antegrade nails is limited by the proximity of the fracture to the joint surface because sufficient length in the distal fragment is required to place distal locking screws. Furthermore, control of the distal fracture fragment is more difficult to achieve with antegrade nails. Inadequate control of the distal fragment may result in permanent malalignment, non-union, and failure of fixation. Benefits of antegrade nailing include a small incision and minimal soft-tissue damage near the fracture site. Of note, approximately 50% of elderly patients with supracondylar femur fractures in one study had implants in the proximal femur which made antegrade nailing of the distal femur impossible [1].

13.4.2.3 Retrograde Intramedullary Nailing

Retrograde IM nailing allows distal locking screws to be placed more precisely, and therefore, closer in proximity to the joint. This allows for fixation of shorter distal fragments. Because the surgical approach through the knee joint can also allow visualization of the joint surface and precise reduction of the articular surface, retrograde nailing can be used for intra-articular fractures. Furthermore, unlike antegrade nails, the smaller distal fragment is more easily controlled with a retrograde rod. Current implants also employ multiple trajectory distal fixation screws in multiple planes, which provide better fixation of the smaller distal femoral fragment.

While retrograde nails provide certain advantages over antegrade devices, they are not without their shortcomings. Driving the retrograde IM nail up through the joint can lead to greater comminution and displacement, and retrograde nails are not commonly used for intra-articular fractures. The insertion site is thought to be outside of the articulating surface of the distal femur, but erroneous placement or prominence of the nail can lead to damage of the joint surface. The theoretical risk of delayed septic arthritis of the knee from the retrograde nail also exists.

All nails, despite their starting location, provide relative rather than absolute stability. If the distal fracture fragment is not reasonably stable, motion and weight bearing at the knee may result in loss of reduction and likely malunion or nonunion. Therefore, proper attention to implant stability and fixation in the distal fragment is a key element in using intramedullary fixation for osteoporotic distal femoral fractures.

The decision regarding the use of antegrade versus retrograde nailing is dependent upon a few factors including the presence of additional proximal or distal hardware, the location of the fracture, and the relative ease of implantation of the proposed implant. Generally, antegrade nailing can be performed in patients with more proximal fractures, a pre-existing total knee prosthesis, and a fracture pattern amenable to distal interlock screw fixation. Retrograde nailing can be performed in patients with more distal fractures, pre-existing total hip arthroplasties, and a fracture pattern amenable to proximal interlock screw purchase. When using either antegrade or retrograde femoral nails, distal interlocking bolts should be placed into metaphyseal bone. Placing these interlock screws into the shaft results in a significant stress riser, which can lead to fracture especially in the elderly osteoporotic patient.

13.4.2.4 Lateral Femoral Plating

The standard lateral femoral plate has historically been used for the treatment of comminuted intra-articular fractures of the distal femur. The advantages are relative ease of placement, the pre-contoured shape which fits the distal femur well, and ability to place multiple screws in the distal femoral fragment. Failure of these constructs typically occurred in the distal fracture fragment where hardware subsidence or screw pullout occurred resulting in varus collapse. This type of failure was more common in patients with osteoporotic bone and those with comminution or impaction of the medial metaphyseal bone. Varus collapse and subsequent non-union were typically treated with correction of the deformity, bone grafting, and revision of the fixation. As time went on, some authors began bone grafting during the primary internal fixation in the setting of medial comminution or impaction [12]. Some authors went so far as to add a medial plate to the bone graft and lateral femoral plate [13]. With the advent of locking plates and their improved stability, standard lateral femoral plates are used less frequently.

13.4.2.5 Fixed Angle Devices and Locking Plates

Fixed angle blade plates and fixed angle dynamic condylar screw plates resist varus collapse because the angle between the distal fixation and proximal portion of the plate is fixed. The key in placement of either device is the correct placement of either the blade or screw in the distal femur. Imperfect placement is difficult to adjust and malposition is a problem. Fixed angle blade plates (Fig. 13.2a) require precise fixation in all planes and are therefore more technically demanding. Dynamic condylar plates are more forgiving in the sagittal plane fracture alignment.

Locking plates, unlike traditional plates and screws, have threaded holes in the plate, which accommodate screws with threaded heads. By locking the head of the

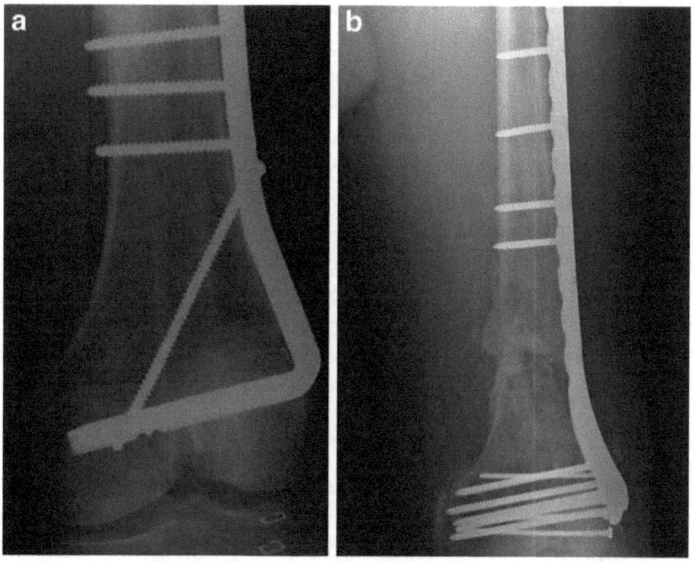

Fig. 13.2 (**a**) The blade plate was utilized for fixation of a type A distal femur fracture. (**b**) The Smith & Nephew distal femoral locking plate provides fixation for a type C distal femur fracture. Several screws were inserted outside of the plate prior to plate application to obtain a reduction of the joint surface (these images are courtesy of UPenn Orthopaedic Trauma Service)

screw into the plate, the locking plate construct acts as a fixed angle device and results in angular stability and increased load-carrying capacity while resisting screw toggle and pullout. One of the main indications for locking plates is the presence of osteoporosis. Locking plates have largely obviated the need for traditional medial and lateral distal femoralplating. The lateral distal femoral locking plate (Fig. 13.2b) has been shown to provide improved distal fixation, especially in osteoporotic bone, compared to the blade plate and retrograde intramedullary nail [14]. It has also been shown to be advantageous in preventing varus collapse of the distal femur [15].

13.4.2.6 Total Knee Arthroplasty

Total knee arthroplasty has also been utilized in elderly patients with distal femur fractures due to the detrimental effects of non-weight bearing and failure of fixation that are associated with internal fixation in the osteoporotic patient. In order to remove the fracture a larger portion of the distal femur is removed. Aside from the removal of bone, the anterior cruciate, posterior cruciate, medial collateral, and lateral collateral ligaments are also removed with the distal femoral fragment. This loss of length and stability must be built into the knee replacement. Typically to provide stability, a constrained total knee arthroplasty is used. By design, a constrained total knee arthroplasty offers additional knee stability over conventional knee arthroplasty because the design allows them to resist varus and valgus forces, which are normally resisted by the lateral and medial collateral ligaments. In one study of patients over 75 years of age [16] the advantages of knee replacement were more rapid rehabilitation, better knee flexion, and better chance of returning to independent walking at medium-term follow-up. Rosen et al. [17] found that 71% of patients treated with total knee arthroplasty resumed their pre-operative level of ambulation at a mean follow-up of 11 months. Disadvantages were increased need for blood transfusion and increased reports of knee pain. Furthermore, results of constrained total knee prosthesis for distal femoral replacement are not as good as primary total knee arthroplasty for degenerative joint disease. Another significant disadvantage of using the knee arthroplasty is that the distal femur fragments and associated ligaments are excised and replaced with metal. A segmental replacement prosthesis utilizes metal segments to replace large segments of bone that are excised. If this type of implant needs revision in the future, even further distal femur bone loss results; this severely limits revision options.

13.4.2.7 Treatment of Distal Femur Periprosthetic Fractures

Distal femur periprosthetic fractures are typically found in those older than 70 years of age. Retrograde nailing is an attractive option if the knee arthroplasty design allows for placement of a retrograde nail through it; plates may yield satisfactory results in those knee prostheses that cannot accommodate retrograde intramedullary fixation [18]. Locking plates (Fig. 13.3) are preferred over conventional plates

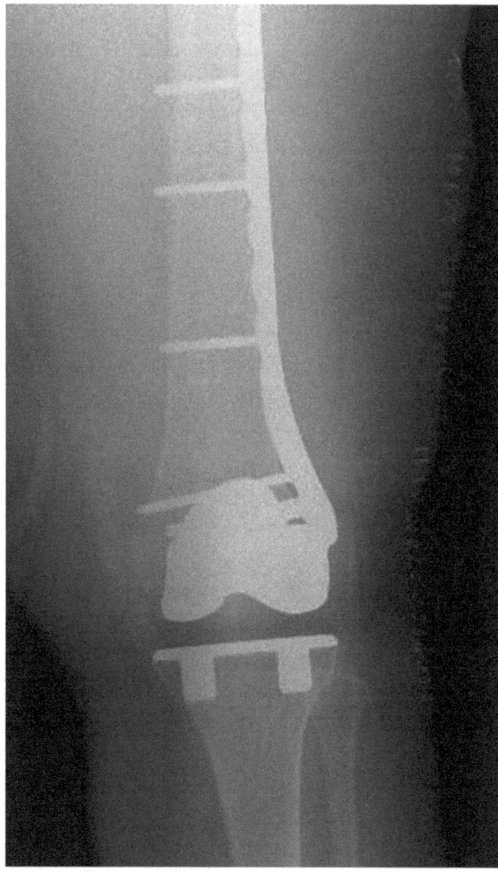

Fig. 13.3 A periprosthetic distal femur fracture after fixation with a lateral locking plate (this image was provided through the courtesy of Dr. Craig Israelite and is property of UPenn Orthopaedic Trauma Service)

because multiple fixed angle screws give optimal fixation near the femoral component. Advantages of the locking plate appear to include maintenance of distal femoral fixation, low infection, and decreased need for bone grafting [19].

13.4.2.8 Summary of Operative Intervention

The fracture pattern largely dictates the type of implant used. Intra-articular fractures require visualization, reduction, and fixation of the joint surface. If the fracture extends into the joint surface, the use of an intramedullary nail may displace the articular fragments or make them hard to reduce and fixed-angle devices such as distal femoral locking plates may be a better option for fixation. Intra-articular fractures that are isolated unicondylar fractures are uncommon, and may be repaired with lag screw fixation alone.

If there is no intra-articular extension, the use of an intramedullary nail would be indicated. If the length of the distal segment is long enough to comfortably allow the placement of distal interlock screws and the distal fragment can be properly aligned during antegrade reaming, then antegrade nailing is a viable option. Otherwise, retrograde nailing would be used to obtain precise positioning of the distal interlocks and aid in the alignment of the distal fragment. A total knee arthroplasty may be indicated for an elderly person with existing knee arthritis and a comminuted intra-articular distal femur fracture.

13.5 Complications

The mortality rate at 1 year in distal femur fractures has been reported as high as 30% [1]. The complication rate including non-union, malunion, infection, cardiopulmonary complications, and decubitus ulcerations has been reported as high as 40% [3, 20]. In one study of 112 frail elderly patients with supracondylar femoral fractures, the medical complication rate was 22.4% and included respiratory infection, UTI, and stroke [2].

Acute infection following surgical fixation of the distal femur has been reported as high as 10% [21] with one large systematic review showing an average rate of 2.7% [11]. The treatment is straightforward in the acute setting and consists of evacuation of the purulent material and necrotic tissue. If the fracture has not yet healed and the fixation is stable the hardware is retained, antibiotics are initiated, and a stable soft-tissue envelope is developed with either soft-tissue flap coverage or delayed closure. If needed, debridement and/or hardware removal is later performed after fracture union. In the presence of unstable fixation or severe infection, temporary external fixation may be placed until the infection is controlled with debridement and antibiotics. When the soft-tissue envelope allows, revision of internal fixation is performed [22].

Malunion (defined as greater than five degrees of varus or valgus, greater than 10 degrees of sagittal plane angulation, greater than 15° of rotational deformity, or greater than 2 cm of shortening) is most common in the varus direction; however, the incidence in either the young trauma or elderly fragility fracture population is not well documented. One study of 123 distal femur fractures reported a malunion rate of 6% [15]; however, only 30 patients were over the age of 65.

Non-union was found to occur in approximately 6% of patients in a recent systematic review of distal femur fractures [11]. However, with more advanced types of minimally invasive locking plates, which reduce damage to soft-tissue and blood supply, union rates approaching 100% have been reported [22]. In patients with non-union and stable fixation, bone grafting of the non-union site is the preferred treatment. In non-unions with associated loss of fixation and reduction, bone grafting and revision of fixation are necessary. Augmentation of fixation with polymethylmethacrylate (bone cement) may help to provide stable fixation in very osteoporotic patients. Distal femoral replacement with a total knee arthroplasty is also an option, especially in patients with small distal segments, pre-existing arthritis, and joint destruction.

Joint stiffness after surgical treatment of distal femoral fractures has many causes. Intra-articular prominence of hardware, heterotopic ossification, malunion, and abundant scar tissue can limit knee range of motion [22]. Early joint motion should be instituted when fixation stability and soft-tissue conditions allow.

13.6 Functional Outcomes

There is no consensus on the long-term advantages of any type of operative treatment. However, it is clear that operative treatment has considerable advantages over non-operative treatment. Although good or excellent results have been reported in approximately half of all operative patients and one-third of non-operative patients [10, 23], no functional outcome studies focus on the elderly, osteoporotic population. With newer techniques which minimize soft-tissue damage, good or excellent results as high as 84% have been reported [24].

13.7 Rehabilitation

The goal of surgical intervention in distal femur fractures is early mobilization in order to avoid complications of prolonged immobilization. Prevention and treatment of these complications through medical management is vitally important. This includes DVT prophylaxis, incentive spirometry, decubitus ulcer prevention, and treatment of UTI. Adequate nutrition is also important in preventing complications and promoting wound healing.

The rehabilitation process is dependent on the surgeon's assessment of fixation. Early range of motion is key to preventing significant loss in knee range of motion. Therefore, knee range of motion is immediately begun if the soft-tissue condition and fixation allow. Initially, this can involve the use of a continuous passive motion (CPM) machine in addition to physical therapy. Quadriceps strengthening exercises are added. For extra-articular fractures treated with internal fixation, the patient is usually partially weight bearing for 4–6 weeks, after which progressive weight bearing is allowed. For intra-articular fractures, non-weight bearing or longer periods of partial weight bearing may be instituted depending on the preference of the surgeon. Rehabilitation following surgical treatment with knee arthroplasty can progress to full-weight bearing soon after surgery, similar to knee arthroplasty patients treated for osteoarthritis, assuming the soft-tissue condition and other injuries allow. Gait training is also valuable to this elderly population that may have underlying weakness and problems with balance.

References

1. Dunlop DG, Brenkel IJ. The supracondylar intramedullary nail in elderly patients with distal femoral fractures. Injury 1999;30:475–484.
2. Karpman RR, Del Mar NB. Supracondylar femoral fractures in the frail elderly. Fractures in need of treatment. Clin Orthop Relat Res 1995;(316):21–24.

3. Neer CS, Grantham SA, Shelton ML. Supracondylar fracture of the adult femur. A study of one hundred and ten cases. J Bone Joint Surg Am 1967;49:591–613.
4. Shaltzker J, Home G, Waddell J. The Toronto experience with the supracondylar fracture of the femur. Injury 1975;6(2):113–128.
5. Kolmert L, Wulff K. Epidemiology and treatment of distal femoral fractures in adults. Acta Orthop Scand 1982;53:957–962.
6. Shewring DJ, Meggitt BF. Fractures of the distal femur treated with the AO dynamic condylar screw. J Bone Joint Surg Br 1992;74:122–125.
7. Nork SE, Segina DN, Aflatoon K. The association between supracondylar-intercondylar distal femoral fractures and coronal plane fractures. J Bone Joint Surg Am 2005;87:564–569.
8. Orthopaedic Trauma Association (OTA) Fracture and Dislocation Classification Compendium. http://www.ota.org/compendium/compendium.html Accessed 15 June 2010.
9. OTA Committee for Coding and Classification. Fracture and dislocation compendium. J Orthop Trauma[AU3] 1996;10(Suppl 1):1–154.
10. Butt MS, Krikler SJ, Ali MS. Displaced fractures of the distal femur in elderly patients. Operative versus non-operative treatment. J Bone Joint Surg Br 1996;78:110–114.
11. Zlowodzki M, Bhandari M, Marek DJ. Operative treatment of acute distal femur fractures: systematic review of 2 comparative studies and 45 case series (1989 to 2005). J Orthop Trauma 2006;20:366–371.
12. Kolb K, Grutzner P, Koller H. The condylar plate for treatment of distal femoral fractures: a long-term follow-up study. Injury 2009;40(4):440–448.
13. Sanders R, Swiontkowski M, Rosen H. Double-plating of comminuted, unstable fractures of the distal part of the femur[AU4]. J Bone Joint Surg Am 1991;73(3):341–346.
14. Zlowodzki M, Williamson S, Cole PA. Biomechanical evaluation of the less invasive stabilization system, angled blade plate, and retrograde intramedullary nail for the internal fixation of distal femur fractures. J Orthop Trauma 2004;18:494–502.
15. Kregor PJ, Stannard JA, Zlowodzki M. Treatment of distal femur fractures using the less invasive stabilization system: surgical experience and early clinical results in 103 fractures. J Orthop Trauma 2004;18:509–520.
16. Pearse EO, Klass B, Bendall SP. Stanmore total knee replacement versus internal fixation for supracondylar fractures of the distal femur in elderly patients. Injury 2005; 36:163–168.
17. Rosen AL, Strauss E. Primary total knee arthroplasty for complex distal femur fractures in elderly patients. Clin Orthop Relat Res 2004;(425):101–105.
18. Bezwada HP, Neubauer P, Baker J. Periprosthetic supracondylar femur fractures following total knee arthroplasty. J Arthroplasty 2004;19:453–458.
19. Kregor PJ, Hughes JL, Cole PA. Fixation of distal femoral fractures above total knee arthroplasty utilizing the Less Invasive Stabilization System (L.I.S.S.). Injury 2001;32(Suppl 3):64–75.
20. Schatzker J, Lambert DC. Supracondylar fractures of the femur. Clin Orthop Relat Res 1979;(138):77–83.
21. Zlowodzki M, Obremskey WT, Thomison JB. Functional outcome after treatment of lower-extremity nonunions. J Trauma 2005;58:312–317.
22. Kregor PJ, Morgan SJ. Fractures of the distal femur. In: Baumgaertner MR, Tornetta P, editors. Orthopaedic knowledge update, 3rd edn. Rosemont, IL: AAOS, 2005, 397–408.
23. Schatzker J, Home G, Waddell J. The Toronto experience with the supracondylar fracture of the femur, 1966-72. Injury 1974;6:113–128.
24. Bolhofner BR, Carmen B, Clifford P. The results of open reduction and Internal fixation of distal femur fractures using a biologic (indirect) reduction technique. J Orthop Trauma 1996;10:372–377.

Chapter 14
Tibial Plateau Fractures in the Elderly

John Alan Scolaro and Gwo-Chin Lee

Abstract Fractures of the tibial plateau in elderly individuals can occur following a low energy mechanism. Frequently, the fractures are depression-type injuries which cause articular incongruity and may have associated soft tissue or ligamentous injury. Definitive treatment of these fractures is often delayed because of the soft tissue envelope and requires a period of external fixation to maintain limb alignment and provide stability. The goals of operative fracture fixation are restoration of the articular surface and stable fixation. This can be accomplished through a variety of operative techniques with recent emphasis on preservation of the soft tissue envelope surrounding the proximal tibia and less invasive surgical exposures. In some circumstances, when the patient has significant degenerative joint disease, acute fracture fixation and total knee arthroplasty has been described for this condition. The management of these fractures can also be complicated by osteopenia and medical comorbidities which are more prevalent in the elderly population.

Keywords Proximal tibia • Tibial plateau • Total knee arthroplasty • Fragility fracture • Elderly

14.1 Introduction

Tibial plateau fractures are complex injuries especially when they occur in the elderly patient. These fractures may be considered compression fractures of the proximal tibia involving the articular surface that supports the opposing femoral condyle [1]. While most of these injuries result from high energy falls and/or motor vehicle collisions, in the elderly, the amount of energy required to cause such a fracture is significantly lower due to age-related changes in both cortical

G.-C. Lee (✉)
Department of Orthopaedic Surgery, University of Pennsylvania, 3400 Spruce Street, 2 Silverstein Pavilion, Philadelphia, PA 19104, USA
e-mail: Gwo-Chin.Lee@uphs.upenn.edu

R.J. Pignolo et al. (eds.), *Fractures in the Elderly*, Aging Medicine,
DOI 10.1007/978-1-60327-467-8_14,

and cancellous bone. In addition to changes in bone architecture, treatment of these injuries has to take into account factors such as patient comorbidities, fracture comminution, and the presence of pre-existing joint arthrosis [2]. The purpose of this chapter is to develop a systematic approach towards the management of tibial plateau fractures in the elderly patient.

14.2 Anatomy

The proximal tibia is formed by both a medial and lateral condyle. The articular surface of the medial condyle is larger than that of the lateral condyle and its surface sits lower than that of the lateral condyle. In addition, the shape of the articular surface is also different between the two sides, as the medial surface is concave in shape while the lateral is convex. The tibia carries a 10–15° anterior to posterior slope to its surface. These geometric differences are important to remember when looking at radiographic studies of the proximal tibia and assessing articular congruence.

On the femoral side, both the medial and lateral femoral condyles are larger anteriorly than they are posteriorly, creating a large wedge-like surface that impacts the proximal tibia when there is directed injury force. This often results in anterior or lateral split fragments or central depressions in the tibial surface. With the knee flexed, the femur rolls back on the articular surface of the tibia and the smaller posterior femoral condyles have less contact with the tibia. The knee is less likely to be in full flexion at the time of injury but attention should always be given to the presence of a posterior fracture component.

Between the tibial plateaus is the non-articular intracondylar eminence which serves as the attachment point for the anterior cruciate ligament (ACL). Avulsion fractures of the intracondylar eminence represent an injury to the ACL but these injuries are usually not included in the discussion of tibial plateau fractures in the elderly patient unless they occur in conjunction with another intra-articular fracture of the medial or lateral plateau. In the elderly population, such an avulsion fracture may be a sign of a greater degree of instability. Since most elderly patients can function without a competent ACL [3], a ruptured ACL is usually not of primary concern.

The normal anatomic axis of the knee joint is approximately 7° of valgus angulation in the coronal plane. It is for this reason that tibial plateau fractures more frequently involve the lateral plateau than the medial plateau. In additional, direct trauma more commonly occurs on the lateral aspect of the knee. When medial plateau fractures are seen, they likely represent a higher energy injury and attention must be paid to the soft tissues as well as other injuries which may be present. In elderly patients, the normal anatomic axis of the knee may be distorted because of medial or lateral arthritis leading to a varus or valgus deformity of the extremity [4]. Restoration of pre-injury anatomy is the goal when treating these fractures as correction of deformity is outside of the scope of the acute fracture surgery [5].

14.3 Diagnosis

Fractures of the tibial plateau typically occur as a result of a valgus force imparted onto the lateral aspect of the knee. However, elderly patients can sustain significant injuries as a result of falls from standing height. In these cases, the circumstances surrounding the fall should be thoroughly evaluated. Syncopal episodes may signal underlying cardiac or cerebrovascular disease. A comprehensive physical examination must be performed. The pelvis, hips, spine, and upper extremities should be inspected for evidence of instability and deformity.

The knee should be evaluated for abrasions, lacerations, or gross deformity. An intra-articular effusion, often a lipo-hemarthrosis, may be both visible and palpable on the affected extremity with a tibial plateau fracture. The range of motion is often diminished and there maybe associated valgus or varus instability depending on the tibial plateau involved. A depressed lateral plateau fracture may be associated with valgus instability of the knee. Lower energy injuries may also be associated with meniscal injuries, specifically the lateral meniscus, in as many as 90% of cases [6]. Higher energy injury mechanisms and split fracture patterns tend to have a higher incidence of associated ligamentous injuries, often as high as 30% [4]. Fractures of the anterior portion of the medial tibial plateau have been strongly associated with injury to the posterolateral structures and possibly even the posterior cruciate ligament [7]. In the elderly, the collateral soft tissue injuries must be recognized and factored into how the patient is managed after fracture fixation.

A complete motor and sensory exam should be carried at the time of presentation to confirm that both the tibial and peroneal nerves are intact. Peroneal nerve injuries have been reported to occur in approximately 3% of patients with tibial plateau fractures [8]. A careful vascular exam should also be performed for each patient. If pulses are unequal between extremities, and/or the ankle-brachial index is <0.9, further imaging and vascular consultation should be obtained. Evaluation of the lower extremity compartments should be carried out on each patient to look for the presence of compartment syndrome. Measurement of the compartment pressures should take place if the patient is unconscious, sedated or unable to give a reliable clinical exam.

Radiographic evaluation of the knee should include AP, lateral and oblique radiographs of the knee. Traction radiographs may be useful in highly comminuted fractures to show individual fragments and aid in defining fracture patterns. A CT scan is essential for cases when there is fracture displacement, depression of articular fragments, or comminution (Fig. 14.1). Computed tomography allows for sagittal, coronal and 3-D reconstructions which are extremely useful for pre-operative planning [9]. It is important to recognize that in the elderly, insufficiency fractures of the proximal tibia may occur and not be visible on plain radiograph. Prasad et al. described a cohort of eight elderly females (mean age 74, range 70–80 years) who presented with fractures of the tibial plateau. In five patients, diagnosis was made by CT or MRI as the fracture could not be identified on plain radiographs alone [10]. Therefore, in an elderly patient who has knee pain or difficulty ambulating

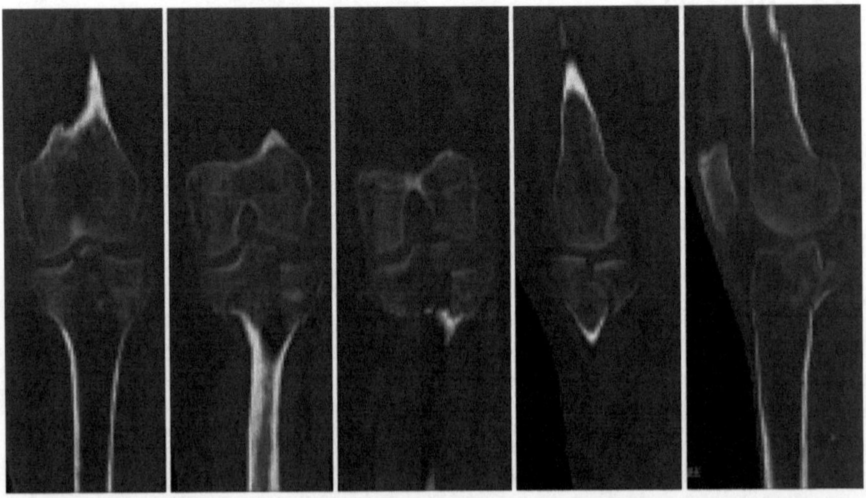

Fig. 14.1 Pre-operative coronal and sagittal CT cuts from an 82-year-old female with advanced knee degenerative arthritis who sustained a bicondylar tibial plateau fracture after a fall from height

after a fall or traumatic event, there should be consideration for advanced imaging of the knee if symptoms persist despite normal plain radiographs. MRI is a useful study if there is concern for collateral ligament injury and significant periarticular soft tissue disruption.

Tibial plateau fractures are not routinely considered alongside distal radius fractures and vertebral compression fractures as fragility fractures, but they may be the first presentation of severe osteopenia or osteoporosis in an elderly patient. Lab studies have shown that the proximal tibia in an estrogen deficient rat model required a significantly lower fracture load and had a significantly lower structural stiffness as compared to control animals [11]. This may be analogous to a postmenopausal woman who has severe osteopenia secondary to estrogen deficiency. Therefore, a fracture of the tibial plateau in an elderly patient should also raise concern to the treating physician that the patient may have poor bone mineral density and medicinal or dietary treatment may be warranted to help prevent subsequent fragility fractures.

14.4 Classification

Under the AO/OTA classification system the proximal tibia is designated as 41. Type A fractures are extra-articular and include avulsions to the tibial spine and both simple and comminuted proximal tibia fractures which do not involve the medial or lateral condyle. Type B fractures are have partial articular involvement and are subdivided into three categories: B1 are pure split fractures, B2 are pure depression fractures and B3 are mixed split–depression type fractures. Type C

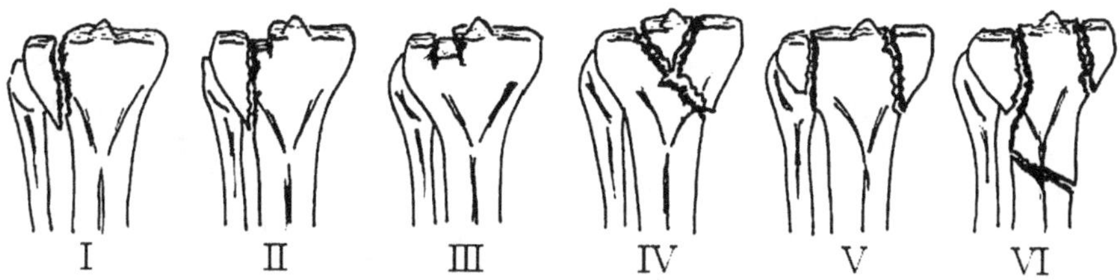

Fig. 14.2 Schatzker classification system (adapted from [13])

fractures are complete articular fractures and divided into type 1 or 2 based on whether the metaphyseal fracture is simple or comminuted; type 3 fractures have articular comminution with metaphyseal extension [12].

The Schatzker classification system is widely used in describing tibial plateau fractures. Type I fractures are pure lateral plateau cleavage fractures that often displace distally and laterally. As mentioned, these fractures tend to occur in younger patients with stronger subchondral bone and have a high incidence of associated ligamentous injury. This facture pattern is also associated with incarceration of the lateral meniscus in the fracture site. Type II fractures are split–depression type injuries where the tibial condyle is first split and then the medial articular edge is depressed inferiorly into the metaphysis. Type III fractures involve a pure central depression with an intact osseous rim. These are usually lower energy injuries and occur more often in elderly individuals who have weaker subchondral and cancellous bone. Type IV injuries are medial tibial plateau injuries which are further described as A or B depending on whether the fracture is a split or depression type injury. These are also considered high energy injuries and both the status of the soft tissues and neurovascular structures around the knee must be examined thoroughly. Type V fractures are bicondylar with involvement of both plateaus. The fracture pattern is usually a split with some degree of articular depression as well. Finally, Type VI fractures are defined by dissociation between the metaphysis and diaphysis in the proximal tibia. There is a high degree of comminution and attention again must be paid to the neurovascular structures coursing through the zone of injury [13]. Recently, Type VI fractures have been divided into those which are angled medially and those which are angled laterally (Fig. 14.2).

14.5 Treatment

The treatment indications for tibial plateau fractures are still controversial and treatments vary based in part on surgeons' preferences. The only definite surgical indications are open fractures, those with vascular injury or those with a developing or diagnosed compartment syndrome [14]. Recommendations regarding the amount of acceptable articular depression at the tibial plateau vary from 2 mm to 1 cm. While this discussion relates primarily to non- or minimally displaced fractures, some authors have described successful non-operative treatment of displaced fractures where others may have advocated surgical restoration of articular congruency and internal fixation. It is generally agreed that fractures, which result in greater than 10° of instability in the extended knee (as compared to the contralateral side), require operative intervention [15]. If there is a fracture of the tibial diaphysis as well as the plateau, non-operative management is difficult since traction on the extremity usually causes greater displacement at the shaft rather than alignment of the proximal plateau fracture fragments. Finally, the type of fracture pattern can also help guide treatment. Pure depression-type injuries are more stable than split-type injuries because the cortical rim of the tibia is not violated which provides stability to varus and valgus stress.

Non-operative management of tibial plateau fractures is best reserved for non-displaced and/or stable fractures. Treatment includes protected weight bearing in a hinged cast brace and early range of motion. Progression to full weight bearing on the injured extremity usually takes place around 8–12 weeks with appropriate clinical and radiographic follow-up. Unrestricted activities are not usually allowed until 4–6 months [4]. Range of motion and strengthening exercises should focus on isometric quadriceps sets and progression from passive to active-assist to active range of motion. Displacement of the fracture at any point during this time period is an indication for operative intervention. In the patient where strict partial weight bearing and adherence to a rehabilitation program may not be a viable option, a long leg cast with the knee bent at 45° of flexion is another non-operative treatment option. Historically, 6 weeks of skeletal traction, with periods of range of motion, were utilized in non-operative treatment of these fractures but this is rarely, if ever, still employed for multiple medical, financial and logistical reasons.

14.5.1 Surgical Fixation

14.5.1.1 Pre-operative Planning

The goal of operative treatment in tibial plateau fractures is reconstruction of the articular surface, stabilization of fracture fragments and restoration of tibial alignment. This undertaking begins with appropriate pre-operative planning and templating from the appropriate radiographs and imaging studies. As mentioned, CT scans, along with various image reconstructions, are tremendously helpful in understanding these often complex fracture patterns. Next, an operative plan, with all potential pitfalls and complications in mind, should be created.

The timing of surgery with tibial plateau fractures often rests on the condition of the soft tissue envelope. Increased rates of infection and wound complications occur when swelling, blistering or trauma-related soft-tissue injury are not handled appropriately [16]. Within hours after the initial injury, fracture hematoma and swelling begin to appear in the area of injury. Depending on the energy of the initial injury and resultant swelling, definitive surgical intervention may be delayed up to 8–10 days. In highly comminuted or unstable fractures where soft tissue swelling and/or delayed fixation is anticipated, knee spanning external fixation is frequently used. This strategy allows for relative maintenance of limb length, alignment and rotation while providing a stable construct until soft tissue swelling resolves.

14.5.1.2 Surgical Anatomy and Approaches

Exposure of the proximal tibia for surgical fixation can be accomplished through a variety of means. Regardless of the approach, adequate visualization with a minimal amount of soft tissue stripping is the goal. Full thickness flaps should be created which include subcutaneous fat and go down to the fascia/retinaculum. Incisions should be made in a longitudinal fashion and as close to the midline as possible. The lateral lazy "S" or "L" shaped incision is often used since the majority of plateau fractures involve the lateral side.

When there is involvement of the medial side, a medial parapatellar incision is made or the posteromedial approach is used. The posteromedial approach is carried out between the medial gastrocnemius and semimembranosus tendons and then between the medial collateral ligament and posterior oblique ligament (Fig. 14.3). When an arthrotomy for visualization of the articular surface is used, it can be

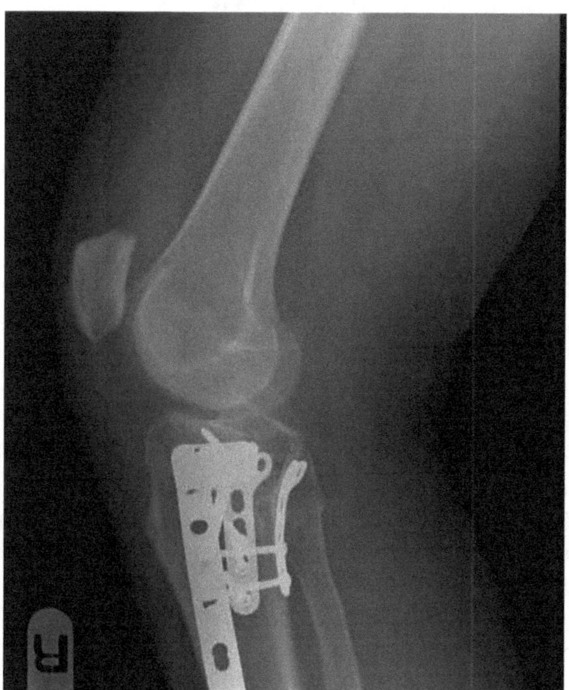

Fig. 14.3 Lateral radiograph of bicondylar tibial plateau fracture with medial buttress plate supporting posteriomedial fracture fragment

performed either submeniscal or in a vertical orientation. Division of the anterior horn of the lateral meniscus has been shown to heal reliably when a second-look arthroscopy has been performed following fracture fixation and healing. This technique ensures that fracture reduction and elevation of subchondral bone restore articular congruence.

Severe bicondylar fractures may require a midline incision that allows access to both the medial and lateral knee compartments. This incision can therefore be used at a later time if joint reconstruction is to be performed and avoid the potential complications of leaving an insufficiently sized skin bridge. When the fracture is reached, if the tibial tubercle is a separate fragment, it may be reflected along with the patellar tendon for adequate exposure. The patellar tendon can also be incised (Z-plasty) yielding the same exposure. If this is performed, the tendon must be repaired and then reinforced with a tension band construct for adequate healing. Depending on the fixation technique chosen, both a medial and lateral incision may be used to avoid a midline incision and excessive periosteal stripping. An adequate skin bridge must be left between incisions to avoid skin necrosis and wound healing problems but this technique has gained popularity with continued emphasis on protecting the soft tissue envelope surrounding the proximal tibia [17].

14.5.1.3 Alternative Methods of Surgical Fixation

Recently, some authors have advocated alternative means of open surgical fixation which utilize smaller incisions and indirect methods of reduction with the goal of protecting the soft tissues. This approach also minimizes soft tissue stripping and damage to any periosteal blood supply. This approach is more beneficial in pure split-type fractures where there is not a depressed articular portion which requires elevation. Using this surgical strategy, incarcerated soft tissues or cartilage are unable to be appreciated unless a direct window of visualization or arthroscopy is used to assess the fracture. In addition, if the soft tissues are not amenable to a full open exposure and the fracture is unable to be adequately reduced and fixed using a "mini open" approach, the patient is placed at higher risk for complication because of the additional procedure.

Minimally invasive percutaneous plate osteosynthesis (MIPPO) or the less invasive stabilization system (LISS) is a technique which utilizes a single incision for fixation of simple split and split–depression fractures confined to the lateral tibial plateau [18]. A single incision, created anterolaterally, is utilized to obtain initial reduction of the fracture fragment. Then, locking plates can be introduced submuscularly and extraperiosteally to bridge the fracture and obtain fixation. Distal screws are placed through percutaneous incisions to minimize soft tissue dissection and protect any vascular contributions to the fracture fragments (Fig. 14.4). If there is a medial wound which requires fixation then a medial antiglide or buttress plate may be added to ensure adequate stability.

Surgical arthroscopy has been utilized to assess the joint line during fracture reduction. Some surgeons are proponents of arthroscopy when treating even

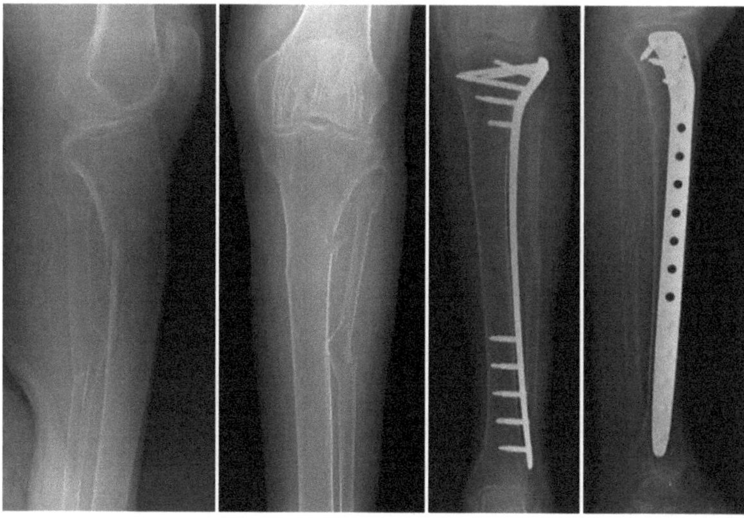

Fig. 14.4 Pre- and post-operative radiographs of a 75F with a history of osteoporosis who sustained a fall from standing height and presented with this proximal third tibia fracture. She was treated with a Less Invasive Stabilization System (LISS) plate. She was allowed immediate full weight bearing on the extremity after surgery

minimally displaced split fractures since there is a risk of meniscal entrapment in the fracture line [19]. The position of the arthroscopic portals and the presence of the menisci make evaluation of the cortical rim difficult, which is a potential limitation in using this technique. In addition, there have been reports of compartment syndrome following arthroscopy of tibial plateau fractures. The movement of fluid from the artificially pressurized intracapsular space during arthroscopy, through the fracture, to the soft tissues is thought to cause this phenomenon. Current recommendations advocate low pressure/flow arthroscopy, if at all, to visualize the joint line [20]. Direct visualization of the chondral surface through an open incision is still the most reliable method of ensuring adequate restoration of the joint surface.

The use of external fixation in the treatment of tibial plateau fractures follows the same principles in the elderly as it does in younger individuals. Following injury, if soft tissue swelling prohibits immediate fixation or if joint alignment needs to be restored, joint spanning external fixators should be utilized. Krappinger et al. reported use of an external fixator, in addition to definitive internal fixation, for approximately 9 weeks in two elderly patients with severe AO 43-C3 type fractures. Their rationale for using both stabilization techniques was based upon the poor bone quality and metaphyseal comminution present in both patients [21]. This technique goes against the principle of early range of motion after fracture fixation and the authors noted that such an approach would not be appropriate in a younger patient.

The management of plateau fractures in the elderly patient who may already have pre-existing degenerative joint disease is slightly different than in the younger patient. Although emphasis is placed on restoration of the articular surface, creating a well-aligned and well supported tibia is also of importance. By ensuring that the limb is well aligned and healed, treatment with joint arthroplasty at a later point, if needed, is less complicated. In some instances, total joint arthroplasty has been used in the acute/sub-acute setting for tibial plateau fractures in the elderly individual [22]. Although this is not common, an elderly individual who has a minimally displaced fracture that does not compromise bone stock and who would be at risk of peri-operative complications from being made non-weight bearing on the affected extremity post-operatively, would be a candidate.

14.6 Outcomes

In the elderly population, surgical fixation of tibial plateau fractures is more challenging because of the poor bone quality present in these patients and the complexity of the fracture patterns. There is only limited data, especially long term, on treatment algorithms or outcomes in elderly patients with tibial plateau fractures. This is partially due to the fact that these injuries were often treated non-operatively in the elderly. In addition the demographic of patients older than 65 years has never been larger or more active than it is today which has led to a greater incidence and frequency of these fracture types. Finally, total joint arthoplasty is one of the most successful orthopaedic procedures available, which has led to an increase in the utilization of this treatment option following plateau fractures in the elderly. It is clear that more information is needed on the treatment and long term outcomes of patients greater than 65 years old who sustain a fracture of the proximal tibia.

Treatment of fractures in the elderly can often be challenging and some believe that these patients are best treated non-operatively or with limited interventions. For example, Ali et al. reported on 11 patients, mean age of 72, with displaced bicondylar tibial plateau fractures (OTA-41C) treated with limited articular reductions and external ring fixators. All patients went on to bony union with three cases experiencing further displacement after initial treatment, and 9 of 11 reporting satisfactory results according to Rasmussen's radiographic and functional scoring system. Despite the limited number of patients the authors concluded that ring fixator placement for complex tibial plateau fractures was a safe and effective way to treat these fractures in the elderly [23].

Improvements in periarticular fracture care and locking technology have led others to treat the elderly in a manner similar to a younger patient with the same injury. Frattini et al. retrospectively looked at 49 patients between the ages of 66 and 88 who had sustained tibial plateau fractures and found that 75% experienced satisfactory results both functionally and radiographically at 2–11 years of follow-up [2]. Biyani et al. retrospectively looked at 32 patients with tibial plateau fractures (Schatzker Type 2 being the most common) with a mean age of 71.7 years and found similar results both clinically and radiographically using the Rasmussen criteria at an average follow up of 3.7 years [24]. Su and colleagues, in their series of plateau fractures in patients older than 55 who had been treated with open reduction and internal fixation, determined that Shatzker classification and pre-existing degenerative joint disease were not predictive of results. They correlated use of external fixation and increasing age as predictors of poor clinical outcome [25]. It is still unclear exactly which patient or injury factors predict the success of operative fixation but these studies show that elderly patients benefit from operative intervention. The rate of progression to post-traumatic arthritis in these patients and the complications from hardware implantation has yet to be defined.

Total knee arthroplasty has a role in the management of patients with these fractures, both in the acute and in the delayed setting (Fig. 14.5). In the acute time period following a tibial plateau fracture, a limited role for total knee arthroplasty exists when there is significant pre-injury arthritis, periarticular comminution and osteoporosis present. In a select subset of these patients, when condylar support can be maintained, fracture fixation can be accomplished and joint stability ensured, total knee arthroplasty allows for full weight bearing and early mobilization in this

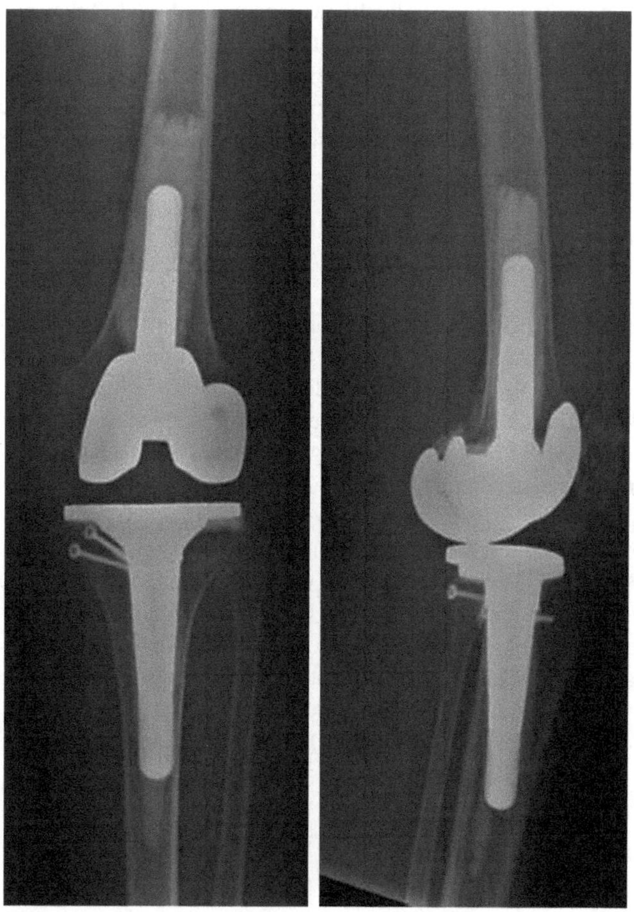

Fig. 14.5 Post-operative AP and lateral radiographs following open reduction and internal fixation of a tibial plateau fracture followed by total knee arthroplasty

patient population. Hsu et al. described their approach for non-hinged total joint arthroplasty in patients with periarticular fractures around the knee. They emphasize the fact that this treatment option applies to a very select group of patients but that when indicated, it can be performed successfully [26].

The most common scenario involving total knee arthroplasty and tibial plateau fractures is when joint reconstruction takes place after post-traumatic arthritis from a plateau fracture has developed. Saleh et al. looked at 15 patients with a previous plateau fracture at an average of 6.2 years after total knee arthroplasty. They found that although TKA decreased pain and improved functional range of motion, there was a much higher rate of complications (three deep infections, two patellar tendon disruptions, three patients requiring closed manipulation) in patients with a history of fracture [27]. Weiss et al. reported their results on 62 patients treated with total knee arthroplasty who had developed post-traumatic osteoarthritis secondary to a previous fracture of the tibial plateau. The authors stated good to excellent clinical results in 78% of these patients noting specifically the technical difficulties they encountered at the time of surgery to optimize component positioning. The authors stressed that the most important factor in the outcome of patients treated with TKA after tibial plateau fracture is initial fracture treatment: meticulous soft tissue handling, fracture reduction and maintenance of range of motion following fracture treatment [28].

14.7 Conclusions

The management of tibial plateau fractures in the elderly must take into account the type of fracture, the health status of the patient, the quality of the host bone and functional expectations. Non-displaced or minimally displaced stable fractures can be treated with brief periods of immobilization and restriction of weight bearing. Operative treatment for these fractures should focus on restoring continuity of the tibial plateau/metaphysis to the diaphysis and restoration of the articular surface. In rare instances when there is significant pre-existing joint arthrosis, osteopenia, and fracture comminution, primary TKA may be warranted if there is sufficient cortical support for placement of a knee prosthesis. Generally speaking though, the emphasis when treating tibial plateau fractures in the elderly is restoration of tibial length and alignment while respecting the often fragile soft tissues surrounding the proximal tibia. The surgical approach to treating these fractures must take into consideration the risks of what is often a large operation, the medical co-morbidities of many elderly patients and the fact that a subsequent operation (such as a total knee arthroplasty) may be needed.

References

1. Moore TM, Patzakis MJ, Harvey JP. Tibial plateau fractures: definition, demographics, treatment rationale, and long-term results of closed traction management or operative reduction. J Orthop Trauma 1987;1(2):97–119.

2. Frattini M, Vaienti E, Soncini G, et al. Tibial plateau fractures in elderly patients. Musculoskelet Surg 2009;93(3):109–114.
3. Seng K, Appleby D, Lubowitz JH. Operative versus nonoperative treatment of anterior cruciate ligament rupture in patients aged 40 years or older: an expected-value decision analysis. Arthroscopy 2008;24(8):914–20.
4. Koval KJ, Helfet DL. Tibial plateau fractures: evaluation and treatment. J Am Acad Orthop Surg 1995;3(2):86–94.
5. Weiss NG, Parvizi J, Hanssen AD, et al. Total knee arthroplasty in post-traumatic arthrosis of the knee. J Arthroplasty 2003;18(3 Suppl 1):23–6.
6. Gardner MJ, Yacoubtian S, Geller D, et al. The incidence of soft tissue injury in operative tibial plateau fractures: a magnetic resonance imaging analysis of 103 patients. J Orthop Trauma 2005;19:79–84.
7. Chiba T, Sugita T, Onuma M, Kawamata T, Umehara J. Injuries to the posterolateral aspect of the knee accompanied by compression fracture of the anterior part of the medial tibial plateau. Arthroscopy 2001;17:642–7.
8. Bennett WF, Browner B. Tibial plateau fractures: a study of associated soft tissue injuries. J Orthop Trauma 1994;8(3):183–8.
9. Chan PS, Klimkiewicz JJ, Luchetti WT, et al. Impact of CT scan on treatment plan and fracture classification of tibial plateau fractures. J Orthop Trauma 1997;11(7):484–9.
10. Prasad N, Murray JM, Kumar D, et al. Insufficiency fracture of the tibial plateau: an often missed diagnosis. Acta Orthop Belg 2006;72(5):587–91.
11. Lotz JC, Kroeber MW, Heilmann M, et al. Tibial plateau fracture as a measure of early estrogen-dependent bone fragility in rats. J Orthop Res 2000;18(2):326–32.
12. Ruedi TP, Murphy WM, editors. AO principles of fracture management. New York, Stuttgart, Arbeitsgemeinschaft fur Osteosynthesefragen; 2000. p. 45–58.
13. Schatzker J, McBroom R, Bruce D. The tibial plateau fracture. The Toronto experience 1968–1975. Clin Orthop Relat Res 1979;(138):94–104.
14. Wiss DA, editor. Master techniques in orthopaedic surgery: fractures. Lippincott, Williams and Wilkins; 2006, pp. 407–37.
15. Rasmussen PS. Tibial condylar fractures. Impairment of knee joint stability as an indication for surgical treatment. J Bone Joint Surg Am 1973;55(7):1331–50.
16. Mills WJ, Nork SE. Open reduction and internal fixation of high-energy tibial plateau fractures. Orthop Clin North Am 2002;33(1):177–98, ix.
17. Barei DP, Nork SE, Mills WJ, et al. Complications associated with internal fixation of high-energy bicondylar tibial plateau fractures utilizing a two-incision technique. J Orthop Trauma 2004;18(10):649–57.
18. Cole PA, Zlowodzki M, Kregor PJ. Less Invasive Stabilization System (LISS) for fractures of the proximal tibia: indications, surgical technique and preliminary results of the UMC Clinical Trial. Injury 2003;34(Suppl 1):A16–29.
19. Caspari RB, Hutton PM, Whipple TL, et al. The role of arthroscopy in the management of tibial plateau fractures. Arthroscopy 1985;1(2):76–82.
20. Belanger M, Fadale P. Compartment syndrome of the leg after arthroscopic examination of a tibial plateau fracture. Case report and review of the literature. Arthroscopy 1997;13(5):646–51.
21. Krappinger D, Struve P, Smekal V, et al. Severely comminuted bicondylar tibial plateau fractures in geriatric patients: a report of 2 cases treated with open reduction and postoperative external fixation. J Orthop Trauma 2008;22(9):652–7.
22. Nau T, Pflegerl E, Erhart J et al. Primary total knee arthroplasty for periarticular fractures. J Arthroplasty 2003;18(8):968–71.
23. Ali AM, Burton M, Hashmi M, et al. Treatment of displaced bicondylar tibial plateau fractures (OTA-41C2&3) in patients older than 60 years of age. J Orthop Trauma. 2003;17(5):346–52.
24. Biyani A, Reddy NS, Chaudhury J, et al. The results of surgical management of displaced tibial plateau fractures in the elderly. Injury 1995;26(5):291–7.
25. Su EP, Westrich GH, Rana AJ, et al.Operative treatment of tibial plateau fractures in patients older than 55 years. Clin Orthop Relat Res 2004;(421):240–8.

26. Hsu JE, Pappas N, Lee G. A systematic approach to primary non-hinged knee replacement in patients with comminuted periarticular fractures about the knee. Unpublished.
27. Saleh KJ, Sherman P, Katkin P, et al. Total knee arthroplasty after open reduction and internal fixation of fractures of the tibial plateau: a minimum five-year follow-up study. J Bone Joint Surg Am 2001;83-A(8):1144–8.
28. Weiss NG, Parvizi J, Trousdale RT, et al. Total knee arthroplasty in patients with a prior fracture of the tibial plateau. J Bone Joint Surg Am 2003;85-A(2):218–21.

Part IV
Rehabilitation, Post-fracture Evaluation, and Prevention

Chapter 15
Rehabilitation

Keith Baldwin, Derek J. Donegan, and Mary Ann Keenan

Abstract In contrast to most injuries in younger individuals, fractures in elderly patients represent life-threatening and life-altering events. The individual and societal costs of these injuries are immense. Management of these conditions represents an important public health concern. In order to successfully navigate a rehabilitation program for these injuries, both surgical and medical concerns must be adequately planned for and adequately addressed. Often the care of these patients requires a multidisciplinary approach in order to be successful. A comprehensive rehabilitation plan for most fractures includes consideration of underlying physiological status and specific goal directed therapy for all major activities of daily living. It is also important for geriatricians and orthopaedic surgeons alike to understand the role of other professionals in the rehabilitation of their patients.

Keywords Fracture • Elderly • Geriatric • Rehabilitation • Therapy

15.1 Introduction

Osteoporosis, impaired balance, and medical problems make the geriatric population highly susceptible to bony injury. By unhappy coincidence, it is the same balance issues, poor bone stock, and medical comorbidities that make fractures poorly tolerated injuries in this population. Immobility is the common denominator that results in many of the poor outcomes associated with fractures in the elderly. It is because of this fact that acute, often surgical treatment is critical to rehabilitation from these injuries. Similarly, since these patients often have an array of medical conditions, a parallel, but often competing need is acute medical management. Medical management of these patients is at least as important to both survival of

K. Baldwin (✉)
Department of Orthopaedic Surgery, Hospital of the University of Pennsylvania,
2 Silverstein Pavilion, 3400 Spruce Street, Philadelphia, PA 19104, USA
e-mail: keith.baldwin@uphs.upenn.edu

R.J. Pignolo et al. (eds.), *Fractures in the Elderly*, Aging Medicine,
DOI 10.1007/978-1-60327-467-8_15, © Springer Science+Business Media, LLC 2011

the patient and final outcome of rehabilitation from these injuries. The goal of surgical and medical management in the rehabilitation of elderly patients with fractures is to safely achieve maximum mobility.

15.2 Consequences of Injury

Falls and fractures in the elderly represent an important source of pain and suffering, as well as monetary cost in nearly all developed countries [1, 2]. The majority of these costs, both economic and personal are due to lower extremity fractures. Nearly half of these fractures occur about the hip. These fractures particularly are associated with a 1-year mortality of 20%. In addition to mortality, about half of these patients are unable to walk without assistive devices postinjury, and 20–40% requires some level of formal care or supervision that they did not require pre-injury.

Medical and neurological comorbidities tend to worsen when an elderly patient experiences a long bone fracture as a result of the underlying changes in physiology [3, 4]. For example, elderly cardiac patients poorly tolerate the anemia that results from a significant fracture haematoma. This can result in orthostatic hypotension, syncope, or cardiac ischemia. Neurological conditions common in the elderly such as the sequelae of cerebrovascular accident (CVA) tend to worsen in the face of long bone fractures [5]. Patients may experience increased tone or spasticity that may worsen in the face of anaesthesia and surgery. The increase in tone is observed regardless of whether or not the fracture occurs on the side of the neurologic insult or the uninvolved side. Because of this increased tone and spasticity, its associated pain, and the challenging nature of these issues for medical staff, patients are at further increased risk for muscle contracture.

Often, the immobilization associated with these injuries results in medical and orthopaedic complications that can be avoided if a skilled multidisciplinary approach is undertaken. Prolonged immobilization or inadequate mobilization will result in osteoporosis, muscle weakness, and increased risk of thromboembolic disease. Decubitus ulcers may result due to immobility and lack of proper positioning. Pneumonia from decreased inspiratory volume, urinary tract infection from prolonged foley catheter usage, and other infectious complications can result from the immobility resultant from injury.

15.3 Barriers to Rehabilitation

Success of any fracture management and rehabilitation protocol should be defined as returning a patient to the safest highest level of function possible after their injury. Several pitfalls in rehabilitation exist, and steps should be taken to avoid or minimize those potential setbacks [6].

15.3.1 *Thromboembolic Complications*

Thromboembolic complications are among the most widely known complications in orthopaedic trauma and include symptomatic deep vein thrombosis (DVT) and pulmonary embolism (PE). In elderly patients, immobilization predisposes to increased risks of thromboembolic complications. Multiple underlying medical problems and poor physiologic reserve both result in poor tolerance of embolic events.

Elderly people often have atypical presentations of PE, which can manifest as a change in mental status. Clinical suspicion for a PE may warrant consideration of a ventilation perfusion (V/Q) scan or spiral computed tomography. In addition, prophylactic anticoagulation should be initiated with low molecular weight heparin, or coumadin, either as a solitary intervention or in combination with sequential compression devices. The decision for how aggressive anticoagulation should be is made by weighing the patient's relative risk of thromboembolic complications versus their propensity for bleeding complications. For details of the risk versus benefit profiles of various anticoagulation regimens, see Chap. 5.

15.3.2 *Decubitus Ulcers*

Decubitus ulcers are a pitfall in any hospitalized geriatric patient population. Bony prominences should be well padded and protected. Nursing care must be vigilant and fracture patients should have their heels protected by soft foam or have pillows placed under their calves in such a way to reduce pressure on the heels. In addition, frequent position change must be employed so that sacral ulcers do not develop. In cachectic patients, the scapula and occiput must be attended to as well, as these areas are also vulnerable to decubiti. If a patient is immobilized, and appears as if they will take some time to mobilize, or if their nutritional status is poor, a pressure relieving air mattress should be considered. Decubitus ulcers are a complication that is better prevented than treated, because often elderly people have compromised blood flow, and as such these ulcers are difficult to treat.

15.3.3 *Pneumonia*

Following surgery, elderly patients often have difficulty taking deep breaths. Part of this difficulty is simply due to atelectasis attributable to anaesthesia, however often times these patients have a certain degree of generalized weakness, which contributes to the development of pneumonia. Occasionally, when rib fractures are present or when fractures are proximal in the upper limb, deep breaths are painful, so patients have difficulty taking deep breaths. In addition, some patients have neurologic compromise that places them at increased risk for aspiration. All of these factors increase the likelihood of pneumonia. Instruction in incentive spirometry is mandatory. In the case of patients that have decreased mental status, chest physical therapy is often useful to clear secretions. The lungs should be carefully auscultated to listen for early signs of lung consolidation. In addition, a chest X-ray should be obtained if the patient is showing signs of fever. If multiple rib fractures are present in an elderly patient, ICU level care should be considered, as these patients can decompensate quickly as a result of poor air movement.

15.3.4 Loss of Joint Range of Motion

Loss of joint range of motion (ROM) is a barrier to rehabilitation that physical and occupational therapists strive to prevent. Immobility that results from injury typically prompts patients to find a comfortable position. Geriatric patients have tissues that are less supple and less plastic than their younger counterparts. As a result, these patients lose ROM quickly. In the upper extremities, loss of ROM results in a decreased ability to perform activities of daily living (ADL). In the lower extremities, loss of ROM results in a less efficient gait and patients lose their ability to walk distances and suffer pain with ambulation. Specifically, prolonged bed rest tends to allow the foot and ankle to rest in an equinus position which, if prolonged, can lead to a contracture of the ankle in a plantarflexed position [7]. If this occurs, gait abnormalities such as toe drag and genu recurvatum can occur, leading to further orthopaedic complications and altered gait mechanics. Several boots are commercially available which keep the foot neutral or dorsiflexed if the patient is in bed. These boots help to prevent this equinus deformity, provided they are correctly applied.

15.3.5 Acceleration of Degenerative Joint Disease

The altered mechanics due to decreased joint ROM, and occasionally from intra-articular fractures, result in an acceleration of degenerative joint disease (DJD). In addition, patients who already have DJD in one limb may be forced to rely on that leg if their weight-bearing status is limited on the opposite leg due to injury.

15.3.6 Delirium

Dementia is present in some form or another in a large proportion of the geriatric population and tends to increase in incidence with increasing age. Dementia at baseline places a patient at increased risk for incidences of delirium that can occur with the disorientation of being in the hospital or the administration of narcotic pain medication. In addition, much of physical and occupational therapy depends on teaching the patient exercises or methods of using assistive devices and/or equipment. When a patient's ability to learn is compromised due to dementia, it substantially impedes their rehabilitation.

Postoperative delirium in older patients is not uncommon [8, 9]. The balance between pain control and retaining adequate mental status is delicate. When postoperative delirium occurs, close attention should be paid to the patients' neurological exam. Other organic sources of delirium such as hypoglycaemia, hypoxia, and vascular issues should be ruled out clinically before attributing the patient's mental status to effects of pain medication. Chapter 6 outlines in detail the approach to the elderly fracture patient at high risk of delirium.

15.3.7 Loss of Strength

Strength is decreased the longer the length of stay in the hospital. Physical and occupational therapists strive to prevent this loss of strength that results from immobility. Often loss of strength results in abnormalities in gait and in difficulty performing ADLs because these activities depend on a coordinated firing of muscle groups with a certain amount of force to be efficient. Physical therapists should concentrate their efforts on hip extensors, hip abductors, knee extensors, and ankle dorsiflexors, as these muscles are the most important for maintaining upright posture, enhancing gait velocity and efficiency, and decreasing the cardiac stress that results from inefficient gait.

15.3.8 Cardiopulmonary Deconditioning

Cardiopulmonary deconditioning is a serious problem in the elderly population. This is especially true in the case of patients with COPD and/or CHF. These patients are less able to tolerate fluid shifts than the average population and have less physiologic reserve than even age-matched cohorts. When these baseline problems are coupled with the anaemia associated with fracture haematoma and surgery, the problem becomes amplified. Physical and occupational therapists can use arm bicycles and repetitive exercise to improve the conditioning of these patients and aid in their overall rehabilitation efforts.

15.3.9 Bowel and Bladder Incontinence

Bowel and bladder incontinence is not uncommon in elderly patients, particularly those who were institutionalized prior to injury. In addition to representing a larger burden to nursing care, patients who suffer from bowel or bladder incontinence run the risk of contaminating their surgical incisions. Care must be taken to keep the surgical incision clean and dry. In addition, if any decubitus ulcers or open wounds are present, they should be covered in an effort to prevent contamination. Strong consideration should be given to the risks of continued foley catheterization versus the risk of wound soiling in this population. It may be prudent to consider keeping the foley catheter if there is a high risk of wound contamination, particularly prior to adequate wound healing. Skin sealants and occlusive wound dressings may be necessary if there is a high risk of contaminating the surgical wound.

15.3.10 Pain Control

Pain control is often an important issue both to the rehabilitation of a patient who has suffered a fracture as well as to that patient's satisfaction with his or her hospital care. Regional blocks may be considered prior to surgery to help control acute surgical pain. These blocks, however, are short lived. Patient-controlled analgesia (PCA) is popular in orthopaedics because it allows a patient to self-regulate their pain control, but these are often not ideal for elderly patients with cognitive impairment or arthritic problems. Nonsteroidal anti-inflammatory drugs (NSAIDS) are popular for pain control, however, they have fallen out of favour due to recent studies that show that they impede fracture healing in animal models. In addition, NSAIDS may not be the best choice for patients with renal insufficiency.

Muscle relaxers such as diazepam can be useful in cases where fractures cause increased spasticity, such as in patients with a history of CVA. In addition, they can help relieve muscle guarding which can interfere with therapy. It should be kept in mind, however, that these medications have an additive effect with narcotics in terms of sedation, and close attention is required to make sure that patients do not get too sedated. Overall, pain control in elderly patients can be challenging and should be carefully monitored by all members of the healthcare delivery team. Additionally, delirium can result from overaggressive attempts to control the patient's pain.

15.3.11 Weight-Bearing Status

Orthopaedic surgeons select the patient's weight-bearing status typically on the basis of the relative instability of the fracture and the relative stability of their repair. In addition, they factor in whether or not the construct they use is load bearing or load sharing. Due to the relative osteopenia of elderly individuals along with the tendency of older people to fracture in patterns that are unstable (e.g., subtrochanteric and intertrochanteric hip fractures), orthopaedic surgeons frequently make patients nonweight bearing or toe touch weight bearing. These weight-bearing statuses require a great deal of balance and come at an immense energy cost. Often the geriatric population cannot tolerate them. If this is the case, physical and occupational therapists must find ways to accommodate these restrictions, including creative ways to mobilize the patient during transfers and for wheelchair mobility [10]. Elderly patients will often autoregulate their weight bearing by pain regardless of what restrictions their physicians place on them.

15.3.12 Neurologic Compromise

Neurologic compromise is present in a variety of ways in the aged population. CVA is common in the elderly population and often patients have residual deficits. If a patient has difficulty speaking due to a past CVA, their needs and communication with the healthcare delivery team can be compromised. Communication boards, picture exchange communication, or other nonverbal methods of communication may become necessary.

In addition, varying levels of weakness will be present, and often spasticity and abnormal gait mechanics exist at baseline. These factors make rehabilitation more challenging and require a greater degree of creativity on the part of the healthcare delivery team. Patients with Parkinson's disease provide an interesting challenge to rehabilitation professionals. They possess a typical gait pattern characterized by difficulty initiating, shuffling steps after gait is initiated, and difficulty stopping (so-called fenestrating gait). This gait can become even more difficult in the presence of a lower extremity fracture and nearly impossible with a limited weight-bearing status. Setting therapy sessions to music in order to time movements may activate different neural pathways and allows these patients to ambulate more easily. With a decreased weight-bearing status, many patients with more severe Parkinson's disease or neurologic involvement may find themselves confined to a wheelchair until the fracture heals and weight-bearing restriction is lifted. In this case, aggressive ROM exercises and functional bracing are often necessary to prevent contractures. Neurosurgical or medication alteration may be considered to alter the brain's dopaminergic input in this population.

15.3.13 Vascular Insufficiency and Diabetes

Vascular insufficiency and diabetes produce additional challenges. Healing bones, skin, and other tissues require uncompromised blood supply for adequate delivery of oxygen, nutrients, and immune factors. Diabetics and patients with vascular insufficiency have longer healing times, increased likelihood of infection, and more complications. In addition, when diabetes or vasculopathy results in microvascular changes, neuropathy often results. When physical therapists train a patient to walk with a walker, crutches, or learn a new gait pattern, the motor learning requires functional posterior column proprioceptive fibres that exist in feet and ankles. In the presence of diabetic neuropathy or vasculopathy, these systems are compromised or absent. Sometimes when the neuropathy is mild or moderate, high stockings can be used to transmit some of the ground reaction force further up the ankle where proprioceptive fibres still work properly. A lightweight ankle–foot orthosis can produce the same effect as long as enough sensation is present to prevent ulcers from forming in areas of increased pressure.

Diabetics particularly offer a challenge to the treating physician. Some patients with long-standing diabetes have issues with neuropathy that can render a delayed union or nonunion insensate. This is problematic as these patients can develop Charcot joints even in the setting of minimal fracture or injury or potentially disrupt their hardware construct by walking on it prior to fracture healing.

15.3.14 Vision or Hearing Problems

Vision and hearing problems are among the most common complaints of the elderly community. Often the geriatric population feels increasingly isolated due to these disabilities. Therapists and physicians must keep these limitations in mind when devising a set of rehabilitation parameters for a patient. Safety is the ultimate goal. When decreased mobility or a decreased weight-bearing status is added upon these baseline disabilities, progress toward rehabilitation goals may be delayed. Consider obtaining speech and hearing evaluations and/or using alternative means of communication (such as writing on a dry erase board) or simple methods to enhance hearing (such as portable amplification devices).

Along with limiting rehab itself, these issues cause problems with safety in settings outside of rehabilitation. Consideration must be given to safety in those patients with visual difficulties and mobility issues may be in greater danger in common activities, such as crossing the road or walking in other public settings.

15.4 Goals of Rehabilitation

Early mobilization is the primary goal of fracture fixation. Physical and occupational therapists help by providing guidance and strengthening muscles required for gait and ADL. Restoration of function is unique to each individual [11–14]. Some patients may be wheel chair ambulators at baseline, and to restore their function means only to enable them to transfer from one surface to their chair, where they will self-mobilize. Other patients may have been community ambulators or even participants in sports-related activities prefracture, and thus their goals will differ with the level of function they wish to achieve toward returning to their pre-injury status. In order to achieve restoration of function, strength and joint ROM must be

Table 15.1 Functional progression of rehabilitation

1. Bed mobility: rolling, scooting, supine to sit
2. Sitting balance
3. Transfers: sit to stand, bed to wheelchair
4. Ambulation: wheelchair, gait, assistive devices

returned. Specific goals are set for different joints, so that strength and ROM can be improved. Specific goals for therapy vary with specific fracture type and personality, however, a typical functional progression is outlined in Table 15.1.

15.5 Common Fractures

15.5.1 Upper Extremity Fractures/Dislocations

Upper extremity fractures and dislocations, although common in an elderly population, do not necessarily mandate admission to the hospital. However, if a patient has an upper extremity fracture, and normally s(he) walks with a walker, then s(he) needs to be admitted to have the fracture stabilized, or learn to ambulate with a platform walker or another assistive device. Similarly, if a patient is right-hand dominant, and lives alone, a fracture of the right upper extremity should be stabilized to allow that patient function. In addition, s(he) should be evaluated by physical and occupational therapy to determine the appropriateness of returning directly home versus spending time in a rehabilitation facility. Occasionally, a home evaluation may be appropriate to determine if adequate resources exist in the patient's home environment, or if modifications or assistive equipment is warranted.

15.5.1.1 Proximal Humerus

Proximal humerus fractures in the elderly typically occur as a result of a fall on outstretched hand, and thus may be accompanied by other upper extremity fractures. These fractures are nondisplaced or minimally displaced 80% of the time, and in these cases the treatment is nonweight bearing on the involved upper extremity, with a sling to be used at all times. If the fracture is displaced, many surgeons will consider open reduction and internal fixation (ORIF). When this is the case surgeon preference usually dictates rehabilitation, and this will vary based on perceived stability of the bone–metal construct. If the bone stock is compromised, or if the fracture is too comminuted, a hemiarthroplasty or total shoulder arthroplasty may be indicated.

From a rehabilitation standpoint, the function of the shoulder is to put the hand in an appropriate position to manipulate tools and assist with dressing and toileting.

Tasks such as feeding require mostly shoulder internal rotation. Reaching, grasping, and dressing, however often require combined movements of flexion, abduction, and varying degrees of internal/external rotation. Often ROM lost at the shoulder can be compensated by distal joints; however, it is important to gain as much range as is possible because its loss of range results in pain and certain contractures, such as internal rotation contractures which in turn can predispose to spiral fractures of the humerus.

In elderly patients, rotator cuff tears are common pre-existing injuries, but may also result from greater tuberosity fractures. Both types of patients will require rotator cuff rehabilitation protocols; however, it is important in patients with nondisplaced fractures of the proximal humerus to delay aggressive rotator cuff rehabilitation until the fracture is stable enough to avoid displacement.

Although bones will typically unite in 6–8 weeks, rehabilitation can last from 12 weeks to 12 months. Elderly patients are at increased risk of stiffness compared to young patients. The involved upper extremity should be nonweight bearing. Shoulders treated nonoperatively are typically immobilized, and gentle ROM of the elbow, wrist, and fingers should be prescribed immediately. In 2–4 weeks, most fractures can withstand gentle pendulum exercises. In 4–6 weeks, patients can begin limited active assisted range of motion (AAROM) exercises in all planes, and the involved extremity can be used for dressing and personal care as tolerated. At 6–8 weeks, gentle active, active assisted, and passive ROM, as well as isometric strengthening are tolerated. At 8–12 weeks and beyond, the majority of patients can tolerate progressive strengthening and stretching.

15.5.1.2 Shoulder Dislocation

The incidence of shoulder dislocations is bimodal; in men, the peak incidence is in the 21–30 age group and in women peak incidence is in the 61–80 age group. Ninety percent of the time these dislocations occur anteriorly. The treatment of these injuries consists of closed reduction and immobilization for 2–5 weeks. Often the shoulder is unstable prior to that, and it is thought that earlier mobilization may result in recurrent dislocation. However, stiffness tends to be a huge problem in the elderly population and recurrent dislocations are less common in this age group. Pendulum exercises as well as wrist, finger, and elbow ROM are allowed almost immediately; shoulder ROM is allowed earlier than in other groups. Shoulder dislocations are associated with rotator cuff tears in as many as 80% of these injuries by some estimates. Aggressive physical and occupational therapy to increase strength and ROM is mandatory following the period of immobilization. In addition, since rotator cuff tears are highly associated with shoulder dislocation in the elderly patient, it is prudent to progress the patient from isometric rotator cuff exercises to light exercises and then to progressive strengthening.

15.5.1.3 Fractures About the Elbow

Functionally, ROM about the elbow is important for activities in which the arm must be shortened. Specifically, tasks such as feeding and bathing are tasks which use the elbow's ability to flex. Flexion ROM is therefore more important than extension ROM for most activities. The exception is when the arm is used in a closed chain fashion for activities such as crutch ambulation or transfers. If the elbow cannot fully extend, it becomes difficult to perform these activities.

Humeral shaft fractures in elderly patients often result from a fall on outstretched hand. A careful neurovascular exam is essential, with special care to rule out radial nerve injury. Most often, these fractures are treated nonoperatively, the exceptions being if there is an open fracture, soft tissue compromise, vascular injury, or polytrauma. If nonoperative treatment is selected, typically a coaptation splint is placed followed by a functional Sarmiento brace.

Most commonly, fractures about the elbow exist as supracondylar humerus fractures or radial head fractures. Supracondylar humerus fractures often result from a fall on outstretched hand or direct blow in an osteoporotic arm. A thorough neurological exam must be conducted in patients with these fractures because of the plethora of neurovascular structures that traverse this region. Frequently, these fractures are treated nonoperatively if they are nondisplaced or if they are severely comminuted in an elderly patient with low baseline functional capacity. However, if there is vascular injury or if the fracture is displaced, ORIF is carried out. If the fracture is severely comminuted, and the individual had a high degree of premorbid function, a total elbow arthroplasty can be considered. If nonoperative treatment is selected, a posterior splint is placed and ROM exercises are initiated in 1–2 weeks. The splint may be discontinued in 6 weeks after radiographic evidence of healing is evident. Similarly, early ROM is typically encouraged with surgically treated patients due to fear of stiffness about the elbow. Radial head fractures if nondisplaced can be treated by sling placement for 24–48 h, after which ROM exercises are begun. If the fracture is displaced or comminuted, often the treatment is ORIF, radial head excision, or radial head arthroplasty. In any case, the goal is early ROM, though the timing is somewhat surgeon dependant.

15.5.1.4 Forearm, Wrist, and Hand Fractures

The majority of forearm and wrist fractures are a result of falls on outstretched hand and can be treated with closed reduction and casting. Occasionally when closed reduction fails, or when too extreme a wrist position is necessary to maintain adequate reduction, open reduction with a plate and screws or percutaneous pinning with Kirschner wires is performed. In either case, early finger and shoulder ROM is required to maintain function in the extremity and avoid excessive stiffness. Reflex sympathetic dystrophy is a feared complication in these fractures. Similarly, most fractures in the hand can be treated with closed methods provided adequate reduction can be achieved and maintained. In addition, noncontiguous joints should be subjected to ROM exercises to avoid stiffness.

The forearm, wrist, and hand are responsible for tasks that require fine manipulation and dexterity. Any loss of ROM in this region requires a larger compensation from the shoulder and elbow. In addition, the loss of nerve function, or ROM in the fingers or hand, becomes more problematic than a loss more proximally because of the fine movements that are required at these joints. Although specific skilled rehabilitation is often not necessary for many injuries about the hand and wrist, all patients should receive a home exercise program that should focus on finger flexion and extension, and grip strength. If a patient fails home therapy or seems to be lagging behind in ROM, it is appropriate at that point to consult a hand therapist who will motivate the patient to regain critical ROM and strength. Nerve damage is a particular concern in this region and special utensils to eat as well as other assistive devices may be required.

15.5.2 Spine Fractures

In elderly patients, 60% of vertebral fractures are the result of a fall. There are a vast array of types of spinal fractures, and many considerations for each individual fracture. For the purposes of rehabilitation, fractures can be considered to be stable or unstable. In the geriatric population, fractures will commonly be compression fractures that occur as a result of osteoporosis. The vast majority of these fractures are stable. However, occasionally these fractures can result in stress on the posterior elements and cause progressive deformity and eventual neurologic compromise.

Physical therapy in the first couple of weeks postoperatively consists of bracing with ambulation, lower extremity strengthening, and log rolling in bed. After 6 weeks, active extension is allowed for compression fractures; 8–12 weeks after surgery or injury, flexion, extension, and rotatory movements are encouraged. After 12 weeks, progressive resistive exercises are permitted.

15.5.2.1 Stable Spinal Fractures

As previously mentioned, the majority of these fractures are compression type fractures of the body of the vertebrae. Often these fractures are associated with a significant amount of pain. This pain impedes rehabilitation, and if present in the thoracic spine can inhibit rib excursion and ability to breathe deeply. Patients should therefore be carefully monitored for signs of atelectasis and pneumonia. These patients are candidates for early mobilization, although a thoracolumbosacral orthothosis is often warranted for patient comfort. In addition, these patients often require assistive devices to ambulate. These patients should undergo assessment of osteoporosis and bisphosphonate or other therapy should be considered. See Chap. 16 for medical approaches to the evaluation of patients with osteoporotic fractures and fracture prevention.

15.5.2.2 Unstable Fractures

Unstable fractures of the spine can be associated with neurologic compromise. Often these patients are treated with steroids acutely if neurologic deficit is discovered within 8 h of injury. The majority of such patients will require rigid stabilization of their spinal column. These patients tend to be extremely complex patients regardless of their age. Varying severity of spinal cord compromise may exist as a result of these injuries. Incomplete injuries may vary from sensory (no motor) to weak motor deficits. Often the extent of neurologic injury will determine the course of rehabilitation. Patients with high spinal cord injuries may be confined to a wheelchair with almost complete dependance on caregivers for IADLs. By contrast, as a spinal cord injury gets lower, more functional recovery is possible. Patients with low cervical spinal cord injuries, particularly those below C7, may be able to transfer independently because they will have use of their triceps. Patients with C6 injuries may also be able to perform transfers, however, these transfers depend on locking out the arm using shoulder internal rotation, a task which is often too complex and difficult to understand even for younger spinal cord injury patients. It is important for patients with high spinal cord injuries to get a good wheelchair seating system, because without this the patient will be at high risk for developing decubitus ulcers. Lower spinal cord injuries, such as those that occur in the lumbar spine, will still have mostly intact sitting balance and trunk control. If the injury occurs low enough (below L3) the patient will still have hip flexors and knee extensors, so ambulation may be possible with knee–ankle–foot orthosis. This ambulation would be reserved for an otherwise healthy patient because of the vast amount of energy this gait consumes. A full discussion of the rehabilitation of these patients is beyond the scope of this chapter, and often therapists and physicians that specialize in these types of injuries are required for maximum rehabilitation potential to be reached.

15.5.3 Lower Extremity Fractures

In contrast to patients with upper extremity fractures, elderly patients with lower extremity fractures will most often need to be admitted for acute fracture treatment. The majority of patients with lower extremity fractures will require surgery to maximize their functional potential.

15.5.3.1 Pelvis Fractures

The majority of pelvic fractures that occur in elderly individuals are secondary to a low energy mechanism and are stable. These fractures are treated by protected weight bearing, usually with crutches or a walker. Radiologic follow up is required after weight bearing is initiated to assure that fracture fragments do not displace. Stool softeners may be helpful as straining with defecation may be painful and may lead to constipation.

The pelvis functions as the base by which weight is shifted from one side to the other during gait. As such, the pelvis has a critical role during weight-bearing activities. Fractures that involve the weight bearing "dome" are particularly problematic for gait training. Often, even when a fracture does not involve a weight-bearing surface, it causes significant pain with weight bearing. Hip extensor and knee extensor strength should be of primary concern early in rehabilitation, as these muscle groups will assist in sit-to-stand transfers. Upper body strength is also important when patients will be reliant on sliding board transfers and wheelchair mobility. Triceps strength is particularly important and should be a focus in this subgroup of patients. In addition, rolling and scooting exercises should be performed while in bed to assist the patient in autoregulating the pressure on their skin and also to become more independent.

15.5.3.2 Hip Fractures

Fractures about the hip are among the most common fractures in the elderly population. They are associated with a high degree of morbidity and mortality. It has been estimated that about 20% of elderly patients will die within a year of their fracture. In addition, it is difficult to estimate the emotional toll on patients who may lose much of their independence as a result of these fractures. Hip fractures are important to rule out in elderly patients. It is important to note that when an elderly patient has groin pain and cannot ambulate, a negative X-ray does not rule out a hip fracture. Those patients should be admitted, and an MRI of the hip should be obtained as soon as possible to rule out fracture. Femoral neck fractures are treated surgically with in situ screw fixation or a fixed-angle device if they are nondisplaced. A displaced femoral neck fracture was historically treated by hemiarthroplasty, but because many patients complain of hip pain following hemiarthroplasty, there has been a recent shift in practice to perform total hip arthroplasty in the case of displaced femoral neck fractures. Typically, subtrochanteric and intertrochanteric fractures are unstable by their nature, and are repaired by ORIF.

It is crucial to repair these fractures early in order to minimize immobility and the deleterious sequelae associated with immobilization. Following repair, early mobilization with physical therapy is essential. The orthopaedic surgeon will dictate the weight-bearing status, and the therapists will devise methods of mobilizing the patient in the framework of their weight-bearing status. Orthopaedic surgeons work to achieve the goal of a construct that will allow a patient to be weight bearing as tolerated, as non- or toe-touch weight bearing is poorly tolerated by the elderly.

Muscles that are instrumental in functional activities, such as gait and transfers are critical to strengthen early in the rehabilitation process. Of particular importance are hip extensors, hip abductors, and quadriceps muscles. Early isometric knee and hip exercises are essential and ankle-pumping exercises are encouraged several times a day. Later, straight leg raises, gravity eliminated abduction exercises, and heel slides are performed. Functional activities are started early, with the primary focus on transfers, gait, and manipulation of stairs. In the case of total hip arthroplasty for fracture, hip extensor and abductor exercises are emphasized. Hip protocols restrict patients to less than 90° of flexion, neutral internal rotation, and zero degrees of adduction. Although assistive equipment including hip chairs, abduction pillows, sock grabbers, and elevated toilet seats are available to decrease the risk of dislocation, recent research calls into question whether these measures are necessary.

The primary goal of rehabilitation as it pertains to lower extremity fractures is the optimization of ambulation or the ability to move from one place to the next safely with as little assistance as possible. Gait in particular is a highly stylized and highly efficient combination of movements that allows weight to shift from one limb to the next while making forward progress. When patients have fractures, often their weight-bearing status is limited by pain or by physician order, and gait becomes more metabolically costly. To be precise, two- and three-point partial weight-bearing patterns and cane walking are 33% more costly than normal gait, and non-weight-bearing gait patterns require 78% more energy than normal gait. Because of this increased energy expenditure, many elderly individuals have difficulty tolerating non-weight-bearing status, and may be relegated to wheelchair ambulation until their fracture is stable. If this is the case, steps must be taken to prevent contractures by skilled physical therapy, nursing, and possibly bracing.

15.5.3.3 Distal Femur

Distal femur fractures in the elderly tend to occur as a result of falls from standing height on a flexed knee. The distal portion is typically flexed as a result of pull from the gastrocnemius, and the extremity is typically shortened by the quadriceps and hamstrings. If the fracture is stable and nondisplaced, the knee should be placed in a hinged knee brace with partial weight bearing. Most displaced fractures require surgery, and if surgery is to be delayed, a traction pin should be considered. If the patient has extremely osteoporotic bone, methylmethacrylate cement may be used to augment ORIF. Often postoperatively, a continuous passive motion machine will be employed, and physical therapy will begin with active ROM devices. The patient will be made partial or nonweight bearing depending on the stability of fixation and quality of bone. In 6–12 weeks, with evidence of radiographic healing, weight bearing can be advanced.

Distal femur fractures are important from a rehabilitation standpoint because knee flexion is important for many functional activities. Eighty-three degrees of ROM of the knee are required for stair climbing, 93° are required for rising from a seated position, and 106° are necessary to tie one's shoes. In addition, gait becomes more inefficient if the screw home mechanism (locking of the knee at the end of knee extension) is unavailable secondary to a flexion contracture. For this reason, aggressive ROM exercises are necessary with these injuries to prevent further morbidity.

15.5.3.4 Tibia, Ankle, and Foot Fractures

Fractures about the tibia, ankle, and foot represent difficult problems for elderly patients. Often these fractures require periods of nonweight bearing which are difficult for patients to tolerate. In addition, many of these bones are very superficial, and given patients' tenuous skin quality, vigilance must be observed to make sure that skin breakdown does not occur. When the tibia is fractured close attention is warranted to assure that there is no compartment syndrome. When the foot or ankle is fractured, the patient's bed should be adjusted to 30° or pillows placed under the involved extremity to assure that the involved extremity is above the level of the heart and will not get excessively swollen. Because of the limited weight-bearing status, patients may require wheelchair mobility and transfer training.

Functionally, the ankle must have 10° of dorsiflexion in order to ambulate with a normal gait pattern. Upon heel strike, the ankle must achieve neutral dorsiflexion, and upon mid-stance as the weight shifts to the ball of the foot, the ankle must rock into 10° of dorsiflexion. This becomes problematic if the ankle is casted in equinus. If this occurs, toe strike can occur instead of heel strike, and toe drag can occur during swing phase. This makes gait less efficient and increases the risk of falls. Hence it is important to observe the attitude of the cast and make sure that it is in neutral or dorsiflexion. When the fracture is united, vigorous stretching may be necessary to regain the dorsiflexion necessary to achieve normal gait.

15.6 Polytrauma

Elderly patients who sustain multiple fractures require special care by a trauma team. Seemingly innocuous injuries in younger patients can be life threatening in elderly patients. Rib fractures, if multiple and contiguous for example, may warrant ICU observation, and possible fixation as patients will not be able to take deep breaths and can decompensate quickly.

From a rehabilitation standpoint, these patients require a comprehensive plan. The impact of all injuries together is usually greater than the sum of the individual injuries. In elderly patients, this often means that for a period of time ambulation may not be possible. This is particularly true if the patient suffers long bone fractures in two different extremities. Often patients can be instructed in sliding board transfers. In addition, a motorized or specialized wheelchair may be considered if the duration of disability is expected to be protracted. Bed mobility is particularly important for these patients because if they can scoot and roll independently then they can autoregulate the pressure on sensitive parts of their bodies and reduce the risk of pressure sores. Trunk strengthening and upper extremity strengthening exercises can make it easier to transfer from surface to surface independently. Overall, each polytrauma patient requires an individualized therapy program that takes into account each individual injury as well as the injuries as a sum total [6, 15].

15.7 Acute Care Hospital

15.7.1 *Team Approach*

Care of an elderly fracture patient requires a team approach to handle the many pitfalls that can arise as a result of this population's multiple medical problems and often difficult social situations [16–18]. Social workers should get involved at the time of admission and provide a tentative discharge plan that is adjustable to fit changing medical and social circumstances. There are many members of the team, and each has their own important role in patient care. The two central decision makers in the acute phase of a patient's management are the orthopaedic surgeon and geriatrician. The geriatrician often will handle the medical management of the patient, and the orthopaedic surgeon will take care of the patient's acute surgical needs. The decision regarding which will be the primary decision maker will depend on the patient's medical comorbidities, social situation, and general medical/psychological condition weighed against the complexity of their acute surgical needs. Some have advocated the usage of combined-specialty orthogeriatric services that focus on these types of problems [16, 18]. Recent studies have suggested that in hospital outcome is determined more by pre-existing medical condition than type of surgery done. Often, team meetings are essential in order to determine what the changing priorities are with patients in different phases of recovery from injury. These meetings allow team members to voice their individual priorities, and to determine which priority takes precedence in any given day.

Physical medicine and rehabilitation physicians are important contacts to make in the acute phase of a patient's hospitalization to identify early barriers to rehabilitation, and to make sure the primary team treats these barriers prior to admission to rehabilitation. In addition, they make suggestions regarding wheelchair seating, assistive equipment, and have input regarding placement.

Physical and occupational therapy services are integral to a patient's early recovery. These services devise therapy regimens for patients, and assess their functional mobility, muscle strength, and ROM. They provide useful information regarding ability to perform ADL. In addition, they conduct functional training and strengthening, as well as make recommendations regarding disposition of patients in the postoperative period.

Social workers are indispensable members of the team as they assist with patient placement and home equipment needs. Often these members of the team are attuned to a patient's home situation and can be indispensable in assisting in community re-entry. These team members are also aware of different rehabilitation centres and community resources available to elderly patients. Social workers are the architects of the discharge plan and individually tailor a plan to a specific patient.

Nursing services are vital to the care of elderly patients. This is particularly true in the case of fracture patients. Excellent nursing care can improve outcomes by preventing decubitus ulcers, administering pain medication in a timely fashion, instructing patients in incentive spirometry, and making the medical or surgical team aware of any changes in patient status. In addition, good nursing care can contribute immensely to the satisfaction of the patient and family with their medical care.

Occasionally, psychiatry and other services will be necessary to evaluate patients. Psychological comorbidities that require specialized care may be exacerbated in the setting of an acute bony injury. In addition, pain management specialists are often useful if patients were taking pain medication prior to injury, since it is often more difficult to control pain in this setting.

15.7.2 Optimization of Pain Control

There is often a delicate balance in elderly patients between pain control and oversedation or delirium [19]. Narcotic pain medications are the mainstay of pain control in surgery in general and orthopaedic surgery, in particular. PCA devices are systems by which a patient can press a button within prescribed amount of time to get a dose of pain medication. These PCAs are popular in orthopaedic populations because the patient can autoregulate how much pain medication they receive, and it is difficult to overdose a patient because the patient will fall asleep before that occurs. In elderly patients in whom cognitive status is an issue, the PCA may not be the ideal choice. These patients may forget to press the button, lose the button, or may not even be able to see the button. If this is the case, a different regimen of oral or intravenous pain medication may be administered. In addition, intravenous narcotic pain medication often causes delirium in older patients, which may be mistaken for a more serious problem or mask the evolution of a more serious problem.

Epidural pain management may be an option with certain lower extremity fractures. These pain medications consist of epidurally administered opioids and anaesthetics. Typically, there will be a baseline level of analgesia administered, and administration of demand doses as needed. Some of the same problems with this type of analgesia exist as with PCAs. In addition, these pain control systems can sometimes drop a patient's blood pressure substantially. Overly vigorous epidural pain control must be considered in the differential of a patient with low blood pressure postoperatively. In addition, the administration of DVT prophylaxis must often be withheld when these catheters are in place to avoid the risk of epidural haematoma. Also, foley catheters should be left in until after the epidural is discontinued to avoid the risk of urinary retention.

In general, narcotic pain medications (whether oral or intravenous) produce some unwanted side effects. Nausea is a common side effect of narcotic pain medication that can be countered with anti-emetics, though many of these medications have untoward side effects themselves, particularly in elderly patients. Constipation is another concern with narcotic pain medication. Patients on narcotic pain medication should be given a bowel regimen starting with stool softeners. Urinary retention is also an unwanted complication of narcotic pain medication, and patients should be able to void less than 6 h after their foley catheter is discontinued. If the foley needs to be re-inserted more than once for urinary retention, a urologic consultation should be considered.

The NSAIDS have recently fallen out of favour in fracture care due to animal studies that suggest that they may impede fracture healing. In addition, care should be taken when considering these medications in patients with chronic kidney disease or a history of gastrointestinal bleeding.

Diazepam and other muscle relaxing medications are often underused medications for pain control. Fractures often result in muscle spasm. This is particularly true in patients who have suffered CVA or other neurologic insults in the past. Muscle relaxing medications decrease muscle spasm, which aids in decreasing overall pain. It should be noted, however, that the sedation caused by these medications is additive with narcotics, so care should be exercised that these patients not get over-sedated. Patients with a large anxiety component to their pain may also particularly benefit from this type of medication.

Acetaminophen is another useful medication for pain, and although it is not as powerful as the above medications, it is an alternative for patients sensitive to narcotics.

Overall, the pain control strategy employs two goals. First to adequately control the patient's pain, so they may participate in physical and occupational therapy, and second, to keep the patient as minimally sedated as possible to reduce postoperative delirium and maximize mobilization. Pain control is discussed in detail in Chap. 7.

15.7.3 Evaluation of Physical Capabilities

Postoperatively for any fracture, particularly any lower extremity fracture, the first step toward rehabilitation is evaluation of physical capabilities [6, 20]. When a patient suffers a fracture, there is decreased weight bearing on that extremity that is imposed either by the operating surgeon or by the patient's discomfort. Limitations of joint ROM are also possible, though in the acute phase they are usually as a result of pain instead of true joint contractures. In addition, limited weight bearing and altered gait mechanics require more energy expenditure by patients. In fact, non-weight bearing with crutches for 5 min increases even young patients' heart rates by 53%, and after 10 min anaerobic metabolism occurs to a significant degree. For this reason ambulation in the acute phase may not be feasible in elderly patients with limited weight-bearing status. If this is the case, the patient should be trained to transfer from bed to wheelchair. If the period of non- or limited weight-bearing will be protracted, a customized wheelchair seating system should be considered to avoid decubitus ulcers. Baseline level of function tends to be a good pretest predictor of what level of activity a patient will be capable of in the future. Neurologic conditions such as CVA, brain injury, or Parkinson's disease may be negative predictors of functional return.

Early physical training consists of joint mobilization, muscle strengthening, and ADL assessment and training. Joint mobilization assures adequate ROM and joint excursion during functional activities. Maintaining joint ROM is particularly important in certain intra-articular fractures such as distal femoral fractures. In addition, fractures about the elbow that are operatively repaired are at high risk for stiffness, and should be treated with judicious ROM exercises within the framework of fracture stability and patient tolerance. In the upper extremity, limitation in ROM in one joint can be compensated by other joints; for example, limitation of forearm supination can often be compensated to a certain extent by increased shoulder external rotation. By contrast, in the lower extremity limitations in joint ROM can result in pathologic gait patterns which require increased energy expenditures that the elderly cannot afford [21]. These gait patterns can create uneven wear, because the lower extremity joints are weight bearing, and this can produce an acceleration of DJD.

Muscle strengthening is an integral part of early fracture care. Hip and knee extensor strengthening is essential to activities, such as gait and sit-to-stand manoeuvres. Typically during transfer from a sitting to standing position, the hip extensors and knee extensors are activated to get a patient to a standing position. However, with one-sided injuries of the lower or upper extremity, the patient will have to perform this transfer without the assistance of the other leg or without the assistance of his or her upper extremities, respectively. Therefore, additional strength is required. Similarly, additional strength is required to deal with the altered weight-bearing status associated with lower extremity fractures. Patients also require upper extremity strengthening and endurance in order to negotiate functional situations using assistive devices. Triceps and grip strengthening exercises are useful in this respect.

The ultimate purpose of rehabilitation is to allow a patient to return to their premorbid functional status, or as close to it as possible. In patients with upper extremity fractures, activities such as feeding, toileting, and bathing are of paramount consideration. Since the goals and assistive equipment selected will vary by patient functional needs and limitations, handedness is an important consideration. A variety of assistive equipment is available to aid patients with IADLs in the setting of upper extremity fractures. Fracture braces and splints can also be useful adjuncts. As previously mentioned, ambulation with a limited weight-bearing status comes at an increased metabolic cost, and may be prohibitive to elderly patients, many of whom have cardiac or respiratory co-morbidities. Wheelchair and transfer training must be kept in mind for these patients.

15.8 Follow-Up Care

Fracture patients must follow up with orthopaedic surgery after they leave the acute care hospital. A follow-up care plan must be intact prior to discharge. Periodic X-rays are necessary to monitor for fracture healing, displacement of fragments, and failure of fixation. This information is used to make decisions regarding advancement of weight-bearing status. In addition, close attention should be paid to all surgical incisions and staples should come out when wound healing is apparent, usually in 2–3 weeks. Geriatric medicine should have follow up as well to manage osteoporosis care, fall prevention, all chronic medical issues, and to confirm that no acute issues have been overlooked. Patients who have suffered a fragility fracture should have vitamin D levels, calcium, magnesium, and phosphorus levels checked, and follow up with an endocrinologist. Additionally, these patients should be followed with bone density scans and consideration for bisphosphonate therapy should be given.

15.9 Nursing Home Care

Long-term nursing home patients typically have self-care issues that surpass those of the average patient. Physical and occupational goals are more modest than for patients in skilled nursing facilities or acute rehabilitation facilities. Typically some variety of recreational therapy is employed to promote socialization. Physical therapy consists of modest ambulation and transfer goals, and directed strengthening programs. Occupational therapy consists of directed IADL goals and muscle strengthening related to those goals.

15.10 Skilled Nursing Facility

Patients in skilled nursing facility have the goal of returning home or to some form of independent or modified independent living situation. Thus, goals are slightly more aggressive than nursing home therapy goals. Patients participate in skilled therapy programs for about 2 h/day, and so a prerequisite of admission to skilled nursing facilities is that the patient must be able to tolerate this level of rehabilitation. Physical therapy goals consist of functional mobility training, including gait, transfers, wheelchair training, and functional strengthening related to these functions. Occupational therapy consists of performance of basic IADLs that a patient will need to do when they return home. Social workers at the skilled nursing facility arrange for whatever home care, home therapy, and home equipment needs that the therapy and medical staff deem necessary, and strive to make community re-entry as seamless as possible.

15.11 Acute Rehabilitation

The primary difference between skilled nursing facility care and acute rehabilitation care is the intensity and duration of therapy. Often patients at acute rehabilitation facilities have two to three sessions of physical and occupational therapy per day. This amounts to four or more hours of therapy per day. Obviously, most elderly fracture patients would not be able to tolerate this intensity. It is for this reason, along with various insurance industry-related limitations, that the majority of elderly fracture patients who would enter rehabilitation go to skilled nursing facilities.

Physical and occupational therapy have similar goals to what they would hope to achieve in skilled nursing facilities, but are more aggressive about their pursuit of those goals, and patients who are able to tolerate this level of care often achieve their goals in a shorter time period. Social work also provides a similar function to what they provide at a skilled nursing facility.

15.12 Home and Beyond

The eventual goal of many patients is to return home. To do so, many patients require home equipment such as those pieces mentioned in other parts of this chapter. In some cases, patients require a home assessment. This is particularly true if a patient will have to go home in a wheelchair, and wheelchair accessibility must be assessed. Sometimes patients have wound care needs and require home nursing. Still others require home therapy services that go beyond the acute care or rehabilitation settings. Occasionally, patients will require outpatient physical or occupational therapy to fine-tune their strength and ROM following injury. This takes place after the orthopaedic surgeon provides parameters by which therapy should proceed.

15.13 Conclusion

Fracture rehabilitation in elderly patients is a complex subject that does not lend itself easily to one quick final statement. A team approach is vital in the care of these complex patients. Medical issues are often as important in the rehabilitation of elderly fracture patients as are the implications of the fracture itself. Pain control can often be difficult because of competing issues of comfort and mental agility. If a team approach is employed and basic principles of care are followed, it is possible to reach optimal outcomes in most patient circumstances.

References

1. Brainsky A, Glick H, Lydick E et al. The economic cost of hip fractures in community dwelling older adults: a prospective study. Journal of the American Geriatric Society. 1997; 45: 281–7.
2. Wilkins, K. Health care consequences of falls for seniors. Health Reports. 1999; 10: 47–5.
3. Petrella RJ, Payne M., Myers A., Overend T., Chesworth B. Physical function and fear of falling after hip fracture rehabilitation in the elderly. American Journal of Physical Medicine and Rehabilitation. 2000; 79(2): 154–60
4. Shah MR, Aharonoff GB, Wolinsky P, Zuckerman JD, Koval KJ. Outcome after hip fracture in individuals ninety years of age and older. Journal of Orthopaedic Trauma. 2001; 15(1): 34–9.

5. Youm T, Aharonoff G; Zuckerman JD, Koval KJ. Effect of previous cerebrovascular accident on outcome after hip fracture. Journal of Orthopaedic Trauma. 2000; 14(5): 329–34
6. Hoppenfeld S, Murthy VL. Treatment and Rehabilitation of Fractures. 2000; Lippincott, Williams and Wilkins, Philadelphia.
7. Tiberio D. Evaluation of functional ankle dorsiflexion using subtalar neutral position: a clinical report. Physical Therapy. 1987; 67: 955–7.
8. Edelstein DM, Aharonoff GB, Karp A, Capla EL, Zuckerman JD, Koval KJ. Effect of postoperative delirium on outcome after hip fracture. Clinical Orthopaedics and Related Research. 2004; 42(2): 195–200.
9. Heruti RJ, Lusky A, Barell V, Ohry A, Adunsky A. Cognitive status at admission: does it affect the rehabilitation outcome of elderly patients with hip fracture? Archives of Physical Medicine and Rehabilitation. 1999; 80: 432–6.
10. Ingemarsson AH, Frandin K, Hellstrom K, Rundgren A. Balance function and fall-related efficacy in patients with newly operated hip fracture. Clinical Rehabilitation 2000; 14: 497–505.
11. Arinzon Z, Fidelman Z, Zuta A, Peisakh A, Berner YN. Functional recovery after hip fracture in old-old elderly patients. Archives of Gerontology and Geriatrics. 2005; 40: 327–36.
12. Cameron L, Crotty M, Currie C, et al. Geriatric rehabilitation following fracture in older patients: a systematic review. Health Technology Assessment. 2000; 4(2): 1–107.
13. Diamond TH, Thornley SW, Sekel R, Smerdely P. Hip fracture in elderly men: prognostic factors and outcomes. Medical Journal of Australia. 1997; 167: 412–5.
14. Koval KJ, Skovron ML, Aharonoff GB, Zuckerman JD. Predictors of functional recovery after hip fracture in the elderly. Clinical Orthopaedics and Related Research. 1998; 348: 22–28.
15. Koval KJ, Zuckerman JD. Handbook of Fractures, Third Edition. 2006; Lippincott, Williams and Wilkins, Philadelphia.
16. Adunsky A, Lusky A, Arad M, Heruti RJ. A comparative study of rehabilitation outcomes of elderly hip fracture patients: the advantage of a comprehensive orthogeriatric approach. Journal of Gerontology: Medical Sciences. 2003; 58A(6): 542–7.
17. Stenvall M, Olofsson B, Nyberg L, Lundström M, Gustafson Y. Improved performance in activities of daily living and mobility after a multidisciplinary postoperative rehabilitation in older people with femoral neck fracture: a randomized controlled trial with 1-year follow-up. Journal of Rehabilitation Medicine. 2007; 39: 232–8.
18. Thwaites J, Mann F, Gilchrist N, McKie J, Sainsbury R. Older patients with hip fractures: evaluation of a long-term specialist orthopaedic medicine service in their outcomes. New Zealand Medical Journal. 2007; 120: 1254.
19. Arinzon Z, Gepstein R, Shabat S, Berner Y. Pain perception during the rehabilitation phase following traumatic hip fracture in the elderly is an important prognostic factor and treatment tool. Disability Rehabilitation. 2007; 29(8): 651–8.
20. Laubenthal KN. A quantitative analysis of knee motion during activities of daily living. Physical Therapy. 1972; 52: 34.
21. Waters RL, Mulroy S. The energy expenditure of normal and pathologic gait. Gait and Posture. 1999; 9: 207–31.

Chapter 16
Evaluation of Bone Fragility and Fracture Prevention

Robert J. Pignolo

Abstract Patients with osteoporotic fractures are much more likely to sustain additional fractures; therefore both appropriate treatment and prevention of future fractures (which takes into account the method of injury) need to be addressed. These patients are also much more likely to have underlying secondary causes for bone loss that need to be diagnosed and treated, as well as other multiple risk factors that should be uncovered and modified if possible. Finally, clinical pathways that unite orthopedic surgeons and medical specialists in osteoporosis care are necessary to target patients with osteoporotic fractures for evaluation and treatment.

Keywords Osteoporosis • Risk factor assessment • Bone mineral density • Fragility fracture • Calcium • Vitamin D • Bisphosphonates • Prevention

16.1 Introduction

According to a prevalence report update by the National Osteoporosis Foundation, one in two women and one in four men over age 50 will have an osteoporosis-related fracture in their lifetime, accounting for more than 1.5 million fractures annually [1]. Nationally, a women's risk of hip fracture is equal to her combined risk of breast, uterine, and ovarian cancer [2].

Individuals who sustain fractures may experience pain, dependence, depression, and skeletal deformity [3]. Only about 40% of hip fracture survivors are able to return to their prior level of activities of daily living (ADL), and even fewer (~25%)

R.J. Pignolo (✉)
Departments of Medicine and Orthopaedic Surgery, University of Pennsylvania School of Medicine, 424B Stemmler Hall, 36th Street and Hamilton Walk, Philadelphia, PA 19104-6081, USA
e-mail: pignolo@mail.med.upenn.edu

R.J. Pignolo et al. (eds.), *Fractures in the Elderly*, Aging Medicine,
DOI 10.1007/978-1-60327-467-8_16,

return to their prefracture level for instrumental ADL. Between ~15 and 25% of patients with hip fractures will require institutionalization [1].

Among those hospitalized, up to 95% of fractures in patients greater than 75 years old and 80–90% of fractures in those 60–74 years old are attributable to osteoporosis [4, 5]. However, currently less than 15% of those with recent fragility fractures, defined here as fractures sustained from low-level trauma (such as a fall from standing height), are evaluated and treated for osteoporosis. This is a disquieting statistic given that the risk of future fracture increases 1.5–9.5-fold following a fragility fracture [4, 6, 7].

16.2 General Approach to Evaluating Patients with Osteoporotic Fractures

The approach to the patient with an osteoporotic fracture incorporates the same basic clinical principles as one would undertake in the evaluation of an individual with known or suspected osteoporosis, but with added considerations. Based on current data, the vast majority of patients with fragility and vertebral compression fractures is not likely to get evaluated for underlying causes of bone loss [6, 8–10], and so their presentations should be viewed as opportunities to reduce future morbidity and mortality as well as to preserve function.

16.2.1 Skeletal History

A complete skeletal history includes the history of previous fractures, how they were sustained (traumatic versus minimal trauma), and if delayed fracture healing occurred. A history of multiple falls, even in the absence of previous fracture, should also be obtained. Previous diagnosis of osteoporosis, extent of bone loss, time since initial diagnosis, and previous or current treatments should be explored. Other components of the skeletal history should include inquiries as to the presence of known bone deformities, complaints of bone or musculoskeletal pain, reduced mobility, height loss, and known primary bone disorders. Other details with bearing on bone fidelity and fracture risk is formally obtained by a risk factor assessment.

16.2.2 Risk Factor Assessment

The assessment of risk for continued bone loss and fractures can arbitrarily be divided into categories of personal risk factors, medical conditions known to cause bone loss, and medications that adversely affect mineral metabolism and/or bone turnover. Risk factors associated with osteoporosis are also risk factors for fractures. Independent risk factors for fractures include impaired neuromuscular function, decreased visual acuity, sedative/hypnotic drug use, and frequent falls.

There is a synergistic interaction between bone mineral density (BMD) and risk factors for the prediction of hip fracture [11]. In women, when the number of risk factors exceeds four, there is an increase in the rate of hip fracture at any BMD, representing more than an additive effect. There is also a dramatic rise in hip fracture rate in women with greater than four risk factors who are concomitantly in the lowest third percentile of BMDs, compared to those in the highest third.

Predisposing and precipitating factors also act synergistically, especially in vulnerable individuals, to cause minimal trauma or fragility fractures. For example, a predominantly bed-bound patient with a prior history of fracture, poor nutritional status, low weight, and advanced age (predisposing factors) may sustain a fracture with seemingly benign movements such as transfers out of bed and positional adjustments, or even spontaneously [12].

16.2.2.1 Personal Risk Factors

Many personal risk factors [13, 14], such as family history, personal history of fracture, age, timing of menses and menopause, history of prolonged periods of bed rest (or immobilization), female sex, and race are not modifiable (Table 16.1). However, they are useful to review in order to accurately evaluate an individual's risk for future fracture. As reflected by their inclusion in multiple algorithms that predict the need for BMD testing, age and body weight, as well as lifetime exposure to estrogen in women, are among the most important personal risk factors [15–20].

Table 16.1 Major personal risk factors associated with osteoporosis

Family history of osteoporosis or fracture
Lifelong low calorie intake
Personal history of fracture as an adult
Poor health/frailty
Increasing age
Immobilization/prolonged bed rest
Early menopause (<45 years old)
Late menarche (>16 years old)
History of amenorrhea or irregular menstrual periods
Thin body frame or low body weight
Tallness
Sedentary lifestyle
Calcium/vitamin D deficient diet
Female sex
Heavy alcohol use
White or Asian ancestry
Cigarette smoking, especially current

Immobilization, especially in the form of bed rest greater than 1 week, is also a significant personal risk factor for substantial bone loss (see Sect. 16.6.6). Weightlessness, as experienced by astronauts, is an extreme example, but this situation is approximated on earth by prolonged bed rest, spinal cord injury or stroke, and by other situations where immobilization occurs.

Although osteoporosis and fractures are less common in men due to their larger skeletons, bone loss starting later in life, slower progression, and the absence of a rapid phase of bone loss as occurs in menopause, men have much higher mortality and chronic disability rates after a hip fracture [21]. They are also more likely to have a secondary cause of bone loss compared to women. Thus, although being female is a personal risk factor for osteoporosis and fracture, this does not exclude males from being at increased risk.

16.2.2.2 Medical Conditions

As illustrated in Table 16.2, a number of co-existing or past medical conditions can predispose older individuals to continued bone loss [22]. Although elderly patients are not a priori excluded from any predisposing condition, they are unlikely to present with genetic conditions that otherwise would present much earlier in life or limit life expectancy. Conversely, there are predisposing medical conditions that are more likely to contribute to bone loss because of advanced age, such as vitamin D deficiency, postmenopausal status, and chronic kidney disease.

16.2.2.3 Medications

Bone loss attributable to medication use is common [23, 24], especially in the elderly. However, the extent to which evidence supports a clear etiological role for

Table 16.2 Secondary medical conditions that alter bone turnover and mineral homeostasis

Endocrine	Hyperthyroidism, hyperparathyroidism, Cushing's syndrome, diabetes mellitus, prolactinoma, estrogen deficiency, hypogonadism (men)
Rheumatologic	Rheumatoid arthritis, ankylosing spondylitis, idiopathic scoliosis, sarcoidosis
Gastrointestinal/nutritional	Malabsorption, hepatobiliary dysfunction, vitamin D deficiency, parenteral nutrition
Hematological/oncological	Mastocytosis, hemolytic anemia, malignancy (general)
Renal	Idiopathic hypercalciuria (on low calcium diet), renal osteodystrophy
Psychiatric	Eating disorders (anorexia, bulimia), depression
Other	Paget's disease, amyloidosis, epidermolysis bullosa, hemochromotosis, hypophosphatasia, multiple sclerosis

Note that genetic conditions which predispose to osteoporosis and fracture are intentionally omitted because they are rare in the elderly

Table 16.3 Major pharmacologic causes of secondary osteoporosis

Glucocorticoids	Anticonvulsants
Lithium	Tamoxifen (premenopausal)
Antacids (chronic use)	Vitamin A, excessive intake
Prolonged anticoagulation	Methotrexate
Gonadotropin-releasing hormone	Antidepressants
Agonist or antagonist	Excessive thyroid supplementation
Phenothiazines	Aluminum-containing medications
Cytotoxic drugs (chemotherapy)	Immunosuppressive therapy
Proton-pump inhibitors	

certain medications is variable. A list of medications with clear contributions to bone loss is shown in Table 16.3. Glucocorticoid-induced osteoporosis [25] and bone loss due to immunosuppressive therapy after solid organ transplant [26] remain challenging problems.

16.3 Physical Exam

The physical examination is focused on detecting the sequelae of osteoporosis (fractures), secondary medical causes of bone loss, and an initial assessment of fall risk. In the absence of exam findings for vertebral compression fractures or occult nonvertebral fractures, physical signs cannot confirm the diagnosis of osteoporosis.

16.3.1 Detection of Vertebral Fractures and Occult Nonvertebral Fractures

Physical findings that support the diagnosis of vertebral fractures include the presence of kyphosis (Dowager's hump) where strict upright posture becomes impossible [27]. This is accompanied by height loss, and depending on severity, narrowed gapping between the ribs and ilium with or without 12th rib resting on the iliac crest. Other suggestive findings include a protruding abdomen, paravertebral muscle spasm, and vertebral tenderness. Pulmonary volume loss due to anterior wedging of spine may be approximated by assessment of diaphragmatic excursion or by estimation of chest expansion by palpation. Nonspecific complaints of abdominal distension, constipation, early satiety, or frequent belching may also be associated with signs of vertebral compression fractures on physical exam.

Occult nonvertebral fractures may be accompanied by bony tenderness and difficulty with weight bearing as well as joint positioning or movement. Multiple chapters in this volume address the spectrum of common fractures in the older adult.

16.3.2 Secondary Medical Causes of Bone Loss

The number of medical disorders that can cause bone loss precludes any complete description of physical exam findings for each condition. However, examples of obvious signs to prompt further inquiry include the bony deformities of rheumatoid arthritis, stigmata of chronic alcoholism and liver disease, scars suggesting thyroid or parathyroid surgery, and skin changes consistent with particular endocrinopathies.

16.3.3 Assessment of Fall Risk

A minimal fall assessment on physical exam should include the ability to rise from a chair without using the upper extremities, measurement of resting pulse, gross visual testing, walking facility, and heel-to-toe ambulation. Difficulty in rising from a chair without the use of the arms, a resting pulse > 80, poor visual acuity, and gait dysfunction, including imbalance, all suggest increased fall risk. Chapter 3 elaborates on the details of assessment.

16.4 Laboratory Testing

The primary purpose of screening laboratory studies in the initial work-up of patients with osteoporotic fractures is to rule out medical causes of secondary bone loss (Fig. 16.1). Serum electrolytes, liver and kidney function tests, albumin, total protein, calcium, intact PTH, 25(OH) vitamin D, phosphorus, magnesium, thyroid-stimulating hormone, serum testosterone (in men), and a complete blood count serve to eliminate most secondary causes of bone loss or suggest further studies. If screening lab tests are unrevealing and there are no obvious contributing medical conditions by history or exam, a 24-h collection for urinary calcium, sodium, and creatinine may be helpful. A low 24-h urinary calcium suggests vitamin D deficiency, osteomalacia, or malnutrition (e.g., celiac sprue). High urinary calcium suggests renal tubular calcium leak, absorptive hypercalciuria, high sodium diet, or excessive bone resorption secondary to malignancy, hyperparathyroidism, hyperthyroidism, or Paget's disease.

Although the approach to screening lab studies in elderly patients with osteoporosis should be individualized, attempts have been made to assess the yield of testing to identify secondary causes of bone loss in otherwise healthy postmenopausal women. In women without a history of diseases or medications known to adversely affect bone, 32% had disorders of calcium metabolism (hypercalciuria, malabsorption, hyperparathyroidism, vitamin D deficiency) [28]. Measurement of 24-h urine calcium, serum calcium, PTH, and TSH (in those on thyroid replacement) would

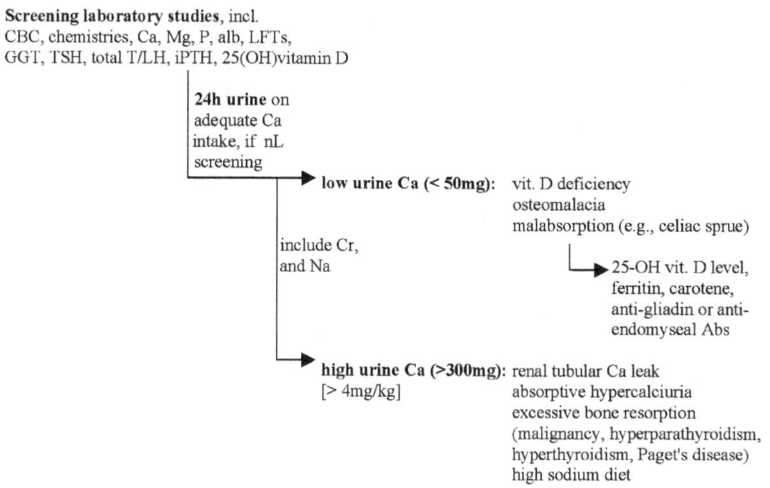

Fig. 16.1 Use of screening laboratory testing to detect secondary causes of bone loss. *CBC* complete blood count; *Ca* calcium; *Mg* magnesium; *P* phosphate; *alb* albumin; *LFTs* liver function tests; *GGT* gamma-glutamyltranspeptidase; *TSH* thyroid stimulating hormone; *T* testosterone; *LH* leutinizing hormone; *iPTH* intact parathyroid hormone; *nL* normal; *Na* sodium; *vit.* vitamin; *Abs* antibodies

have been sufficient to diagnose 85% of underlying causes in this group [28]. In another study, except for measurement of TSH, routine laboratory tests were not found to be useful [29].

In patients at high risk for subsequent fracture, more specialized tests should also be considered based on clinical suspicion, including serum and urine protein electrophoresis, and a 24-h urinary free cortisol or an overnight dexamethasone suppression test. Markers of bone turnover, including various collagen breakdown products, may also serve to distinguish between high and low turnover bone loss. Bone biopsy is not routinely performed in the setting of fracture repair and currently has little practical value in dictating treatment.

16.5 Bone Mineral Density Testing

Dual-energy X-ray absorptiometry (DXA) is currently the gold standard for measurement of BMD. After a fragility fracture, however, measurement of BMD is not necessary to make the diagnosis of osteoporosis. Because bone strength is determined by mineral content as well as bone microarchitecture, and deficits in both of these structural determinants increase the likelihood of fracture, any minimal trauma fracture confirms the clinical diagnosis of osteoporosis regardless of BMD score. However, current T-scores are useful to establish a baseline for purposes of monitoring treatment efficacy and should be performed as part of the initial evaluation after a fragility fracture. Relative BMD at nonfracture sites also provides important information about risk of fracture at these locations. A very low Z-score may indicate either the failure to obtain adequate peak bone mass during an individual's formative years or the presence of secondary cause(s) that have contributed to bone loss.

DXA and similar radiographic techniques only provide information about BMD and do not evaluate bone microarchitecture. The near future of bone imaging awaits MRI-based techniques that can be used to construct 3D volumes, akin to virtual bone biopsies, which can be sampled repeatedly in time and in the identical location. For example, the same trabecular bone volume was measured before and after treatment of a hypogonadal man with testosterone to demonstrate a 33% increase in surface-to-curve ratio and 22% decrease in erosion index, results which suggested microarchitectural improvement in response to treatment [30]. Application of this technology to fracture care and prevention will be tremendous.

16.6 Treatments and Prevention

The treatment of osteoporosis as the major cause of fragility fractures requires a multipronged approach: changing modifiable personal risk factors, management of secondary medical causes of bone loss, reduction or elimination of medications that adversely affect mineral homeostasis and bone turnover, improving fall and injury risk, and initiating pharmacological and nonpharmacological interventions that increase bone mass and improve skeletal structural fidelity (Fig. 16.2). Prevention of subsequent fractures requires the early identification and evaluation of patients that sustain an initial fragility fracture, adequate and sustained treatment and monitoring of osteoporosis, as well as environmental and activity modifications that address the circumstances and mechanics of the presenting fracture.

It is sometimes helpful to qualify the type of bone loss as high- or low-turnover, as a general approach to select pharmacological agents for minimizing further bone loss and recouping lost bone. High-turnover conditions, where bone resorption exceeds bone formation, such as hypogonadism, thyrotoxicosis, hyperparathyroidism, conditions of cytokine excess, skeletal metastases, Paget's disease, rheumatoid arthritis, and periodonitis, may be best treated with agents that inhibit the resorptive process. Low-turnover conditions, including aging, disuse, and steroid-induced osteoporosis may be most responsive to anabolic agents.

16.6.1 Fragility Fracture Clinical Pathways

Despite convincing research that has detailed the relationship between osteoporosis, fragility fractures, morbidity and mortality, there continues to be a significant gap between known guidelines and actual treatment algorithms [8, 31].

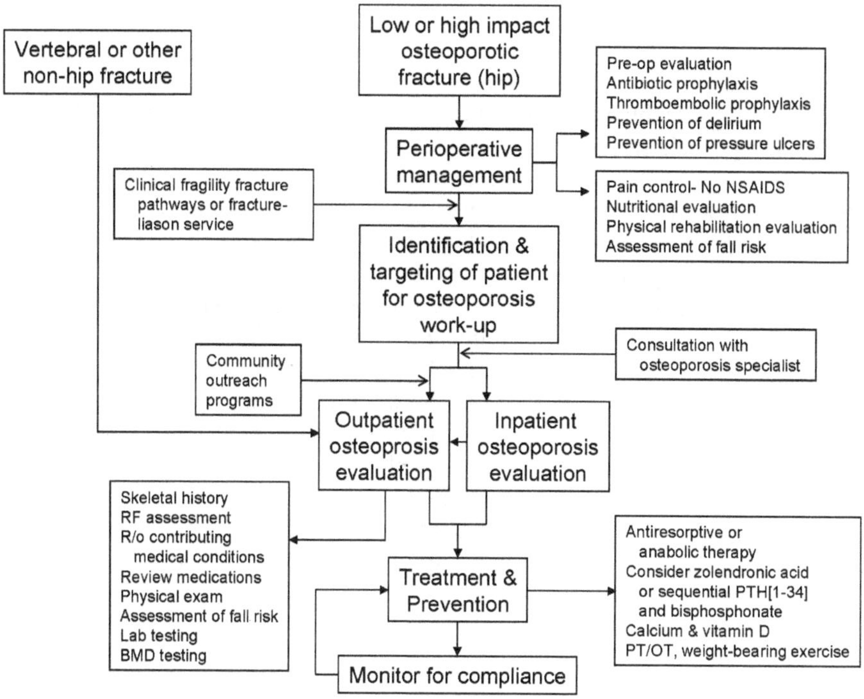

Fig. 16.2 Algorithmic approach to the patient with osteoporotic fracture. *RF* risk factor; *NSAIDS* nonsteroidal anti-inflammatory agents; *BMD* bone mineral density; *PTH* parathyroid hormone; *PT* physical therapy; *OT* occupational therapy; *R/o* rule out

Osteoporosis prevention and treatment guidelines are among the standards proposed by the National Committee of Quality Assurance. The American Academy of Orthopaedic Surgeons (AAOS), in its "Recommendations on Enhancing the Care of Patients with Fragility Fractures" has established recommendations for the care of persons with fractures that recognize the need for high quality prevention and postsurgery medical care [6]. Among these recommendations are the following: (1) consider osteoporosis as a predisposing factor; (2) advise patients that evaluation and treatment of osteoporosis can reduce the risk of future fractures; (3) initiate an investigation of osteoporosis; (4) establish partnerships within the medical community to facilitate evaluation and treatment; and (5) establish clinical pathways that ensure optimal care.

Recent studies have shown that dedicated interdisciplinary collaboration among orthopedic surgeons, medical specialists in metabolic bone disease, screening coordinators, nurse educators, and information technologists can play important roles in improving osteoporosis care and therefore potentially help decrease the risk of subsequent fragility fractures [32–37]. The national demand for improved quality of care of older adults aligns with this interdisciplinary collaboration between the medical, surgical, and other specialties.

Barriers to initiating treatment of patients who have or are at risk for osteoporosis exist and must be overcome. They include lack of patient and primary physician knowledge of the subject, lack of awareness and use of current osteoporosis guidelines, the perception by orthopedic surgeons that evaluation and treatment of osteoporosis is not their responsibility, cost of therapy, time and cost of diagnosing osteoporosis, side effects of medications, confusion about medications or their effectiveness, complex medical conditions in elderly patients, reluctance of elderly patients to add more medications, lack of access to BMD testing, and lack of time to address secondary prevention [34, 38]. Even if these barriers are overcome, the clinical challenge still remains that a proportion of patients, even when followed by dedicated interdisciplinary teams, refracture in spite of being placed on osteoporosis treatment after their incident fracture [39]. Patients who are likely to refracture are older, are more likely to sustain another hip fracture after an incident hip fracture, and are likely to refracture early, particularly when the incident fracture is of the hip; they are often already on treatment for osteoporosis. This underscores the importance of not only identifying these high-risk patients, but offering them a combined approach of early drug treatment through an interdisciplinary approach as well as interventions aimed at reducing any reversible predisposition to falls or other environmental risk factors.

16.6.2 Calcium, Vitamin D, and Nutritional Considerations

Adequate calcium and vitamin D intake from diet and supplementation is an essential part of osteoporosis care and fracture prevention. Clinical trials that have evaluated many of the currently available osteoporosis therapies included calcium and vitamin D supplementation in both the treatment and control groups, thus requiring that patients who receive these therapies also be calcium and vitamin D replete to achieve the same or similar efficacies as study subjects.

There is a decline in calcium absorption with age, likely attributable to vitamin D insufficiency or deficiency. Vitamin D insufficiency is a frequent finding among community-dwelling elderly and practically ubiquitous in the institutionalized elderly [40]. Risk factors for vitamin D depletion in the elderly include deprivation of sunlight, poor nutrition, age-related changes in skin and renal function, darker pigmentation, living at higher latitudes, community-dwelling status, institutionalized status, and previous hip fractures. There is a positive correlation between 25(OH) vitamin D levels and BMD, with the risk of fractures increased at values <30 ng/ml [41].

Calcium supplementation alone slightly lowers the risk of vertebral but not nonvertebral fractures [42]. Calcium alone does not lower fracture risk in patients with prior fracture, even after about 4 years of supplementation [43]. However, supplemental vitamin D appears to reduce fracture risk when taken in doses sufficient to keep serum 25(OH) vitamin D levels above about 32.5 ng/ml. In trials where 25(OH) vitamin D levels were measured, fracture risk reduction tended to be directly proportional to circulating levels [44]. Fracture risk reduction is thought to be related to the effects of vitamin D on both muscle and bone. Optimal therapeutic benefit is achieved with combined calcium plus vitamin D supplementation and when supplementation exceeds minimum doses [45].

Among other nutritional interventions, dietary protein appears to be an important factor for continued bone health. Age-related bone loss is inversely related to protein consumption [46], an effect that is associated with adequate calcium and vitamin D intake [47]. Although high protein consumption had been considered potentially detrimental to bone due to increases in urinary calcium, this appears not to have an effect on bone turnover [48]. Protein intake of about 1 g/kg body weight/day has been shown to improve patient outcomes posthip fracture, and serum albumin levels appear to be a very reliable predictor of survival after fracture. [49–51]. Thus, adequate dietary protein intake and protein supplementation, with the possible exceptions of those with chronic kidney disease or history of nephrolithiasis, should be prescribed for patients with osteoporosis and previous fracture.

Similar concerns have been raised about the effects of excessive intake of sodium, caffeine, phosphorus, and sugar causing increased urinary calcium losses and altered calcium homeostasis that contribute to bone loss. Although urinary calcium losses are usually followed by reduced renal calcium clearance [52, 53], this may not be efficiently accomplished in the elderly. Further, the beverage sources for caffeine, phosphorus, and sugar usually qualify as being of low nutrient density (LND), and as such, their consumption is often a poor substitute for more calcium- and protein-rich drinks. The recommendation of reduced intake of LND beverages in patients at risk for continued bone loss appears to have merit.

16.6.3 Bisphosphonates

With the exception of once-yearly infusions of zoledronic acid [54], no other controlled clinical trial has to date shown utility in the secondary prevention of fractures. Despite this, oral bisphosphonates are routinely used as standard of care in patients suffering an incident fracture. High rates of refracture may thus be related to the form of bisphosphonate given, but more likely to nonadherence to bisphosphonates due to side effects or to lack of receiving optimal care (including any osteoporosis treatment).

There has long been the theoretical concern that bisphosphonates may contribute to poor fracture healing by inhibiting osteoclast-initiated bone remodeling, especially if given early after fracture. Lyles et al. [54] has shown that this is unlikely to be the case. The risk of hypocalcemia, especially after IV bisphosphonate use, can be avoided by repleting low vitamin D stores common among older adults and particularly in elderly patients who present with hip fracture.

Another potential concern is that the long-term use of bisphosphonates will result in oversuppression of bone remodeling and actually predispose one to fracture [55–57]. Although this is likely to be the case in a subpopulation of patients with a history of long-term bisphosphonate use, it remains unclear how these individuals can be routinely identified. Long-term safety and continued efficacy of alendronate were reported in individuals after as many as 10 years of use [58–60].

The choice of bisphosphonate should be made on the basis of known efficacy data, medical conditions such as gastrointestinal reflux disease that may limit or preclude their use or form, previous medication use for treatment of osteoporosis, major known or suspected cause of osteoporosis, patient adherence factors, and patient preference. Oral and IV bisphosphonates tend to be well tolerated in patients with mild or moderate chronic kidney disease.

Carefully chosen and monitored, the side effects of bisphosphonates can be minimized. Gastrointestinal upset due to esophageal irritation is probably the most common complaint with use of oral bisphosphonates, although this is reduced by following proper instructions for administration by mouth and potentially by increasing the dosing interval.

16.6.4 Estrogens and Selective Estrogen Receptor Modulators

It is clear that estrogen replacement in postmenopausal women, with or without a progestin, reduces vertebral and nonvertebral fractures. The use of hormone and estrogen therapy for this purpose, however, has been limited due to adverse outcomes observed in the Women's Health Initiative (WHI) study [61–63]. Therapy with estrogen plus progesterone was associated with an increased risk of deep venous thrombosis (DVT), pulmonary embolism (PE), stroke, myocardial infarction, and breast cancer. Estrogen therapy alone was associated with an increase in the risk of DVT, PE, and stroke.

Although current guidelines suggest that hormone replacement be used primarily for treatment of menopausal symptoms and for the shortest period of time necessitated for symptom relief, the role of estrogen alone or in combination with a progestin is still far from being adequately defined. In specific populations, such as early postmenopausal women, and under specific regimens, such as low dose estrogen or forms other than conjugated equine estrogens, the risk–benefit ratios for the use of hormones may be different than that seen in the WHI study. Estrogen replacement may currently be considered for osteoporosis treatment after all other alternatives have been considered and when all risks and benefits are fully discussed with the patient.

Selective estrogen receptor modulators, such as raloxifene, increase BMD at the spine and hip, but only reduce the incidence of vertebral fractures and not hip or other nonvertebral fractures [64, 65]. Among the adverse events that are associated with both estrogen and tamoxifen, including DVT, gallbladder disease, endometrial cancer, and cataracts, raloxifene is associated with a higher relative risk for DVT, but not other adverse events [66]. Raloxifene may be considered for use in combination with other medications in selected women with or at risk for vertebral fractures.

16.6.5 Teriparatide and Other PTH Analogues

As the only FDA-approved anabolic agent for bone loss, teriparatide or PTH (1-34) confers a reduction of vertebral and nonvertebral fractures in high risk individuals [67–70]. PTH analogues may also decrease the risk of subsequent fractures in those with severe osteoporosis, vertebral compression fractures, or with other osteoporosis-related fractures, although at present long-term data is lacking. Teriparatide and other PTH analogues may also be useful for individuals who have been on prior antiresorptive therapy, but who have had fractures or continued bone loss despite treatment.

Studies on combination or sequential therapy in previously untreated women and men, where PTH analogues were combined with or followed alendronate treatment, have produced results suggesting no clear benefit to any permutation [68, 71, 72]. Prior long-term alendronate treatment might diminish, but does not eliminate BMD accrual induced by PTH analogues [73, 74]. It is likely that BMD is lost in individuals who do not take antiresorptive agents after cessation of PTH analogues, and that antiresorptive therapy can maintain or further increase PTH-induced gains [72, 75–80].

The combination of PTH (1-34) and hormone replacement results in increased BMD in the spine and to a lesser extent in the hip [75, 81]. Similar results were obtained when teriparatide was combined with raloxifene [82]. The applicability of these findings to fracture prevention is unclear.

All PTH analogues should be avoided in those with an elevated risk for osteosarcoma, including individuals with a history of Paget's disease, irradiation, or unexplained elevations in alkaline phosphatase. Other contraindications include metastatic bone cancer, multiple myeloma, hyperparathyroidism, and hypercalcemia. Treatment with teriparatide is limited to a 2-year course due to concerns over the possibility of osteosarcoma; however, no substantiated case of osteosarcoma has been reported to date [83, 84].

16.6.6 Physical Activity and Exercise

Physical activity is a critically important strategy to reduce osteoporosis and fractures in the elderly. It is well established that increases in BMD or reductions in bone loss occur with sufficient exercise or mechanical loading [85, 86].

A careful history in osteoporotic patients, particularly those who fracture, often reveals failure to optimize skeletal size and strength during the formative years as a result of poor diet and inactivity. Despite potentially missed opportunities to maintain a strong skeleton into adulthood and old age, and minimizing bone loss in peri-menopausal years and later life, physical activity and exercise at virtually any age can still increase BMD and potentially reduce fracture risk with minimal therapeutic harm [86–88].

Mechanical loading, in general, improves bone quality and quantity. However, studies in humans and in animals suggest that physical activity and exercise strategies that allow adequate rest periods between skeletal loads, limit loading cycles to avoid bone desensitization, and incorporate low-level strain protocols can potentially maximize bone formation in patients with osteoporosis [89–91]. Physical rehabilitation after fracture aims at increasing strength and mobility to reduce falls, maintain or build BMD, and in the case of vertebral fracture, at decreasing kyphotic posture [92]. Newer physical modalities, such as whole body vibration, may offer future prospects of nonpharmacologic treatment regimens for fracture prevention [93].

Prolonged bed rest or severely reduced physical activity causes devastating atrophy of trabecular and cortical bone, as well as declines in numerous body systems. BMD may decline as much as 1–2% per week in both weight- and nonweight-bearing bones, with little or unpredictable recoup after re-initiation of ambulation [94–96]. Thus, to the extent possible, bed rest and reduced physical activity should be minimized in patients with a prior history of fracture.

16.6.7 Prevention

Prevention of future fractures begins with in-hospital medical evaluation at the time of the incident fracture, particularly of the hip, spine, and wrist. Because osteoporosis increases the risk of fracture from both low- and high-impact trauma, evaluation should be pursued in both settings [97]. This initial evaluation includes referral of the patient to an osteoporosis specialist for evaluation and treatment, which can be as part of a fragility fracture pathway (see above), as part of a targeted outreach program to primary care physicians [98], or as inpatient or outpatient direct consultations to endocrinologists, rheumatologists, geriatricians, or other specialists with training in bone disorders. In-hospital medical management aimed at prevention should also include adequate pain control without NSAID use, nutritional evaluation with recommendations for adequate protein intake, and initiation of physical rehabilitation.

Prevention strategies in the outpatient setting should incorporate pharmacologic treatment with antiresorptive or anabolic agents, optimal calcium and vitamin D intake, treatment of secondary medical causes of bone loss, approaches to reduce modifiable risk factors, and physical rehabilitation that includes a fall assessment and prescribed exercise for strength, balance, and mobility. Weight bearing and other exercises should be tailored to the individual. Education, environmental modifications, and specific aids should be also be prescribed, ideally by a multidisciplinary team. Hip protectors may not be an effective physical aid to prevent future fracture, both for long-term adherence issues and data suggesting that they are not effective in some populations [98, 99]. Patient adherence to pharmacologic therapy, exercise and dietary regimens, as well as environmental and safety concerns should be regularly monitored.

A new conceptual approach to prevention involves the prophylactic fixation of unfractured hips at the time of the initial hip fracture [100]. Given a 10% risk of breaking the noninvolved hip after a documented hip fracture, it may actually be cost effective to treat the unfractured hip prophylactically, as opposed to waiting until a second hip fracture occurs on the unaffected side. This proposal will remain controversial given the potential for an added operative risk of "fixing" a second hip, difficulty in choosing who would most benefit from a second prophylactic fixation, and perhaps the temptation to avoid or postpone treatment of underlying causes of bone loss that would affect the entire skeletal.

References

1. National Osteoporosis Foundation. America's bone health: The state of osteoporosis and low bone mass in our nation. 2002; Washington, DC: National Osteoporosis Foundation.
2. Riggs BL, Melton LJ 3rd. The worldwide problem of osteoporosis: insights afforded by epidemiology. Bone 1995; 17:505S–11S.
3. Brenneman SK, Barrett-Connor E, Sajjan S, Markson LE, Siris ES. Impact of recent fracture on health-related quality of life in postmenopausal women. J Bone Miner Res 2006; 21:809–16.
4. Klotzbuecher CM, Ross PD, Landsman PB, Abbott TA 3rd, Berger M. Patients with prior fractures have an increased risk of future fractures: a summary of the literature and statistical synthesis. J Bone Miner Res 2000; 15:721–39.
5. van Staa TP, Leufkens HG, Cooper C. Does a fracture at one site predict later fractures at other sites? A British cohort study. Osteoporos Int 2002; 13:624–9.
6. Bouxsein ML, Kaufman J, Tosi L, Cummings S, Lane J, Johnell O. Recommendations for optimal care of the fragility fracture patient to reduce the risk of future fracture. J Am Acad Orthop Surg 2004; 12:385–95.
7. Center JR, Bliuc D, Nguyen TV, Eisman JA. Risk of subsequent fracture after low-trauma fracture in men and women. JAMA 2007; 297:387–94.
8. Siris ES, Bilezikian JP, Rubin MR, Black DM, Bockman RS, Bone HG, et al. Pins and plaster aren't enough: a call for the evaluation and treatment of patients with osteoporotic fractures. J Clin Endocrinol Metab 2003; 88:3482–6.
9. Delmas PD, van de Langerijt L, Watts NB, Eastell R, Genant H, Grauer A, et al. Underdiagnosis of vertebral fractures is a worldwide problem: the IMPACT study. J Bone Miner Res 2005; 20:557–63.
10. Freedman KB, Kaplan FS, Bilker WB, Strom BL, Lowe RA. Treatment of osteoporosis: are physicians missing an opportunity? J Bone Joint Surg Am 2000; 82-A:1063–70.
11. Cummings SR, Nevitt MC, Browner WS, Stone K, Fox KM, Ensrud KE, et al. Risk factors for hip fracture in white women. Study of Osteoporotic Fractures Research Group. N Engl J Med 1995; 332:767–73.
12. Galabova V, Steiner E, Carson L, Schwab EP, Pignolo RJ. Spectrum of minimal trauma fractures. J Am Geriatr Soc 2004; 52:S23–24, Abstract.
13. Anonymous. Osteoporosis prevention, diagnosis, and therapy. JAMA 2001; 285:785–95.
14. Robbins J, Aragaki AK, Kooperberg C, Watts N, Wactawski-Wende J, Jackson RD, et al. Factors associated with 5-year risk of hip fracture in postmenopausal women. JAMA 2007; 298:2389–98.
15. Cadarette SM, Jaglal SB, Murray TM, McIsaac WJ, Joseph L, Brown JP. Evaluation of decision rules for referring women for bone densitometry by dual-energy x-ray absorptiometry. JAMA 2001; 286:57–63.

16. Cadarette SM, Jaglal SB, Kreiger N, McIsaac WJ, Darlington GA, Tu JV. Development and validation of the Osteoporosis Risk Assessment Instrument to facilitate selection of women for bone densitometry. CMAJ 2000; 162:1289–94.
17. Geusens P, Hochberg MC, van der Voort DJ, Pols H, van der Klift M, Siris E, et al. Performance of risk indices for identifying low bone density in postmenopausal women. Mayo Clin Proc 2002; 77:629–37.
18. Lydick E, Cook K, Turpin J, Melton M, Stine R, Byrnes C. Development and validation of a simple questionnaire to facilitate identification of women likely to have low bone density. Am J Manag Care 1998; 4:37–48.
19. Koh LK, Sedrine WB, Torralba TP, Kung A, Fujiwara S, Chan SP, et al. A simple tool to identify Asian women at increased risk of osteoporosis. Osteoporos Int 2001; 12:699–705.
20. Sedrine WB, Chevallier T, Zegels B, Kvasz A, Micheletti MC, Gelas B, et al. Development and assessment of the Osteoporosis Index of Risk (OSIRIS) to facilitate selection of women for bone densitometry. Gynecol Endocrinol 2002; 16:245–50.
21. Center JR, Nguyen TV, Schneider D, Sambrook PN, Eisman JA. Mortality after all major types of osteoporotic fracture in men and women: an observational study. Lancet 1999; 353:878–82.
22. Fitzpatrick LA. Secondary causes of osteoporosis. Mayo Clin Proc 2002; 77:453–68.
23. Lawson J. Drug-induced metabolic bone disorders. Semin Musculoskelet Radiol 2002; 6:285–97.
24. Bannwarth B. Drug-induced musculoskeletal disorders. Drug Saf 2007; 30:27–46.
25. Canalis E, Mazziotti G, Giustina A, Bilezikian JP. Glucocorticoid-induced osteoporosis: pathophysiology and therapy. Osteoporos Int 2007; 18:1319–28.
26. Cohen A, Shane E. Osteoporosis after solid organ and bone marrow transplantation. Osteoporos Int 2003; 14:617–30.
27. Green AD, Colon-Emeric CS, Bastian L, Drake MT, Lyles KW. Does this woman have osteoporosis? JAMA 2004; 292:2890–900.
28. Tannenbaum C, Clark J, Schwartzman K, Wallenstein S, Lapinski R, Meier D, et al. Yield of laboratory testing to identify secondary contributors to osteoporosis in otherwise healthy women. J Clin Endocrinol Metab 2002; 87:4431–7.
29. Jamal SA, Leiter RE, Bayoumi AM, Bauer DC, Cummings SR. Clinical utility of laboratory testing in women with osteoporosis. Osteoporos Int 2005; 16:534–40.
30. Benito M, Vasilic B, Wehrli FW, Bunker B, Wald M, Gomberg B, et al. Effect of testosterone replacement on trabecular architecture in hypogonadal men. J Bone Miner Res 2005; 20:1785–91.
31. Bellantonio S, Fortinsky R, Prestwood K. How well are community-living women treated for osteoporosis after hip fracture? J Am Geriatr Soc 2001; 49:1197–204.
32. Chevalley T, Hoffmeyer P, Bonjour JP, Rizzoli R. An osteoporosis clinical pathway for the medical management of patients with low-trauma fracture. Osteoporos Int 2002; 13:450–5.
33. McLellan AR, Gallacher SJ, Fraser M, McQuillian C. The fracture liaison service: success of a program for the evaluation and management of patients with osteoporotic fracture. Osteoporos Int 2003; 14:1028–34.
34. Bogoch ER, Elliot-Gibson V, Beaton DE, Jamal SA, Josse RG, Murray TM. Effective initiation of osteoporosis diagnosis and treatment for patients with a fragility fracture in an orthopaedic environment. J Bone Joint Surg Am 2006; 88:25–34.
35. Elliot-Gibson VIM, Jain RJF, Beaton1 DE, Bogoch ER, Richie S, F. Samji F. Osteoporosis post-fracture screening program. J Bone Miner Res 2007; 22:S311, Abstract.
36. Nanci V, Berry G, Harvey E, Goltzman D, Morin SN. A novel integrated approach to the management of patients following hip fracture: The Hip Fracture Integrated Intervention Program (HIIP). J Bone Miner Res 2007; 22:S312, Abstract.
37. Glowacki J, Harris MB, Simon JB, Kolatkar NS, Thornhill TS, LeBoff MS. Osteoporosis care pathways for hospital patients with fragility fractures: a paradigm shift. J Bone Miner Res 2007; 22:S334, Abstract.

38. Skedros JG, Holyoak JD, Pitts TC. Knowledge and opinions of orthopaedic surgeons concerning medical evaluation and treatment of patients with osteoporotic fracture. J Bone Joint Surg Am 2006; 88:18–24.
39. Langridge CR, McQuillian C, Watson WS, Walker B, Mitchell L, Gallacher SJ. Refracture following fracture liaison service assessment illustrates the requirement for integrated falls and fracture services. Calcif Tissue Int 2007; 81:85–91.
40. Gloth FM 3rd, Gundberg CM, Hollis BW, Haddad JG Jr, Tobin JD. Vitamin D deficiency in homebound elderly persons. JAMA 1995; 274:1683–6.
41. Ooms ME, Lips P, Roos JC, van der Vijgh WJ, Popp-Snijders C, Bezemer PD, et al. Vitamin D status and sex hormone binding globulin: determinants of bone turnover and bone mineral density in elderly women. J Bone Miner Res 1995; 10:1177–84.
42. Shea B, Wells G, Cranney A, Zytaruk N, Robinson V, Griffith L, et al. Meta-analyses of therapies for postmenopausal osteoporosis. VII. Meta-analysis of calcium supplementation for the prevention of postmenopausal osteoporosis. Endocr Rev 2002; 23:552–9.
43. Grant AM, Avenell A, Campbell MK, McDonald AM, MacLennan GS, McPherson GC, et al. Oral vitamin D3 and calcium for secondary prevention of low-trauma fractures in elderly people (randomised evaluation of calcium or vitamin D, RECORD): a randomised placebo-controlled trial. Lancet 2005; 365:1621–8.
44. Bischoff-Ferrari HA, Willett WC, Wong JB, Giovannucci E, Dietrich T, Dawson-Hughes B. Fracture prevention with vitamin D supplementation: a meta-analysis of randomized controlled trials. JAMA 2005; 293:2257–64.
45. Tang BM, Eslick GD, Nowson C, Smith C, Bensoussan A. Use of calcium or calcium in combination with vitamin D supplementation to prevent fractures and bone loss in people aged 50 years and older: a meta-analysis. Lancet 2007; 370:657–66.
46. Hannan MT, Tucker KL, Dawson-Hughes B, Cupples LA, Felson DT, Kiel DP. Effect of dietary protein on bone loss in elderly men and women: the Framingham Osteoporosis Study. J Bone Miner Res 2000; 15:2504–12.
47. Dawson-Hughes B, Harris SS. Calcium intake influences the association of protein intake with rates of bone loss in elderly men and women. Am J Clin Nutr 2002; 75:773–9.
48. Carter JD, Vasey FB, Valeriano J. The effect of a low-carbohydrate diet on bone turnover. Osteoporos Int 2006; 17:1398–403.
49. Delmi M, Rapin CH, Bengoa JM, Delmas PD, Vasey H, Bonjour JP. Dietary supplementation in elderly patients with fractured neck of the femur. Lancet 1990; 335:1013–6.
50. Rico H, Revilla M, Villa LF, Hernandez ER, Fernandez JP. Crush fracture syndrome in senile osteoporosis: a nutritional consequence? J Bone Miner Res 1992; 7:317–9.
51. Bastow MD, Rawlings J, Allison SP. Benefits of supplementary tube feeding after fractured neck of femur: a randomised controlled trial. Br Med J (Clin Res Ed) 1983; 287:1589–92.
52. Barger-Lux MJ, Heaney RP, Stegman MR. Effects of moderate caffeine intake on the calcium economy of premenopausal women. Am J Clin Nutr 1990; 52:722–5.
53. Heaney RP, Rafferty K. Carbonated beverages and urinary calcium excretion. Am J Clin Nutr 2001; 74:343–7.
54. Lyles KW, Colon-Emeric CS, Magaziner JS, Adachi JD, Pieper CF, Mautalen C, et al. Zoledronic acid and clinical fractures and mortality after hip fracture. N Engl J Med 2007; 357:1799–809.
55. Odvina CV, Zerwekh JE, Rao DS, Maalouf N, Gottschalk FA, Pak CY. Severely suppressed bone turnover: a potential complication of alendronate therapy. J Clin Endocrinol Metab 2005; 90:1294–301.
56. Ott SM. Long-term safety of bisphosphonates. J Clin Endocrinol Metab 2005; 90:1897–9.
57. Goh SK, Yang KY, Koh JS, Wong MK, Chua SY, Chua DT, et al. Subtrochanteric insufficiency fractures in patients on alendronate therapy: a caution. J Bone Joint Surg Br 2007; 89:349–53.
58. Bone HG, Hosking D, Devogelaer JP, Tucci JR, Emkey RD, Tonino RP, et al. Ten years' experience with alendronate for osteoporosis in postmenopausal women. N Engl J Med 2004; 350:1189–99.

59. Rodan G, Reszka A, Golub E, Rizzoli R. Bone safety of long-term bisphosphonate treatment. Curr Med Res Opin 2004; 20:1291–300.
60. Black DM, Schwartz AV, Ensrud KE, Cauley JA, Levis S, Quandt SA, et al. Effects of continuing or stopping alendronate after 5 years of treatment: the Fracture Intervention Trial Long-term Extension (FLEX): a randomized trial. JAMA 2006; 296:2927–38.
61. Rossouw JE, Anderson GL, Prentice RL, LaCroix AZ, Kooperberg C, Stefanick ML, et al. Risks and benefits of estrogen plus progestin in healthy postmenopausal women: principal results From the Women's Health Initiative randomized controlled trial. JAMA 2002; 288:321–33.
62. Cauley JA, Robbins J, Chen Z, Cummings SR, Jackson RD, LaCroix AZ, et al. Effects of estrogen plus progestin on risk of fracture and bone mineral density: the Women's Health Initiative randomized trial. JAMA 2003; 290:1729–38.
63. Anderson GL, Limacher M, Assaf AR, Bassford T, Beresford SA, Black H, et al. Effects of conjugated equine estrogen in postmenopausal women with hysterectomy: the Women's Health Initiative randomized controlled trial. JAMA 2004; 291:1701–12.
64. Ettinger B, Black DM, Mitlak BH, Knickerbocker RK, Nickelsen T, Genant HK, et al. Reduction of vertebral fracture risk in postmenopausal women with osteoporosis treated with raloxifene: results from a 3-year randomized clinical trial. Multiple Outcomes of Raloxifene Evaluation (MORE) Investigators. JAMA 1999; 282:637–45.
65. Delmas PD, Ensrud KE, Adachi JD, Harper KD, Sarkar S, Gennari C, et al. Efficacy of raloxifene on vertebral fracture risk reduction in postmenopausal women with osteoporosis: four-year results from a randomized clinical trial. J Clin Endocrinol Metab 2002; 87:3609–17.
66. Grady D, Ettinger B, Moscarelli E, Plouffe L Jr, Sarkar S, Ciaccia A, et al. Safety and adverse effects associated with raloxifene: multiple outcomes of raloxifene evaluation. Obstet Gynecol 2004; 104:837–44.
67. Neer RM, Arnaud CD, Zanchetta JR, Prince R, Gaich GA, Reginster JY, et al. Effect of parathyroid hormone (1-34) on fractures and bone mineral density in postmenopausal women with osteoporosis. N Engl J Med 2001; 344:1434–41.
68. Finkelstein JS, Hayes A, Hunzelman JL, Wyland JJ, Lee H, Neer RM. The effects of parathyroid hormone, alendronate, or both in men with osteoporosis. N Engl J Med 2003; 349:1216–26.
69. Kurland ES, Cosman F, McMahon DJ, Rosen CJ, Lindsay R, Bilezikian JP. Parathyroid hormone as a therapy for idiopathic osteoporosis in men: effects on bone mineral density and bone markers. J Clin Endocrinol Metab 2000; 85:3069–76.
70. Orwoll ES, Scheele WH, Paul S, Adami S, Syversen U, Diez-Perez A, et al. The effect of teriparatide human parathyroid hormone (1-34) therapy on bone density in men with osteoporosis. J Bone Miner Res 2003; 18:9–17.
71. Black DM, Greenspan SL, Ensrud KE, Palermo L, McGowan JA, Lang TF, et al. The effects of parathyroid hormone and alendronate alone or in combination in postmenopausal osteoporosis. N Engl J Med 2003; 349:1207–15.
72. Black DM, Bilezikian JP, Ensrud KE, Greenspan SL, Palermo L, Hue T, et al. One year of alendronate after one year of parathyroid hormone (1-84) for osteoporosis. N Engl J Med 2005; 353:555–65.
73. Cosman F, Nieves J, Woelfert L, Shen V, Lindsay R. Alendronate does not block the anabolic effect of PTH in postmenopausal osteoporotic women. J Bone Miner Res 1998; 13:1051–5.
74. Cosman F, Nieves J, Zion M, Woelfert L, Luckey M, Lindsay R. Daily and cyclic parathyroid hormone in women receiving alendronate. N Engl J Med 2005; 353:566–75.
75. Cosman F, Nieves J, Woelfert L, Formica C, Gordon S, Shen V, et al. Parathyroid hormone added to established hormone therapy: effects on vertebral fracture and maintenance of bone mass after parathyroid hormone withdrawal. J Bone Miner Res 2001; 16:925–31.
76. Kaufman JM, Orwoll E, Goemaere S, San Martin J, Hossain A, Dalsky GP, et al. Teriparatide effects on vertebral fractures and bone mineral density in men with osteoporosis: treatment and discontinuation of therapy. Osteoporos Int 2005; 16:510–6.

77. Lane NE, Sanchez S, Modin GW, Genant HK, Pierini E, Arnaud CD. Bone mass continues to increase at the hip after parathyroid hormone treatment is discontinued in glucocorticoid-induced osteoporosis: results of a randomized controlled clinical trial. J Bone Miner Res 2000; 15:944–51.
78. Lindsay R, Scheele WH, Neer R, Pohl G, Adami S, Mautalen C, et al. Sustained vertebral fracture risk reduction after withdrawal of teriparatide in postmenopausal women with osteoporosis. Arch Intern Med 2004; 164:2024–30.
79. Kurland ES, Heller SL, Diamond B, McMahon DJ, Cosman F, Bilezikian JP. The importance of bisphosphonate therapy in maintaining bone mass in men after therapy with teriparatide. Osteoporos Int 2004; 15:992–7.
80. Rittmaster RS, Bolognese M, Ettinger MP, Hanley DA, Hodsman AB, Kendler DL, et al. Enhancement of bone mass in osteoporotic women with parathyroid hormone followed by alendronate. J Clin Endocrinol Metab 2000; 85:2129–34.
81. Lindsay R, Nieves J, Formica C, Henneman E, Woelfert L, Shen V, et al. Randomised controlled study of effect of parathyroid hormone on vertebral-bone mass and fracture incidence among postmenopausal women on oestrogen with osteoporosis. Lancet 1997; 350:550–5.
82. Deal C, Omizo M, Schwartz EN, Eriksen EF, Cantor P, Wang J, et al. Combination teriparatide and raloxifene therapy for postmenopausal osteoporosis: results from a 6-month double-blind placebo-controlled trial. J Bone Miner Res 2005; 20:1905–11.
83. Gold DT, Pantos BS, Masica DN, Misurski DA, Marcus R. Initial experience with teriparatide in the United States. Curr Med Res Opin 2006; 22:703–8.
84. Harper KD, Krege JH, Marcus R, Mitlak BH. Osteosarcoma and teriparatide? J Bone Miner Res 2007; 22:334.
85. Dalsky GP, Stocke KS, Ehsani AA, Slatopolsky E, Lee WC, Birge SJ Jr. Weight-bearing exercise training and lumbar bone mineral content in postmenopausal women. Ann Intern Med 1988; 108:824–8.
86. Smith EL, Gilligan C, McAdam M, Ensign CP, Smith PE. Deterring bone loss by exercise intervention in premenopausal and postmenopausal women. Calcif Tissue Int 1989; 44:312–21.
87. Feskanich D, Willett W, Colditz G. Walking and leisure-time activity and risk of hip fracture in postmenopausal women. JAMA 2002; 288:2300–6.
88. Wiswell RA, Hawkins SA, Dreyer HC, Jaque SV. Maintenance of BMD in older male runners is independent of changes in training volume or VO(2)peak. J Gerontol A Biol Sci Med Sci 2002; 57:M203–8.
89. Srinivasan S, Weimer DA, Agans SC, Bain SD, Gross TS. Low-magnitude mechanical loading becomes osteogenic when rest is inserted between each load cycle. J Bone Miner Res 2002; 17:1613–20.
90. Rubin C, Turner AS, Bain S, Mallinckrodt C, McLeod K. Anabolism. Low mechanical signals strengthen long bones. Nature 2001; 412:603–4.
91. Helge EW, Kanstrup IL. Bone density in female elite gymnasts: impact of muscle strength and sex hormones. Med Sci Sports Exerc 2002; 34:174–80.
92. Pfeifer M, Sinaki M, Geusens P, Boonen S, Preisinger E, Minne HW. Musculoskeletal rehabilitation in osteoporosis: a review. J Bone Miner Res 2004; 19:1208–14.
93. Johnell O, Eisman J. Whole lotta shakin' goin' on. J Bone Miner Res 2004; 19:1205–7.
94. Bloomfield SA. Changes in musculoskeletal structure and function with prolonged bed rest. Med Sci Sports Exerc 1997; 29:197–206.
95. LeBlanc A, Marsh C, Evans H, Johnson P, Schneider V, Jhingran S. Bone and muscle atrophy with suspension of the rat. J Appl Physiol 1985; 58:1669–75.
96. Hulley SB, Vogel JM, Donaldson CL, Bayers JH, Friedman RJ, Rosen SN. The effect of supplemental oral phosphate on the bone mineral changes during prolonged bed rest. J Clin Invest 1971; 50:2506–18.
97. Mackey DC, Lui LY, Cawthon PM, Bauer DC, Nevitt MC, Cauley JA, et al. High-trauma fractures and low bone mineral density in older women and men. JAMA 2007; 298:2381–8.

98. Feldstein AC, Vollmer WM, Smith DH, Petrik A, Schneider J, Glauber H, et al. An outreach program improved osteoporosis management after a fracture. J Am Geriatr Soc 2007; 55:1464–9.
99. Kiel DP, Magaziner J, Zimmerman S, Ball L, Barton BA, Brown KM, et al. Efficacy of a hip protector to prevent hip fracture in nursing home residents: the HIP PRO randomized controlled trial. JAMA 2007; 298:413–22.
100. Faucett S, Genuario J, Tosteson A, Koval KJ. Is prophylactic fixation a cost-effective method for prevention of secondary hip fracture? Orthopaedic Trauma Association Meeting 2007; Scientific Poster #137.

Index

R.J. Pignolo et al. (eds.), *Fractures in the Elderly*, Aging Medicine,
DOI 10.1007/978-1-60327-467-8, © Springer Science+Business Media, LLC 2011

FSC
www.fsc.org
MIX
Papier | Fördert gute Waldnutzung
FSC® C083411

Kolibri 360 GmbH
Ferdinand-Jühlke-Straße 7
99095 Erfurt, Deutschland
produktsicherheit@kolibri360.de